Health and Society in Twentieth-Century Wales

Health and Society in Twentieth-Century Wales

Edited by

PAMELA MICHAEL AND CHARLES WEBSTER

*Published on behalf of the
Social Science Committee
of the Board of Celtic Studies*

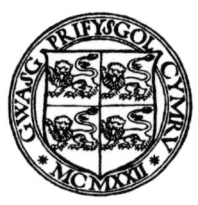

UNIVERSITY OF WALES PRESS
CARDIFF
2006

© The Contributors, 2006

All rights reserved. No part of this book may be reproduced, stored in a retrieval system, or transmitted, in any form or by any means, electronic, mechanical, photocopying, recording or otherwise, without clearance from the University of Wales Press, 10 Columbus Walk, Brigantine Place, Cardiff, CF10 4UP.
www.wales.ac.uk/press

British Library Cataloguing-in-Publication Data
A catalogue record for this book is available from the British Library.

ISBN 0-7083-1908-4

The right of the Contributors to be identified separately as authors of this work has been asserted by them in accordance with Sections 77 and 78 of the Copyright, Designs and Patents Act 1988.

Printed in Great Britain by Cambridge Printing, Cambridge

Contents

    Preface   vii
    Notes on contributors   ix

    An Overview of the History of Health and Medicine in Wales
    PAMELA MICHAEL   1

1. Sickness and Health in Caernarfonshire, 1870–1939
   GLYNNE ROBERTS   60

2. 'Sea Wall against Disease': Port Health in Cardiff, 1850–1950
   NEIL EVANS   78

3. Unemployment, Poverty and Women's Health in Inter-war South Wales
   STEVEN THOMPSON   98

4. 'The Growing Toll of Motherhood': Maternal Mortality in Wales, 1918–1939
   MARI A. WILLIAMS   123

5. 'Teach the Miners Birth Control': The Delivery of Contraceptive Advice in South Wales, 1918–1950
   KATE FISHER   143

6. Nurse Training in the Caernarvon and Anglesey Hospital, 1935–1949
   KATHERINE WILLIAMS   165

7.	The Jewish Medical Refugee Crisis and Wales, 1933–1945 PAUL WEINDLING	183
8.	Part I Dr Julian Tudor Hart: A Profile PAMELA MICHAEL	201
	Part II Storming the Citadel: From Romantic Fiction to Effective Reality JULIAN TUDOR HART	208
9.	What was Wales? Towards a Contextual Approach to Medical History MARTIN POWELL	216
10.	Devolution and the Health Service in Wales, 1919–1969 CHARLES WEBSTER	240
11.	Change the Welsh Way: Health and the NHS, 1984–1994 JOHN WYN OWEN	270
12.	History is What You Live: Understanding Health Inequalities in Wales GARETH WILLIAMS	287
	Index	313

Preface

This collection of essays is the outcome of a conference held on St David's Day, 1 March 2000. The conference was sponsored by a grant from the British Academy and a generous donation from the Research Committee of the University of Wales, Bangor. We wish to express personal thanks to Professor Mark Williams, who at that time was pro vice-chancellor with responsibility for research, for his warm encouragement.

The conference covered a wide-ranging field of topics and expertise and these essays represent only a part of the conference proceedings. It was decided that two important areas addressed by other papers in the conference, namely mental health and occupational health, each warranted a volume in their own right. It is hoped that these themes may form the basis of future volumes.

To all the contributors, who have patiently awaited the publication of this volume, we extend our thanks. A great deal of effort has gone into additional research and presentation of the papers in a form suitable for publication and we believe that the current volume represents a significant advance in our knowledge of health and society in modern and contemporary Wales.

It has been one of the delights of editing this volume that friendships have been cemented and that over a period of some five years we have been fellow-travellers in advancing the history of medicine in Wales. During that time many significant life events have occurred. We would like to congratulate Dr Kate Fisher and Dr Mari Williams, both of whom managed to deliver the definitive version of their papers shortly before they delivered their babies. Mari's baby, Ifan Gruff, was born on 20 November 2003 and weighed 7 lbs 7 ounces and Kate's baby, Edmund, was born on 23 November 2003 and weighed 7 lbs 4 ounces.

Finally, we wish to express our thanks to the University of Wales's Board of Celtic Studies for sponsoring this volume and to staff at the University of Wales Press for their cheerful and highly professional management of the publication process.

Pamela Michael and Charles Webster

Notes on contributors

Neil Evans is an Honorary Research Fellow in both the School of History and Archaeology at Cardiff University and the Welsh Institute of Social and Cultural Affairs in the University of Wales, Bangor. He is joint editor of *Llafur: The Journal of Welsh People's History* and has published widely on the history of modern Wales. He has edited *Networking Europe: Essays in Regionalism and Social Democracy* (with Eberhard Bort, 2000) and *A Tolerant Nation? Exploring Ethnic Diversity in Wales* (with Charlotte Williams and Paul O'Leary, 2003).

Kate Fisher is Lecturer at the University of Exeter. Her book, *Birth Control, Sex and Marriage in Britain, 1918–1960*, will be published in April 2006. She is currently completing a book (with Dr Simon Szreter of the University of Cambridge), *Sexuality, Love and Marriage in England 1918–1960*, and beginning an interdisciplinary research project with Dr Rebecca Langlands of the University of Exeter on the reception of erotic material from ancient civilizations in nineteenth- and twentieth-century Britain.

Julian Tudor Hart qualified in medicine from Cambridge University in 1952. He was a GP for thirty-five years, first in London and then in Glyncorrwg, a coal-mining village in south Wales. He was also trained in epidemiology by Richard Doll at the London School of Hygiene and by Archie Cochrane at the Medical Research Council Pneumoconiosis Research Unit in Cardiff. Based on research in his practice organized by his wife Mary, also trained by Cochrane in research methods, he produced many papers and several books, mostly on continuing care of chronic disease in whole populations and other aspects of social medicine and National Health Service policy. He retired from full-time practice in 1987 and from the MRC Epidemiology and Medical Care Unit staff in 1992. Since then he has held visiting appointments at several medical schools in the UK and overseas, and is a Fellow of Cardiff, Glamorgan, Glasgow and Swansea Universities. He was awarded an honorary D.Sc. at Glasgow University in 1999, the first GP so honoured since Sir James Mackenzie. His most recent book, *The Political Economy of Health Care: a Clinical Perspective*, will be published in February 2006.

Pamela Michael is Lecturer in Health Studies and Social Policy in the School of Social Sciences, University of Wales, Bangor. Her research interests range from the history of psychiatry to contemporary social policy; all have a strong focus on Wales. She is author of *Care and Treatment of the Mentally Ill in North Wales, 1800–2000* (2003) and has published widely on the history of insanity in Wales.

John Wyn Owen is Chairman of the Board of Governors of the University of Wales Institute, Cardiff (UWIC). His career has spanned the public, private and charity sectors. He held various posts in Wales before moving to St Thomas's Hospital, London; he later became Executive Director of United Medical Enterprises (1979), First Director of NHS Wales, Welsh Office and Chairman of the Welsh Health Common Services Authority (1985–94), Director General of the North South Wales Health Department and Chairman of the Australian Health Ministers Council (1994–97) and Secretary of the Nuffield Trust (1997–2005). He has received a number of honorary fellowships and degrees and was awarded Companionship of the Institute of Health Care Management (2004) and the Chartered Management Institute (2005). In 1994 he was awarded Companion of the Order of the Bath in the Queen's Birthday Honours.

Martin Powell is Professor of Social Policy at the University of Stirling. He has written widely on current and historical aspects of health policy. His interest in Welsh medical history goes back to an article on the hospital survey of south Wales during the Second World War which was published in *Local Population Studies* in 1992. He is currently working on research funded by the Wellcome Trust (with John Stewart, Oxford Brookes University) on municipal medicine in inter-war England and Wales. He is author of *Evaluating the National Health Service* (1997) and has published in journals such as *Journal of Social Policy*, *Social History of Medicine* and the *Bulletin of the History of Medicine*.

NOTES ON CONTRIBUTORS

Glynne Roberts completed his doctoral thesis on 'The history of public health in Caernarfonshire, 1870–1939' in 1993. He has published in the *Caernarvonshire Historical Society Transactions* and co-authored a centenary history of Minffordd Hospital. He is currently General Manager for Women and Family Services with the north-west Wales NHS Trust having previously managed cardiology and health promotion services. He has also published in relation to health promotion, contributing articles to the *Health Education Journal* and *Drugs: Education, Prevention and Policy*.

Steven Thompson is a native of Pontardawe in the Swansea valley and was educated at the University of Wales, Aberystwyth, where he is currently Lecturer in History. He has published a number of studies in Welsh medical history in journals such as *Llafur*, *Ceredigion*, *Welsh History Review* and *Social History of Medicine*, and continues to conduct research into various aspects of the social, political and cultural history of medicine in Wales.

Charles Webster has worked in Sheffield, Leeds and Oxford. He has written extensively on health care and welfare since 1900 and on science and medicine in the early modern period. He is author of the two-volume official history of the National Health Service.

Paul Weindling is Wellcome Trust Research Professor in the History of Medicine in the School of Arts and Humanities, Oxford Brookes University. His publications include *Health, Race and German Politics between National Unification and Nazism* (1989), *Epidemics and Genocide in Eastern Europe 1890–1945* (2000) and *Nazi Medicine and the Nuremberg Trials: from Medical War Crimes to Informed Consent 1945–55* (2004). He edited a volume on *International Health Organisations and Movements 1918–1939* (1995) and co-edited the journal *Social History of Medicine* (1992–8). His research interests include international health organizations in the twentieth century, the medical emigration to Britain in the 1930s and 1940s and Nazi medical war crimes. He has compiled a database on medical refugees in the United Kingdom, covering over 4,800 doctors, dental surgeons, medical scientists and biologists, and nurses who came to Britain as a result of Nazism and the Second World War. He can be contacted at *pjweindling@brookes.ac.uk*.

Gareth Williams is Professor of Sociology at Cardiff University where he has worked in the School of Social Sciences since 1999. He is Deputy Director of the Regeneration Institute (a joint initiative with the Department of City and Regional Planning), Associate Director of the Cardiff Institute for Society Health and Ethics, Director of the Welsh Health Impact Assessment Support Unit, acting lead for the south-east Wales section of All Wales Alliance for Research and Development in health and social care (AWARD) and a member of the executive group of QUALITI, a node of the Economic and Social Research Council's National Research Methods Centre. He has published widely in academic and professional journals and has written and edited a number of books. He is a member of the Scientific Committee of the National Prevention Research Initiative and of the Researcher Development Panel of the Department of Health's National Co-ordinating Centre for Research Capacity Development.

Katherine Williams is Lecturer in Nursing in the School of Nursing, Midwifery and Health Studies in University of Wales, Bangor. Katherine began nursing at the Caernarfonshire and Anglesey Hospital in Bangor in 1979. She has been involved in different aspects of nurse education since 1988 and has developed a keen interest in the history of nursing in Wales. She strongly believes that women, such as those whom she interviewed for her research, played an innovative and creative role in developing health care in north Wales and that their experiences needed to be recorded. She hopes to conduct further interviews with former hospital and district nurses in Wales.

Mari A. Williams is currently Project Officer with Culturenet Cymru. She is the author of a number of publications on Welsh women's history and the history of the Welsh language, including *A Forgotten Army: Female Munitions Workers of South Wales, 1939–1945* (2002) and co-editor (with Geraint H. Jenkins) of *'Let's Do Our Best for the Ancient Tongue': The Welsh Language in the Twentieth Century* (2000).

An Overview of the History of Health and Medicine in Wales

PAMELA MICHAEL

The establishment of a National Assembly for Wales and other devolved structures in Northern Ireland and Scotland has stimulated a growing interest in historical difference within the United Kingdom. Opposing interpretations of the historical development of the 'four isles' and the extent to which distinct 'national identities' emerged or were sustained, have fuelled recent debates.[1] Political and cultural differences have hitherto remained centre stage in comparative discussions and it is only of late that historians have begun to consider the nature and extent of difference regarding the evolution of health and welfare provision in the four nations. Already a number of publications have addressed the history of medicine, health and welfare in Scotland and even analysed developments post-devolution.[2] Ireland too is generating a new body of work in the social history of health and medicine.[3] Whilst this volume does not attempt to make direct comparisons it is hoped that the studies presented here may usefully sit alongside the rich vein of work on the other constituent nations of the United Kingdom. On the whole, much less is generally known about Wales than about Scotland or Ireland, and so a few basic parameters may help by way of introduction.

Wales is a country of some 8,006 square miles (or 20,761 square kilometres), with a population of 2,903,085 at the 2001 census. England is a country over six times its size, with a population at least eighteen times greater (England occupies 83.6 per cent of the total land area of the United Kingdom, Wales 4.9 per cent, Scotland 8.6 per cent and Northern Ireland 2.9 per cent). The topography of

Wales, with its north–south mountainous core and coastal plains, has inevitably exerted a powerful influence over the culture and economy, farming and transportation. Communication links historically ran west to east, and although by the middle of the twentieth century a complex network of railways had evolved, there is still no direct route from north to south.

Wales was united with England by the Acts of Union in 1536 and 1543, preceding the unions with Scotland and Ireland respectively. To all intents and purposes 'England and Wales' was henceforth treated as a single legislative and administrative unit. Most commentators therefore recognize that Wales has been more closely allied to England, for both Scotland and Ireland always retained greater political and legislative autonomy. Wales's distinctiveness is to be found in other areas for, as Raymond Williams once observed: 'Lacking a state, the Welsh have been primarily identified by their culture.'[4] Many writers have emphasized the tenacity of the Welsh language in sustaining a strong sense of separate identity, whereas others have argued that the sense of cultural difference endures even where the language is English or 'Anglo-Welsh'.[5]

When the eminent Canadian physician Sir William Osler began advising on medical education in Wales in the early twentieth century, he was struck by the continuing sense of national identity which he encountered on his visits. 'A most interesting people,' he remarked, 'a nation apart in thought and in tongue. I am surprised to find Welsh such a living language.'[6] From 1905 onwards, the year in which he took up the Regius Chair of Medicine in Oxford, Osler took a lively interest in the medical affairs of that 'small and comparatively poor country'.[7]

Even in the early twentieth century the Welsh language remained the dominant medium of communication in many areas of Wales. In the counties of Anglesey, Caernarfonshire and Merioneth in the north-west almost half of the population were unable to speak English in 1901; in some areas, such as the slate-quarrying districts of Llanberis and Nantlle, almost three-quarters of the population spoke only Welsh. However, across Wales as a whole the use of Welsh was declining, as the English language moved into the ascendancy. According to the first language census, taken in 1891, 55 per cent of the population could speak Welsh. By 1951 the proportion had fallen to 29 per cent.[8] By then, monoglot Welsh speaking was confined to very young children and a few elderly residents in rural areas. Usage of the Welsh language continued to decline so that by the last decade of the twentieth century, only 19 per cent of the population of Wales were recorded as Welsh speaking.[9]

A land of dispersed settlements and small market towns, of varied and distinct communities, Wales was transformed by the economic changes associated with industrialization. Pre-industrial Wales had a sparse and relatively evenly distributed population. It was the least urbanized area of Britain and only in areas of lowland, with better soils, could greater densities of people be found. Massive industrialization after 1780 meant that the population quintupled in the century and a half after 1750 – from just under half a million to just under two and a half million – and became notably unevenly distributed. Clusters of hastily erected dwellings crowded around hubs of intense economic activity, such as the ironworks of Dowlais and Cyfartha in Glamorgan. By the 1840s south Wales produced 40 per cent of British iron and had the two largest ironworks in the world. This industry was concentrated in an eighteen mile by one mile strip at the north-eastern rim of the coalfield and there were 150,000 people living there in the 1840s. The area around Swansea was the only other significant pocket of industrial development in the period. Inevitably these dynamic economic changes began to affect the distribution of people in Wales. In 1801 some 20 per cent of the population of Wales lived in the two southern counties of Glamorgan and Monmouthshire where most of the industry was located. By 1851 they had increased their population share to 33 per cent.[10]

In the rest of Wales there was a brief boom affecting many different industries but they were almost all in difficulties by the 1820s. Most areas were by then beginning to experience an outflow of population and for the rest of the century and beyond massive rural depopulation was their fate. The only exceptions were the two industrial regions which emerged in north-west and north-east Wales based on slate extraction and coal mining respectively. These enjoyed modest population growth up to the First World War and small industrial towns grew in both areas. Resorts developed along the north coast, in such places as Rhyl and Llandudno, and attracted both holiday visitors and wealthy settlers from the industrial north-west of England.

In south Wales the iron industry shrank into relative insignificance after 1850 whereas coal production, once largely a subsidiary of iron, became of world importance. As international trade expanded, the need for fuel for shipping created a vast global market for the high-quality steam coal of south Wales. The labour demands of deep mining saw areas like the Rhondda valleys 'transformed into a human warren with twenty-four thousand souls to the square mile'.[11] At the peak of employment in the early 1920s there were well over a quarter of a million miners employed in south Wales. Slate quarrying brought employment to some districts in Caernarfonshire and Merioneth and there was mining and some industrial development around Wrexham, but the two industrial areas of north Wales never employed more than 16,000 quarrymen or miners each. These developments therefore become less significant once they are compared with mining in south Wales. Coal production spread across the northern portions of the counties of Glamorgan and western Monmouthshire and into eastern Carmarthenshire whilst the coastal plains of those counties became the location of major ports like Cardiff, Newport and Swansea, which also had significant metal-producing and metal-working industries. By 1911, 66 per cent of the population of Wales lived in Glamorgan and Monmouthshire. This process of industrialization had produced a country of stark contrasts. In the period 1861–91 the south-eastern counties of Wales rank as the areas of highest population growth in Britain. The mid and west Wales counties, by contrast, share with the Scottish Highlands the distinction of being the only areas of Britain to experience population decline. The two minor industrial regions in the north sustained relatively modest population growth.[12]

The population of the industrial county of Glamorgan grew with extraordinary rapidity. It leapt from 70,879 in 1801 to 231,849 in 1851 and by the beginning of the twentieth century to 859,931, with the result that by 1901 one-third of the population of Wales lived within a twenty-five mile radius of Cardiff. By this time mining was in its final phase of expansion, and still attracting workers into south Wales. Between 1901 and 1911 about 130,000 people moved into the colliery districts of Glamorgan and Monmouthshire, as the coal industry took on an additional 70,000 workers.[13] By 1931 the population of Glamorgan had grown to one and a quarter million. Extractive and heavy industries, so concentrated in this one county, dominated the economy and employment market of the country as a whole. In 1921 mining, quarrying and metal manufacturing employed over a third of the entire male workforce in Wales.[14] This dramatic resettlement of the people of Wales and concentration in heavy industry was of immense significance for the health status of the Welsh people, and had profound implications for public health and medical services provision.

Although not entirely immune to the effect of trade cycles during their expanding phase, the extractive and heavy industries faced serious depressions of trade during the inter-war years. Coinciding with a deep structural decline in the mining and heavy industries of south Wales, this economic crisis brought manifold consequences to the related communities. By the 1930s unemployment was threatening the livelihood of thousands of families, and undermining the standard of living in hard-hit industrial districts. At the same time the depression in farming was adversely affecting the rural counties, adding to the rural exodus and starving local authorities of income and resources. Both industrial and rural communities suffered during the inter-war period, contrasting with other parts of the UK, where modern light industries offered new opportunities for employment and a restructuring of the economy. Such developments were scarce in Wales. Nearly half a million people left south Wales in search of work during the 1930s. The legacy of its heavy industrial base continued to dominate the post-war economy of Wales. Similarly, the health implications of long-term employment in heavy and extractive industries, of lengthy periods of high unemployment during the inter-war years, together with lack of investment in housing and health, were all to present Wales with a unique set of problems during the second half of the twentieth century.

The above synopsis is amplified in the specialist papers contained in this volume. Wales certainly provides ideal territory for case studies relating to health and social conditions in modern society. This makes it surprising, as Anne Borsay and Dorothy Porter have pointed out, that the history of medicine in Wales remains underdeveloped, despite the recent academic growth of the social history of medicine.[15] However, they have perhaps been too hasty in their dismissal of all that has hitherto been written and researched, and therefore risk inviting neglect of the relative wealth of previous studies of numerous aspects of health, medicine and society in Wales. Certainly Borsay's edited volume makes a valuable contribution to the development of the history of medicine in Wales, and is a long overdue complement to the pioneering collection on *Wales and Medicine*, edited by John Cule in 1975.[16] The need for a new publication to meet the growing interest in the history of medicine in Wales was recognized by the compilation of a historical miscellany on health in Wales, edited by Colin Baber and John Lancaster in 2000, which brought together some commissioned and other already published work.[17] Attention has been drawn to the wealth of archival source materials existing on the history of medicine in Wales.[18] However, there is as yet no accessible overview of the history of health and medicine in Wales. This introductory chapter offers a brief résumé of the historiography of health and medicine in Wales, and in general aims to provide a suitable context for the studies contained in the present volume.

As part of its distinctive cultural heritage Wales has its own indigenous medical traditions, intimately associated with its landscapes and folklore. One of its most famous legends relates to the foundation of a medical dynasty, the Physicians of Myddfai. The story of the Lady of the Lake of Llyn y Fan Fach in Carmarthenshire, who bequeathed to her sons her extensive medical knowledge before forsaking her husband and returning to her home beneath the lake, has linked the origins of Welsh medicine to the realm of magic. The oral tale was recorded around the turn of the fifteenth century, and survives in Welsh manuscripts held at the British Museum and Jesus College, Oxford. These early Welsh medical treatises are similar to many other European texts linked with classical sources and take the form of a compendium of herbal remedies, brief tracts describing commonly performed operations, horoscopes and calendars giving lists of lucky or unlucky days for blood-letting and so on. The Myddfai traditions have been central to popular conceptions of Welsh medicine, and the treatises have been published and republished numerous times since the mid-nineteenth century.[19] In 1908, the Celtic scholar Sir John Rhŷs (1840–1915) then principal of Jesus College, Oxford, proudly presented a copy of Pughe's translation of the Myddfai text to Sir William Osler, as proof of Wales's unique traditions.[20] The British Medical Association (BMA) Wales even now celebrates the Myddfai traditions as the epitome of Welsh medical culture.[21] Other elements of ancient Celtic folklore had medicinal associations. The tradition of stone cults (such as the hydrophobic stones believed to be a cure for rabies) and of healing wells had pagan origins but became associated with the ancient Celtic churches and saints.[22] They formed an integral part of the therapeutic landscape that characterized Wales prior to the rapid modernization of the eighteenth and nineteenth centuries.

Many traditional healers used charms and magic, and employed astrology and superstitious rites alongside botanical or physical cures, but by the end of the eighteenth century 'the heyday of the medically inclined polymath, the enchanter, the quack astrologer' was effectively over.[23] The registration of apothecaries in 1815 and the registration of doctors in 1858, associated with a system of recognized medical qualifications, notionally displaced unauthorized practitioners. Yet the renown of some of the Welsh conjurors or cunning folk was such that people continued to consult them, long after the date of their official demise. For instance, the notable Harries family of Cwrtycadno in Cardiganshire established a reputation that drew patients from a wide area during the early years of the twentieth century.[24]

The transition from older methods of medical treatment to modern practice was sometimes fluid; often generations of traditional practitioners merged into modern specialists. Among the leading pioneer orthopaedic surgeons, Hugh Owen Thomas (1834–91) and Robert Jones (1858–1933) came from a lineage of famous Anglesey 'bone-setters'.[25] These were skilled craftsmen; following the Medical Registration Act of 1858, many descendants of these dynasties decided to acquire formal qualifications.[26] Thomas Jones (whose mother was a skilful bone-setter, having learnt the art from her father Richard Evans, Cilmaenan), gained his MRCS (England) and LRCP (London) in 1896. He became Medical Officer and Public Vaccination Officer for the Amlwch District of Anglesey and worked for several insurance companies. He set up practice in Amlwch; when the patients of other doctors on the island suffered fractures they often preferred to consult Dr Jones, due to his reputation as a 'bone-setter'.[27] He was still practising during the 1930s. Arthur Rocyn Jones (1883–1972), who gave many years' service as orthopaedic surgeon at the Royal National Orthopaedic Hospital and acted as consultant surgeon to the Prince of Wales and Glan Ely Hospitals in south Wales and to the North Wales Sanatorium as well as to other hospitals in Wales and England, came from a family of Welsh bone-setters in Pembrokeshire. His eldest brother continued in the traditional practice established by his great-grandfather, whilst another brother served as Medical Officer of Health for Monmouthshire.[28]

The number of qualified doctors in Wales expanded during the latter half of the nineteenth century, but they co-existed with a range of other practitioners. The *Medical Directory* of 1861 listed 523 registered medical practitioners in Wales, of whom 69 were qualified as MD, 52 had qualifications as physicians with the remainder being apothecaries. By 1881 the total number of registered doctors had risen to 594.[29] In some rural areas the distribution of qualified medical practitioners was very thin. In Gower, west Glamorgan, in 1883 there was only one qualified practitioner, Dr Ellis, covering a population of

6,351 persons in an area of more than 49,000 acres.[30] Many rural dwellers continued to take responsibility for their own health care and to grow medicinal plants and prepare home medications late into the nineteenth and even into the twentieth century.[31] Much oral testimony of the medicinal uses of plants in Wales was collected and recorded by staff of the Museum of Welsh Life (then the Welsh Folk Museum) during the 1960s and 1970s.[32]

Early in the twentieth century some unqualified healers claimed to have found a cure for cancer, and many sufferers resorted to their treatments when qualified doctors had little hope to offer. The journalist W. T. Stead drew public attention to the claims of two 'cancer curers' in Cardiganshire, Daniel and John Evans, and this led to an enquiry by the BMA and the Cancer Research Committee in 1907, which found the claims to be bogus.[33] However, people continued to visit lay practitioners, and there is some evidence to suggest that their 'secret remedies' may occasionally have had some success in the treatment of rodent ulcers (*y ddafad wyllt*).[34] Rural people would secretly consult unlicensed healers even into the middle decades of the twentieth century.[35] In the urban and industrial areas alternative practitioners often competed for trade with registered doctors. The Medical Officer of Health for Rhondda Urban District reported to a parliamentary inquiry of 1910 that there were twenty-six 'quacks' practising in the area, including herbalists, chemists, a bone-setter and others. They all gave medical advice and prescribed medicines and at least eight of them made house calls.[36] In Neath market during the 1930s there were six or seven stalls selling herbal remedies.[37] The tenacity of Welsh folk-medicine makes this brief outline relevant to an introduction to health and society in twentieth century Wales. It illustrates the different time rhythms of cultural and social change within Wales. These long-standing traditions have intrigued folklorists and doctor-historians alike, and so have inspired a large component of the writing on the history of medicine in Wales.[38]

The medical profession has played a prominent role in the cultural and institutional life of the nation. Since the mid-nineteenth century doctors have been active members of Welsh cultural bodies such as the Cymmrodorion or the Cambrian Archaeological Society, in the Gorsedd of Bards, and many have been prominent freemasons. Sir John Williams (1840–1926), who was appointed first Professor of Obstetric Medicine at the University College Hospital, London in 1887, retired in 1903 to devote his energies to the establishment of the

National Library of Wales.[39] He donated his rare books and manuscripts to form the foundation of its collection. He was imbued with a strong sense of national consciousness and together with Dr Morgan Davies he succeeded in detaching Wales from the 'England and Wales' section of *The Medical Directory*.[40] Sir Isambard Owen rose through the ranks at St George's Hospital Medical School in London and in 1914 was appointed Principal of Armstrong College in Newcastle-upon-Tyne. His influence in Wales was considerable and he helped to draft the Charter for the University of Wales.[41] A group of prestigious medical men were key benefactors of the University College of North Wales, Bangor during its formative years.[42] In Cardiff many doctors have been active members of the Cardiff Naturalists Society, as well as being magistrates and members of the Medical Society.[43] In market towns, such as Denbigh, Pwllheli and Carmarthen, doctors could play a leading role in municipal life, acting as coroners and magistrates, sitting on town councils and presiding as mayor.[44] In Wales the middle class has been comparatively small, owing to the nature of economic developments described above, and so the medical profession has probably played a more significant role in the country's social and cultural institutions than in England.

Another aspect of these class formations in Wales is the effect it has had on demand for medical services. There was not a sufficiently large upper or middle class to provide a market for specialist services and so the number of consultants in Wales was always very small. However, many renowned Welsh doctors became specialists in London and Liverpool, and the wealthy were able to access their private services. The landed gentry and rich industrial magnates usually owned properties in London, or at least had close connections there. The private market for specialist practice did not really develop outside Cardiff, and Welsh hospitals did not have the range of facilities to support specialist practices. At the same time the medical market for general practitioners was not as lucrative as it would be in many areas of England. People on small incomes would usually attempt self-treatment before they would contemplate incurring a doctor's bill.[45] Chemists' shops provided remedies for many ailments, and customers would seek advice from their local pharmacist in the first instance, only resorting to a doctor if the condition worsened. Lloyd George knew from personal experience of the grief and suffering which could be caused by lack of medical attention, and the impact which the death of the breadwinner could have on the family. His National

Insurance Act of 1911 brought benefit to many in Wales, providing free treatment for that large stratum of the population not impecunious enough to receive poor relief and not rich enough comfortably to afford the services of a doctor. A Welsh-language version of the National Insurance Act, as far as it related to National Health Insurance, was issued in 1912.[46] A more accessible 'free translation' was published in the same year by Lloyd George's brother William George, a solicitor in Criccieth. The latter version explained in more clearly comprehensible language the terms of *Y Ddeddf Yswiriol 1911*, and hailed the new Act as a revolutionary measure of social reform:

> Mesur chwyldroadol ydyw Deddf Yswiriol, 1911, – hynny ydyw, golyga gyfnewidiadau pwysig ym mheirianwaith Cymdeithas, olwynion yr hon pan weithia y Mesur hwn, fyddant yn troi dipyn yn wahanol i'r hyn wnaent cynt. Yn wir, os caniateir i ni ddilyn y gydmariaeth ymhellach gallem ddyweyd fod lle cryf i ddisgwyl y bydd yr Olwyn Fawr newydd hon yn help dirfawr i godi yr isel-radd o ddyfnderoedd afiechyd a thlodi a'u dwyn i gyrhaedd awelon iach a llawnder bywyd.[47]

Translating the Act represented a great challenge, for it contained many terms hitherto not encountered in the Welsh language. Whilst he was preparing the Welsh version William offered a guinea prize to any readers of *Y Brython* or *Yr Herald Gymraeg* who could suggest phrases that would equate to a list of twenty-four terms encountered in the legislation.[48] The fifty-one entries were adjudicated by Professor John Morris-Jones of the University College of North Wales, Bangor. Thus, state intervention in health placed new demands upon the Welsh language, as well as bringing about other significant social and cultural changes.

Health and society in twentieth-century Wales

The above outline introduces some key features of the economic, social and cultural history of Wales, in so far as they affect health and medicine. It indicates the relevant time frames, discontinuities and spatial variations of developments, as well as the cultural context of class formation and language.

The emphasis in this volume is on the relationship between health and health provision and various aspects of Welsh society in the twentieth century. Contributors explore the interplay between health and society from a variety of different standpoints. The first two chapters provide a background to the development of public health in Wales in the nineteenth century and describe the subsequent evolution of public health provision in two very different contexts – one a large commercial port and the other an extensive, predominantly rural county. The following chapters continue with the theme of public health but focus on female health and explore the ways in which the particular industrial and social conditions in Wales had a detrimental influence on the health profile of women. They each offer different ways of understanding and interpreting the evidence for gender variations in health and for differing patterns of mortality and morbidity according to age and sex. Two chapters look at the professions in Wales, one exploring the experience of refugee doctors who came to train and work in Wales before and during the Second World War, and the other exploring the experience of nurses, as seen through the eyes of women who trained in north Wales during this same period. Expert witnesses are then given centre stage, firstly to provide a critique of A. J. Cronin's *The Citadel*, a fictional representation of general practice in south Wales, from the perspective of a distinguished and experienced practitioner in primary care in Wales; and secondly to recount the achievements of the first directorate of NHS Wales during the period 1979–88. By the time this corporate institution had come into being Wales had already achieved a significant measure of devolution in regard to health. The uneasy relationship between the Welsh Board of Health (1919–69) and the Ministry of Health together with the political events leading up to the transfer of executive responsibility to the Welsh Office in 1969 is the subject of another chapter. How distinctive Wales was in regard to health is a theme that runs throughout the book, but it is explored in greater detail with reference to the inadequacy of hospital services as inherited by the NHS in Wales. Another emergent theme is that of health inequalities, an issue of major importance not only in terms of health needs and provision, but also as a preoccupation of policymakers in the new National Assembly for Wales. This is the timely subject of the final chapter.

Public health
The rapid and uneven process of industrialization described above led to huge problems of public health in Wales during the nineteenth century. Assemblages of workers' dwellings were erected with little thought about the sanitary conditions of these new industrial settle-

ments.[49] The town of Merthyr Tydfil was one of the fastest growing towns in Wales in the first half of the nineteenth century. The high density of population and lack of attention to sewerage or clean water supplies made Merthyr a breeding ground for infection. During the year of 1849, when the town was affected by a cholera epidemic, over 3,000 people died, one-third of them children under five. Water was in short supply and there was a conflict between the needs of the inhabitants to obtain supplies of clean water and the need for water in the iron industry. The situation finally improved when the Pantwyn reservoir was opened in 1863 and gradually a town sewerage system was installed during the 1860s.[50] As industry and mining drew more workers into the Rhondda valley, the problems of public health became ever more acute; damp dwellings, imperfect drainage and contaminated water supplies were linked to intestinal and throat infections, diphtheria and enteric fever.[51]

A rapidly growing population and increasing birth rate brought problems to many towns. The population of Cardiff grew fivefold in the period 1801–41, and increased by a further 83 per cent during the next decade. Between 1842 and 1848 the death rate exceeded the birth rate by 4 per cent, with infant mortality accounting for 43.6 per cent of deaths. Following the Public Health Act of 1848 the town council became the statutory public health authority and over the next twenty years a series of measures were carried out to improve water and sanitation in the town.[52] In Neath the poor standard of cottages and diffused ownership patterns made it particularly difficult to implement improvements. There were differences of opinion and animosity amongst town councillors driven by a fear of high rates. Although various schemes of improvement were proposed, little progress was made between 1850 and 1860; it was not until the mid-1870s that any real investment was made in improved sanitation.[53] Towns like Swansea and Wrexham had more ambitious schemes, but the level of improvement varied widely between districts.[54] Studies of towns such as these provide a glimpse of the momentous public health issues that rapid industrialization and urbanization brought to Wales. It was the hope of leading scholars, in particular I. G. Jones, that a programme of research into public health in Wales would be inaugurated. It was with this in view that the Board of Celtic Studies funded a project to transcribe all of the correspondence from the principality to the General Board of Health of 1848–71.[55] A comprehensive research programme is still desirable, but in the meantime contributions of enormous value have been made by the doctoral researches of Steven Thompson and Glynne Roberts, two of the contributors to this volume, both of whom extend our horizons to encompass public health during the first half of the twentieth century.[56]

The chapter by Glynne Roberts examines the state of public health in the county of Caernarfonshire and indicates the variation in conditions that exist within the boundaries of a single county, containing rural districts, urban centres and quarrying districts. The pace of social improvement varied, reflecting the health needs, resources and civic consciousness of residents, with progress being slowest in the slate-quarrying villages of the Gwyrfai district and most advanced in the city of Bangor. By contrast Neil Evans offers a study of port health in the docklands of Cardiff where, faced with the threat of imported epidemics, a highly efficient system of sanitary inspection was developed. Taken together, these two chapters illustrate the crucial role of public health and the wide diversity of health conditions that emerges as one defining characteristic of Wales.

Many previous local studies of early public health in Wales have drawn attention to the importance of cholera in galvanizing local sanitary movements.[57] Evans indicates how successive waves of cholera infection were instrumental in triggering formal measures to deal with port health. Similarly, Roberts shows how outbreaks of cholera, typhoid and smallpox provided an impetus for sanitary improvements in Caernarfonshire. Public health measures in Wales were often reactive rather than proactive, and shortage of finance and lack of zeal often stalled progress. Public health reform in the nineteenth century belonged to local initiative, and was dependent upon collaboration between the middle and working classes, but in Wales class formations were very different from England. 'Hence it was', as Ieuan Gwynedd Jones pointed out in a classic essay on the people's health in nineteenth-century Wales, 'that only places with enlightened middle class leadership could achieve substantial reforms quickly.'[58] This partly explains why the pace of change was so variable across Wales, resulting in a differential and uneven pattern of public health provision by the early twentieth century. Cardiff, with its strong civic consciousness, and the city of Bangor, with its intellectual and business elite, pioneered progressive reforms, whereas many towns and districts lagged sadly behind.[59] Often, in an attempt to overcome lack of resources, local authorities would combine responsibilities, but as Roberts shows in this volume, such attempts could leave the

Medical Officer of Health hopelessly overstretched and render the reforms ineffective.

Roberts also illustrates the crucial importance of securing clean water supplies in preventing the spread of disease. He indicates the difficulties this presented in the Welsh context of dispersed settlements and mountainous areas of heavy rainfall where watercourses were so numerous that it was difficult to trace the source of pollution. Similar problems were faced in the closely populated valleys of Glamorgan, as illustrated by Mabbitt in his comprehensive account of the health services of Glamorgan.[60] Outbreaks of typhoid fever in Neath, Caerphilly, Cowbridge, Pontardawe and half a dozen other villages in 1894 were all attributed to the drinking of polluted water. A succession of Acts of Parliament passed in the early twentieth century gave the County sufficient powers to bring about a general improvement in water supplies, but there could still be dangers if a supply was polluted at its source in the hills. A major outbreak of dysentery in the Ogmore and Garw Urban District in 1921 was caused by the consumption of raw untreated waters, contaminated by faecal discharges. New reservoirs and water schemes continued to be erected during the 1920s and 1930s and the issues of river pollution and floodwater were also addressed. Pure water was fundamental to the improvement of people's health and the significance of Welsh water to public health in both Wales and England, whilst recognized in the past, has recently become the subject of renewed scholarly attention.[61]

Infectious diseases were an important cause of premature death in the early twentieth century, and posed a particular threat to children. Local authorities were required to provide isolation facilities for the treatment of infectious diseases, and they responded with varying levels of enthusiasm. The Minffordd Hospital in Bangor, opened in 1895, was the culmination of the city's ambitious response to the typhoid epidemic of 1882. Between 1903 and 1912 the hospital took in 393 cases of scarlet fever, 81 of diphtheria, 11 of enteric fever and 1 case of measles. Many of the patients were children.[62] A proliferation of small 'isolation hospitals' was erected across Wales, many of them defective in structure and lacking in comfort, often empty, but ready to separate infectious cases from the general population. In Merthyr Tydfil the only hospitals provided by the Local Board of Health in the early years of the twentieth century were the fever hospitals. A corrugated iron building erected at Twynyrodyn in 1902 served as a smallpox hospital. When the new Mardy Isolation Hospital was erected in 1907, the former building was re-erected on Mountain Hare, and continued to provide isolation facilities until it blew down in 1928.[63] These fever hospitals are illustrative of the rudimentary level of hospital provision in Wales in the early twentieth century. With so many small ports and coastal shipping outlets around the shorelines of north, west and south Wales, there was a fear that infection could come from the sea as well as the land. Roberts shows how in some areas the local constabulary kept a watch on shipping and sailors, to guard against epidemic disease. Once a source of infection was detected, isolation was an important strategy adopted for port health; as Evans shows, old vessels were sometimes employed for this purpose.[64] In north Wales a hospital ship was moored in the Menai Straits between Bangor and Beaumaris. During a smallpox epidemic in 1917 the sister and a nurse from the Minffordd Hospital, near Bangor, were sent aboard to nurse the sick.[65] Whereas the geography of Wales often caused problems of public health, as this issue illustrates it could occasionally be employed to positive effect.[66]

Outbreaks of infectious diseases, such as smallpox and diphtheria, whilst dramatic in their effect on local communities were of relatively short duration. Over the longer term a more insidious disease claimed the lives of many more Welsh people. Tuberculosis – *y dicáu* (decay) or *y darfodedigaeth* (perishing/wasting away) as it was known in Welsh – was the scourge of both urban and rural populations in Wales during the nineteenth and first half of the twentieth century. It was often termed the 'white plague' (*y pla gwyn*). Whilst death rates from tuberculosis were generally falling during the early decades of the twentieth century, the decline in Wales was much slower and the four counties in England and Wales with the highest death rates from tuberculosis were in north-west and west Wales (Caernarfonshire, Anglesey, Merioneth and Cardiganshire). Various explanations were advanced for this persistence of tuberculosis in Wales, including a suggestion that it was due to a genetic propensity amongst the Welsh, especially the small dark-haired Celts, to contract the disease.[67] Other hypotheses included the notion that the high incidence of the disease along the western seaboard of Wales resulted from the deleterious effects of the maritime mists. All of the chapters in this volume which deal with public health discuss the problem of tuberculosis, and indicate that there were considerable variations both in the age patterns and between districts. The causes of a high degree of local discrepancy were clearly social, and not racial. However, eugenicist explanations were popular, especially during the inter-war years and, as Neil Evans shows, a racial theory was similarly advanced for the high incidence of tuberculosis amongst Arab seamen in Cardiff, although their working conditions were the more likely cause.

Occupational health

The existence of a connection between tuberculosis and occupational conditions, be it quarrying, maritime occupations or coal mining, was highly contested during the inter-war years. Owing to conflicts of opinion, Wales was the site of a number of significant governmental inquiries and scientific surveys. This volume touches on occupational health in Wales to only a limited extent; the issue is of such importance that it requires a separate volume. However, it is helpful to explain a little of the background, since work-related illnesses have been so significant in determining the health status of the nation and reducing life expectancy, particularly of the male workforce.

The many extractive industries located in Wales have proved particularly hazardous. Lead mining, a significant source of employment in north-east and mid Wales until the First World War, was extremely injurious to health. Workmen were regularly afflicted with heart and lung diseases, to the extent that: 'A miner over the age of forty was rare; one of forty-five had the constitution of an old man.'[68] The most common symptoms associated with lead mining were 'the black spit' and shortness of breath, which made climbing the ladders to the surface at the end of a shift both laborious and painful. Ventilation was often poor and tuberculosis spread easily.[69] This, in addition to accidents and injuries, made the work very hazardous. Copper, nickel and manganese were also mined in Wales, and each presented its own health hazards.[70] Slate quarrying accounted for a much larger sector of employment in north Wales; although in decline, the industry continued to employ significant numbers throughout the inter-war years (13,000 workers in 1910 falling to 3,520 by 1945). Accidents were numerous and a number of works hospitals were established during the nineteenth century to deal with casualties, funded by employers and workmen, each with its own scheme of organization. Some excellent orthopaedic and medical work was conducted in these hospitals, and they made early use of innovations such as X-ray equipment. Dr Edward Davies's recent account of the quarry hospitals has added immeasurably to our knowledge of this unique aspect of Welsh medical history.[71]

The prevalence of tuberculosis amongst the quarrymen of Caernarfonshire became an important national issue and was the subject of a number of inquiries.[72] An investigation by Dr T. W. Wade in 1926, commissioned by the Minister of Health, Neville Chamberlain, concluded that inhalation of slate dust was causing silicosis amongst the slate workers and predisposing them to tuberculosis. This then created a pool of infection which affected the rest of the community and drove up rates of tuberculosis in the quarry districts. However, Wade's report did not lead to inclusion of the industry within the compensation scheme for silicosis and, as Linda Bryder has pointed out, the medical profession in the area did not accept Wade's findings.[73] Further investigations into the high rates of tuberculosis in these areas, conducted by Chalke and published in 1933, paid little attention to the issue of slate dust inhalation, and focused instead on general social conditions.[74] Throughout the 1930s many commentators continued to employ an explanatory framework that emphasized the tendency of the Welsh to resign themselves to their fate rather than seek treatment in a sanatorium. Instead of locating the causes in working and social conditions created by local economies, a personalistic explanation was favoured by the medical profession; consequently, the diet and domestic habits of the quarrymen became the focus of official scrutiny. Particular blame was placed upon the poor housekeeping skills of the women; indeed it was sometimes claimed that inappropriate diet rather than inadequate diet was at the root of the problem.[75]

Other areas of employment associated with high frequency of accidents included roads and railways, construction, shipping and farming. The largest single source of employment in Wales was the coal industry. Here, lack of investment in safety measures exacerbated the difficulties caused by geology. The daily hazards faced by miners working underground included rock falls, haulage accidents, winding shaft failures and problems with pumping equipment resulting in a sudden rise of water levels. The most feared catastrophes were underground explosions, since they could kill, burn and maim large numbers, as happened at the Universal colliery in Senghennydd in 1913, when 439 miners were killed, and at the Gresford colliery disaster, near Wrexham, in 1934.[76] Whilst these major accidents caught the headlines, small accidents such as those vividly described by Bert Coombes in his autobiography *These Poor Hands* were almost daily occurrences in Welsh coalfields.[77] These accounted for five times as many deaths as those caused by major explosions. In addition, a vast number of disabling accidents occurred on the railways and docks that were associated with the mines. However, over the long term it was probably the occupational diseases, mainly in the form of lung diseases, which exacted the heaviest toll. Although less transparent than fatal accidents, the wastage of life was heavy and the impact on the lives of elderly miners devastating.[78]

Medical opinion was slow to recognize the condition of silicosis, as opposed to general chest disease and pneumoconiosis, and some experts continued to argue over a long period that miners were chiefly the victims of tuberculosis.[79] Matters of compensation were involved. It was argued that silicosis could only occur after exposure to silica, and that the mineral composition of coal in south Wales excluded this possibility. However, an investigation by Collis and Gilchrist into the lungs of coal trimmers in Cardiff docks, conducted in 1928, found that, after working in a confined space loading steam coal over a number of years, their lungs showed signs of silicotic fibrosis.[80] A subsequent study of anthracite miners in the western area of the coalfield, carried out by Cummins and Sladden, showed that dust had accumulated in their lungs, causing serious and fatal disease.[81]

Recognition of the condition of silicosis in Wales became a burning political issue.[82] In 1934 the government conceded the rights of all underground miners to compensation under a new silicosis scheme, but as claims rose, the number of refusals, particularly in south Wales, escalated.[83] The mine owners argued that the condition was pneumoconiosis and not silicosis. Expert opinion continued to be divided, J. S. Haldane believing that miners' disease was primarily attributable to tuberculosis, bronchitis and bronchiectasis.[84] In 1936 Jim Griffiths, newly elected as Labour MP for Llanelli, raised the issue in parliamentary question time and called for a special investigation by the Medical Research Council (MRC). The Lord President of the Council, Ramsay MacDonald, was sympathetic and an inquiry was duly set up to look into the incidence and special characteristics of chronic pulmonary diseases amongst coal miners in south Wales.[85] Dr Philip D'Arcy Hart was seconded from the MRC in London to carry out a large-scale clinical and radiological survey.[86] Initially assisted by Dr Edward Aslett of the Welsh National Memorial Association, D'Arcy Hart gradually built up a team of experts, and produced a series of detailed reports.[87] Their work clearly showed that exposure to coal dust over a long period led to disease amongst miners, even in the anthracite fields. The work of this small research unit led to the establishment in 1945 of the MRC Pneumoconiosis Research Unit at Llandough Hospital in Penarth, Cardiff, and to a series of important scientific and epidemiological studies. These surveys expanded and laid the foundations of population-based research in the UK. In 1948/9, D'Arcy Hart was joined by Archie Cochrane, fresh from the Rockefeller Foundation in New York, who participated in a major study of the Rhondda Fach to look at the interaction between dust exposure and tuberculosis in generating pulmonary disease.[88] Tests did not indicate a relationship between tuberculin sensitivity and the type of lesion on miners' lungs.[89] It has been suggested that the effectiveness of streptomycin in reducing the incidence of tuberculosis, together with the improvement in social conditions, prevented this study from generating definitive results.[90] The high participation rates achieved in this study made it a classic in the history of epidemiological research. Cochrane went on to develop his enquiries in south Wales and to expand the use of population-based research and pioneer the method of randomized control trials, making a unique international contribution to the development of epidemiology.[91] The records of the south Wales MRC research unit have recently been transferred to Bristol University and the unit has been the subject of a Wellcome Expert Witness seminar, signalling a recognition of the wider importance of the research work carried out in Wales during this period.[92]

The miners, their wives and the entire valley communities were vital participants in this path-breaking research. For long they had held their own theories and beliefs about the effects of coal dust and about the treatment of ailments relating to work in the pits. It was the custom for miners to suck a piece of coal in order to prevent swallowing the dust that arose from cutting into the coalface, indicating that they were all too aware of the dangers of inhalation. Much folk medicine was based on the idea of treating like with like. Burns would be treated with oil and fire. A special burn bed would be placed in front of the fire, and the afflicted miner laid on a bed of straw soaked in oil.[93] Blacksmiths, widely employed in the iron and tin-plate industries, treated their burns in the same way. Blisters and callouses were everyday problems and new recruits to the industry were instructed to harden the skin on their hands and knees by soaking them in urine. Hernias were another common problem for men in these heavy industries and various types of bandage and corset were employed.[94] Self-help and shared knowledge were all important in negotiating the health risks of this major industry. This is a part of the cultural history of mining communities, which has not received the attention it deserves.

Women's health

Women's history generally was long neglected in Wales.[95] In 1991 a seminal article appeared entitled 'Counting the cost of coal', where Dot Jones posed the crucial question of how the coal industry of south Wales had affected the health of women. She revealed the startling fact that between 1881 and 1911 the number of women dying in childbirth in the south Wales coalfield exceeded the number of men killed in accidents in the mines.[96] Her analysis drew attention to the impact of the industry on the health of miners' wives. Many mothers and their unborn babies were harmed by lifting tin baths full of water for the miners to bathe on their return from the pits. The campaign for pit-head baths was an important cause that united men and women in the labour movement.[97] Although women's role in the professions has received valuable attention of late,[98] women's health status in general remains a relatively neglected area of Welsh medical history. Studies of the health of women and children broaden the picture of health and social conditions in Wales beyond that of occupational health, drawing attention to the wider social processes influencing health. In a closely argued chapter in this collection, Steven Thompson shows how economic conditions and cultural context shaped the experiences of women in districts of high unemployment and low wages in south Wales, rendering them vulnerable to ill health and premature death.

Women's reproductive role formed an important part of the health profile of younger age groups and high rates of maternal mortality are demonstrated and discussed in this volume by both Thompson and Williams. Neonatal mortality and the number of stillbirths in a district are selected by Thompson as reliable indicators of maternal health and nutritional status; these indicate a startling pattern of negative contrast when compared with the average for England and Wales. Comparison of any of the chosen indicators for these economically depressed districts of south Wales with more prosperous districts in south-east England, where women would not only have enjoyed better nutrition but been provided with better antenatal and obstetric care, would of course expose an even greater contrast. Yet the comparison with the average for England and Wales is sufficiently persuasive to support Thompson's conclusion that mortality increased as a direct result of economic depression, unemployment and poverty and that women in industrial south Wales suffered disproportionately, their gendered experience constituting a reflection of their subordinate status within these beleaguered industrial communities.

The problem of high rates of maternal mortality was an issue that attracted the concern of public health specialists and the wider public. The chapter by Mari Williams analyses the findings of a series of important inquiries into maternal mortality in Wales conducted during the inter-war period. The relationship between economic depression and the life-chances of expectant mothers in Wales has remained a subject of controversy ever since the 1920s in Wales, when the Labour Party issued a pamphlet entitled *Distress in South Wales: Health of Mothers and Babies Imperilled*, which argued that economic hardship due to industrial conditions was undermining the health of women and infants.[99] As unemployment and social conditions worsened, voluntary organizations also took a direct interest in the situation in south Wales. During the 1930s the National Birthday Trust Fund carried out an experimental feeding programme with the aim of fortifying the health of expectant mothers and babies. The results of the scheme were strongly contested by medical experts. Susan Williams traced the history of this experiment, showing how women involved in giving assistance demonstrated the evidence for the effectiveness of these programmes, signalling a close link between nutrition and maternal mortality.[100] The schemes were motivated primarily by humanitarian concerns to provide supplementary food to malnourished women during pregnancy. The notion of withholding food from a 'control' sample was regarded as abhorrent by members of the Trust. They refused to adopt such a strategy in order to fulfil the demands of 'scientific validity'. Consequently, the 'findings' of these 'experiments' were scathingly dismissed by members of the Medical Research Council's Nutrition Committee.[101]

In many districts, where financial hardship prevailed, the ability of even Labour-controlled councils to provide maternal and infant welfare clinics was limited by scarce resources. Elizabeth Peretz, in a study comparing Merthyr Tydfil, Tottenham and Oxford, showed that Merthyr compared favourably with Oxford in terms of providing free milk to expectant mothers, but that it was less generous than Tottenham, offering little that was comparable in the way of antenatal or screening programmes, hospital deliveries or convalescence, all of which were prescribed free of charge in Labour-controlled

Tottenham.[102] Generally, however, health provision in Merthyr Tydfil was inferior to that in Oxford. Similarly, the average circumstances of expectant women in Oxford were very much better than those living in Merthyr Tydfil, so by overall comparison the women of Merthyr fared the worst. These types of comparisons are extremely useful in furthering our understanding of how the worst areas of Wales compared with better areas of England.

The chapter by Mari Williams in this volume sets the issue of maternal mortality within the context of Wales as a whole, enabling us to see that the high losses of maternal lives were not confined to a few deprived districts, but constituted a national problem. The weakened constitution of mothers endangered their health whether they were living in impoverished circumstances in rural or industrial Wales. Nevertheless, she suggests that by the beginning of the Second World War significant changes were taking place and that the outlook for women was improving.

Between 1901–10 and 1934 the birth rate in Wales practically halved. Men and women in Wales were undoubtedly taking the decision to reduce family size. However, official advice on birth control was a contentious issue within Wales. Mari Williams argues that there was a strong antipathy toward birth control guidance, deriving from the opposition of religious institutions, especially Welsh Nonconformist chapel communities, who regarded official family planning advice as 'immoral and irreligious'. At a conference on health and society held in Bangor in March 2000 (the proceedings for which formed the basis for this book), Dr Rhoda Jones, a long-serving family planning doctor in north Wales, told how there was no formal provision in north Wales, partly for religious reasons, in the late 1960s when she was asked to establish a clinic. In setting up family planning clinics the Family Planning Association had to overcome a great deal of moral hostility, but when eventually the clinics were opened it became clear that they provided a long unmet need, for both family planning advice and concerning the health needs of women generally. Dr Jones ran busy clinics in Blaenau Ffestiniog, Porthmadog and Pwllheli, serving predominantly working-class communities, and provided advice to women of different ages and backgrounds over a period of more than thirty years. Dr Jones was a well-known member of the community in Blaenau Ffestiniog and would often be asked for medical advice whilst doing her shopping in the local Co-operative store on a Friday morning. Because the local group general practice was staffed by four male doctors, women evidently preferred to take their health problems to the family planning doctor. Over the years Dr Jones saw moral attitudes change considerably and the antipathy to family planning clinics gradually subside. Mari Williams views the antagonism which had formerly obstructed the development of birth control provision in Wales as being essentially based on gender divisions, reflecting a 'conflict between the needs of local mothers and the prejudices of their elected male representatives' (p. 133). This is clearly the impression to be gained from reading political reports and the views of Medical Officers of Health.

On the basis of letters from Wales located amongst the papers of birth control campaigner Marie Stopes and of oral interviews conducted with women who lived in south Wales during the inter-war period, Kate Fisher comes to a rather different conclusion. She argues that working-class women were reluctant to take advantage of birth control advice, preferring to rely on 'traditional' methods of birth control, notably withdrawal, and to 'leave it to the man'. Three-quarters of the forty-one women whom she interviewed in south Wales relied on their husbands practising withdrawal. She notes the frequency with which women who had been prescribed other birth control methods at the clinic (such as the cap, diaphragm or sponge) reported that they abandoned them and returned to a reliance on 'traditional methods'. In some cases, women were encouraged by their husbands to attend the birth control clinics, although clinics did not welcome direct approaches by the men. She concludes on the basis of oral evidence collected in industrial south Wales that we need to rethink our assumptions about female-centred birth control. Such an approach takes us beyond assumptions about moral and religious attitudes, and shifts the emphasis toward one of marital partnership. However, there was a total absence of birth control clinics in large swathes of rural Wales, where arguably religious, moral and financial constraints were stronger. The interpretations offered by Williams and Fisher are not entirely incompatible, but give us two different views taken from different methodological perspectives. Taken together they greatly enrich our understanding of both birth control and the dangers of maternity in inter-war Wales.

The professions
Whilst historians have written about women in education and domestic service in Wales, the role of women in nursing has been

unaccountably ignored. The life of a nineteenth-century Welsh nurse, who served at Scutari under Nightingale and then closer to the warfront at Balaclava, was recorded for posterity by the enterprising work of one of Wales's earliest feminist writers, Jane Williams (Ysgafell), who interviewed Elizabeth Williams and notated her 'oral history'. The manuscript was republished in 1987 with an introduction by Deirdre Beddoe.[103] It tells the life-story of a woman from a Welsh rural background, totally unlike that of Florence Nightingale, and offers a more 'rank-and-file' perspective on the work of nurses in the Crimean War. In this volume, Katherine Williams employs oral history to illustrate the day-to-day experiences of nurses who trained in the Caernarfon and Anglesey (C & A) Hospital in Bangor. This account of nursing at the C & A Hospital corresponds closely to descriptions written by Welsh nurses at other hospitals. They all emphasize the long hours of work and the physical stamina that was required. Zillah Jones, for instance, recalled that 'sound feet were the great essential' in selecting nurses for training, mirroring the recollections of nurses who trained at the C & A in Bangor.[104] Fflorens Roberts, who trained in Liverpool, and another nurse, who trained at the sanatorium in Abergele, north Wales, that was owned by the City of Manchester, described hours of work and conditions of training and discipline entirely comparable with those of the women whose experiences are graphically outlined by Katherine Williams in this volume.[105] This portrait is probably applicable to many provincial hospitals during this period.

The situation of nurses in large parts of Wales was compounded by the issue of the Welsh language, and Williams's study illustrates the subordinate status of both nurses and the Welsh language within the hospital regime. Her portrayal of trainees at the C & A hospital contrasts somewhat with the account provided by Sara Brady of probationers who trained at the King Edward VII Hospital in Cardiff during a slightly earlier period (1911–18).[106] The majority of the Cardiff intakes came from middle-class backgrounds, they were slightly older and appear to have been more career-orientated and driven by personal ambitions. The work of Brady and Williams illustrates the need for further case studies of nursing in Wales to provide a more comprehensive picture. Both of these studies are of voluntary hospitals; long overdue is a study of nurse training in poor law hospitals, as well as studies of Welsh district nursing, health visiting and midwifery. Williams's chapter highlights the importance of combining reminiscence with written records, so underlining the need for a research agenda prioritizing systematic oral history collection. Through her recording of the experiences of former nurses, together with her imaginative reading of the nurse training records, she has recreated the power of the lost institutional role of matron and identified the diligent commitment to duty required among the probationer nurses. Their stories stand as a testament to the heroic contribution of so many 'unsung' women to the health services of Wales.

A recent small-scale project has recorded the oral histories of nurses who trained in a specialist institution, the Prince of Wales Orthopaedic Hospital, Rhydlafar, and who specialized in orthopaedic nursing and the care of sick children.[107] Their voices tell of a similar hierarchical regime, but also describe some of the specific aspects of caring for children (although virtually none of them had received training in nursing sick children) and of nursing patients placed for long periods in plaster casts and in traction. This indicates the wealth and diversity of experience which could yet be retrieved from a period when nursing was very different from what it is today.

Another area of immense significance in terms of the social history of medicine in Wales is the work of district nurses and midwives. During the inter-war period they carried a great deal of responsibility, but also enjoyed much autonomy, as illustrated in a biography of Nurse Mills Evans, who served as district nurse and midwife in a rural area of Montgomeryshire, between 1921 and 1964.[108] An intrepid woman, she would visit a patient even during the most extreme weather conditions, day or night, and, like many district nurses in Wales, would travel fearlessly on a motorbike with her black bag packed full with first aid and medicines to deal with almost any emergency. She also managed to raise a family, do the accounts for her husband's decorating business and run a small village shop. During this period district nurses were responsible for a particular geographical 'patch' and so had a strong relationship with their local constituency. The relationship changed partly with the establishment of the National Health Service, but more so with the health service reorganization of 1974, which moved the employment of district nurses from local authorities to area health authorities. This had implications both for the geographical site of the service and for professional and gender relations. These important shifts have been described by Anthea Symonds, who interviewed health visitors in south Wales in 1996 and produced an insightful account of the way in which these women negotiated their changing roles.[109] Susan Pitt interviewed midwives and doctors who worked in Swansea during the period 1947–74, observing the strong sense of community loyalty which grew out of their attachment to a district; she noted how this changed with the move toward hospital-based midwifery, arguing that the community role shifted to one of surveillance.[110] Professional knowledge, responsibilities and functions have altered dramatically, and with accelerating rapidity during the second half of the twentieth century.

Indeed, it is hard to capture the enormous changes which took place in health and medicine during the twentieth century. One man's career illustrates this well. Dr Emyr Wyn Jones, distinguished cardiologist and polymath, commenced his medical studies at Liverpool in the early 1920s, at a time when certain 'pre-modern practices continued to exist'. In an interview with John Stewart he recalled vestiges of 'almost . . . Georgian medicine', including 'blood letting . . . and cupping, putting the hot cup on the back' as well as the use of leeches.[111] He also noted that digitalis was still commonly prescribed for use by patients with heart conditions during the early days of his career. Later he wrote extensively on the history of medicine in Wales, including papers on the use of *bysedd cochion* or *bysedd y cŵn* (foxglove) in traditional Welsh medicine.[112] In describing his medical training, he emphasized the extent to which doctors were then advised to listen carefully to the individual story which each patient had to tell, and to value the 'personal basis' of the doctor/patient relationship.[113] In effect, he continued to practise a form of 'bed-side medicine' for most of his career, up to his retirement in 1972.[114] He spoke of the importance of 'intuitive skill', of the 'undefinable form of medicine', and whilst this may seem anachronistic in an age of X-rays and laboratory testing, he was of a generation which spanned profound changes in the organization and practice of medicine.

In Wales, these traditions of 'personalistic' or person-centred medicine endured amongst many long-serving practitioners. The individual approach of many doctors left a lasting impression on the communities they served. Dr David Tomos, for instance, provided thirty-five years' service as a family doctor at his surgery in Llansannan, spanning the inter-war years, the Second World War and the early post-war years: 'Ystyriodd, nid y clefyd, ond y claf, nid yr afiechyd, ond yr afiach. Cofiodd am y dyn cyfan, yr enaid byw, y bersonoliaeth' (He considered, not the sickness, but the sick, not the disease, but the sufferer. He remembered the whole person, the living soul, the personality).[115] He would visit dying patients at night, even though there was no hope of prolonging life, in order to comfort them during their final hours. His distinctive appearance (he wore spats) and unusual companions (he always took his two white ferrets with him in the car on his rounds) made him a familiar figure in the local community. He often acted as anaesthetist, and would recite Welsh poetry as he sent his patients to sleep, whilst the surgeon, Mr Owen Thomas of Wrexham, would sing Welsh hymns.[116] With such literary and musical accompaniments the experiences of their Welsh patients must have differed somewhat from those of their neighbours east of Offa's Dyke!

The domesticated aspect prevailed in many aspects of the medical services in Wales well into the twentieth century. Dr Gwyn Thomas of Denbigh recalled as a boy watching his father conduct a post-mortem in the shed at the back of the house, clad in his overcoat and trilby hat, a cigarette dangling from the side of his mouth.[117] Trevor Hughes wrote of his 'eighty years on call', from the times he first accompanied his father as a small boy to the period when he continued to practise well into his eighties, in a community where his knowledge of his patients was long and intimate.[118] Often, the extended kinship networks of doctors as well as their patients reinforced this knowledge and understanding of community. Idris Naunton Davies lived and practised in Cymer, Porth, in the Rhondda valley the whole of his working life. His son, who qualified in 1910, and practised in the Valleys until his death in 1949, could count twenty-six of his relatives simultaneously in practice in the region.[119] It is this strong, community-based aspect of Welsh medicine, certainly prior to the Second World War, which is so distinctive. However, care must be taken not to over-generalize, for there were areas where it was difficult to attract doctors, where the medical market place was not lucrative and where doctors were themselves in open competition. Anne Digby, in her study of general practitioners, referred to five generations of the same family who practised in Fishguard in west Wales, and three generations of families who had practised in towns in Devon and Derbyshire, but warned that these could create a misleading impression, pointing out that her data-set for England and Wales did not support the interpretation that general practice was a 'family practice'.[120] It would be interesting, nevertheless, to compare patterns of general practice in Wales, England and Scotland.

The distinction between the acute and primary services remained much more blurred in Wales during the inter-war period. Many small cottage hospitals were staffed by nurses who would call upon the support of general practitioners, who visited the hospitals when necessary. Staff in general hospitals often worked for medical aid societies and would carry out surgery in the homes of members of these societies. Cornelius Griffiths, who trained at Bristol and St Bartholemew's Hospital, London, became surgeon at the King Edward VII Hospital in Cardiff and surgeon to the Cardiff branch of the Surgical Aid Society. A 'neat, precise operator' who taught surgery for over forty years, 'much of his operating was performed under primitive circumstances in lonely farmhouses and in the poor homes of coal mining districts'.[121] Many tonsolectomies and appendectomies in Wales were carried out on the kitchen table in the patient's home. Large areas of the country were remote from even a small cottage hospital, there were no telephones and road access was poor. Joan Hughes Parry described her daily routine as a doctor in an isolated rural practice on the Llŷn peninsula in the 1930s, where the nearest hospital was twenty-five miles away, and remarked upon the stark contrast between this and her former work in a London hospital. In south Caernarfonshire nearly all babies were delivered at home, and wounds and injuries would be treated and stitched at the patient's house or in the surgery. There were no X-ray facilities and laboratory tests had to be sent away to London or Manchester, so the doctors had for the most part to rely on their own judgement, in order to avoid impossible delays.[122] Much health care was provided by relatives, usually women without any formal qualifications, who devoted themselves to the long-term care of the sick. Joan's husband and practice partner, Robert Hughes Parry, recalled that the person 'who led the most exacting and strenuous life in the community was the district nurse midwife', who served an area of several square miles with a scattered population. She usually travelled by bicycle, although many isolated farms could only be approached on foot, and she carried a bag filled with dressings and necessary medications. The doctors would invariably do their own dispensing and carry medicines on their rounds, as a majority of patients had no easy access to a chemist.

The recollections of general practitioners confirm the conclusion drawn by the Welsh Consultative Council, which in its first report in 1920 pointed out that 'in several parts of Wales many types of institution and of service to be found in other parts of the United Kingdom are entirely absent or exist only to a very imperfect and inadequate extent'.[123] The same remained true at the end of the 1930s.

Compared with England, Scotland and Ireland, Wales was very late in establishing its own officially recognized system of medical education. The School of Nursing at the King Edward VII Hospital in Cardiff dates back to 1888, when it was called the Cardiff Royal Infirmary but, at this time, Wales, unlike England, Scotland and Ireland, had no medical school of its own. A pre-clinical medical school was established in Cardiff in 1893, constituting part of the University College of South Wales and Monmouthshire, founded in 1883.[124] This allowed students to follow the first two or three years of their training in Wales, before moving on to qualify in medicine at the University of London or elsewhere. There were demands within Wales for a fully fledged medical school. In 1893 the University of Wales was established by charter, forming a federal structure, and so when a proposal was put forward to establish a full medical school the issue arose as to whether it should form a separate constituent college within the University of Wales. The University of South Wales and Monmouthshire wished to retain medicine as a constituent faculty within its own institution and was not sympathetic to the creation of a new rival institution. In 1916 a Royal Commission was established under the chairmanship of Lord Haldane to consider the work of the university and the relationship of its constituent colleges. It recommended the establishment of a complete medical school as a separate college, to serve as a national school of medicine for Wales. Largely under the influence of Sir William Osler, the Commission recommended the adoption of the 'hospital unit system', based on the pioneering model of the medical faculty at John Hopkins University. This involved the appointment of full-time professors in each of the clinical departments of the medical school, each with its own laboratories and constituting a unit.[125] Staffs in the associated hospital fulfilled a dual role and became clinical teachers and were to work in association with the professors of the medical school. A certain number of beds were required to be linked to the medical school, in order to provide students with experience of patients in particular specialisms. However, the University of South Wales and Monmouthshire at Cardiff did not welcome the separation of the medical school, and a very difficult period ensued.[126] Finally, in 1931, the Welsh National School of Medicine was established by charter, and won independent status within the federal structure of the

University of Wales, and it became possible for students to complete clinical degrees in Wales.[127] A full-length history of the Welsh School of Medicine is currently being prepared by Alun Roberts. This will provide a valuable addition to the growing body of work on the history of medicine in Wales and a vital record of one of Wales's foremost national institutions.

One little-known aspect of the history of the Welsh National School of Medicine is the facility it offered to medical refugees from Nazi Europe to obtain recognized qualifications in Britain. In a chapter which traces the careers of medical refugees from Austria, Germany, Czechoslovakia and Poland, Paul Weindling indicates the small, but significant, role played by the Welsh National School of Medicine in providing an avenue for requalification. A majority of those who qualified in Wales stayed on to work as general practitioners. Although constituting only about 1 per cent of the medical refugees who came to Britain, their history provides an unusual insight into the general situation of medicine in Wales around the time of the Second World War, as well as a fascinating record of this particular group of refugee doctors.

Ever since the nineteenth century doctors from Scotland, Ireland and England have moved into Wales to help fill gaps in the services, often moving to areas of high need.[128] The refugee doctors strengthened medical provision at a time of shortage. A further wave of immigrant doctors arrived in Wales during the 1960s and 1970s. More than 18,000 doctors came to Britain from the Indian subcontinent. Many of them moved to fill vacancies in deprived south Wales valleys, where some have continued to provide a valuable service over a period of thirty years and more. Occasionally, during the 1990s for instance, they became the victims of racist attacks, but on the whole they were welcomed and their talents appreciated, and they have continued to receive a good deal of support from the communities they serve.[129] A recent investigation showed that in 2003 Asian doctors accounted for 73 per cent of the general practitioners in the Rhondda valley and 71 per cent of those in the neighbouring Cynon valley.[130] What will happen when these doctors retire is an issue currently facing many of these communities and policymakers in the Welsh Assembly Government.

One possible solution for deprived areas facing medical recruitment problems has been advanced by retired general practitioner Dr Julian Tudor Hart. In his scheme 'Going for Gold' he has proposed the introduction of a system of salaried doctors along with support for night and weekend cover and advocated that general practice in these areas should embrace an integrated research function that would assist the advancement of evidence-based medicine.[131] Ever an imaginative thinker and strident critic of the ills of the existing system, in this volume Julian Tudor Hart takes on the 'myth' of general practice in south Wales created by the doctor-novelist A. J. Cronin. Over past decades *The Citadel* has come to represent the essence of received wisdom concerning inter-war health provision in Wales. Martin Powell, for instance, has argued polemically that: 'General history texts on Wales say little about health care. Arguably A. J. Cronin's novel *The Citadel* contains more about health care in Wales than academic writings.'[132] Many historical accounts have cited Cronin's novel as a realistic representation of the general state of affairs in general practice in south Wales during the 1930s.[133] Tudor Hart discusses Cronin's motives and underlying political position and draws on his own experience and knowledge of general practice in south Wales to lay bare some of the problems of taking Cronin's book as documentary. Hart's contribution jolts us into thinking critically about the role of public health and general practice and about the issues facing the medical profession in late industrial society. In particular he focuses our attention on the specific context and needs of the valley communities of south Wales. He devoted his entire career to working in a poorly served area of high need, was one of the 'most notable single-practice researchers' in the UK, and his insights into the health care needs of a declining industrial community are internationally recognized.[134]

Hospital services and health administration in Wales

A comprehensive history of hospital services in Wales has yet to be written, but the work of Martin Powell has made a significant contribution to our knowledge of the overall shape and pattern of inter-war health services.[135] In addition a growing number of histories of individual hospitals are enriching the history of medicine in Wales.[136]

The institutional characteristics and spatial patterning of the hospital services in Wales reflect some of the issues of demography and industrial development discussed at the outset. One of the first initiatives of the Welsh Consultative Council, established in 1919 to make recommendations on the future of health services in Wales, was to commission a full survey of hospital provision in Wales. The

Council were 'impressed by the great need for increased accommodation for the residential treatment of sick persons other than those suffering from mental disease, tuberculosis, and infectious fevers'. They found the provision for general medical and surgical and gynaecological cases (at less than 8 beds per 10,000 of the population) 'seriously insufficient' and urged that the deficiency in Wales 'should be made good immediately', by providing ('on a conservative estimate') an additional 2,000 to 3,000 beds.[137] They also found that the distribution of hospital beds in Wales was extremely uneven. Nearly a half (46 per cent) of the general hospital beds available for the whole of Wales and Monmouthshire were located within the county boroughs of Cardiff, Merthyr, Newport and Swansea. Yet outside the boroughs, the administrative county of Glamorgan, with a population of over 800,000, had only 227 general hospital beds, a ratio of less than 3 beds per 10,000 of the population – 'a state of affairs which ought no longer to be countenanced'.[138]

The concentration of population in Glamorgan and Monmouthshire contrasted starkly with the dispersed populations in more rural counties, with consequent problems for hospital provision. The combined population of eight counties of Wales (Anglesey, Brecknockshire, Cardiganshire, Carmarthenshire, Flintshire, Merioneth, Montgomeryshire and Pembrokeshire) was about 25 per cent of the total population of Wales, whereas the land area of these counties covered about two-thirds of Wales. Yet they possessed only 15 per cent of the total number of hospital beds.[139] Emphasizing the problems created by this uneven dispersal of population, the Council pointed out that the entire population of Wales was greatly exceeded by some individual counties in England (for instance, the population of Wales was 2,568,068 as compared to Lancashire being 4,883,622). The Welsh Consultative Council put forward innovative proposals for the creation of a three-tier system of local, central and national health institutes, for the implementation of basic minimum provision in each area, and for a programme of modernization to include the establishment of medical institutes, providing a laboratory, a library, a statistical and record-keeping service. These proposals were not implemented, and despite the existence of a separate Welsh Board of Health there was no radical restructuring nor significant investment during the inter-war years. Indeed, there was virtual stagnation in hospital provision in Wales during the 1930s. A small decrease occurred in the number of beds provided in institutions under the

Poor Law Act, from 5,170 in 1931 to 5,088 in 1938, although additional ones were provided in general hospitals under the Public Health Acts (there were 504 beds in 1938 compared with only 76 in 1931).[140] One of the most notable characteristics identified by a survey of hospital services in north Wales, conducted during the Second World War, was the lack of specialist facilities. North Wales came under the orbit of specialist services in Liverpool and Manchester, and this helps to explain the decision to conduct separate surveys of the hospital services in north and south Wales.[141] The north-western survey team concluded that 'North Wales is poorly provided with hospital services' and that 'there is at present no general hospital of the requisite size and quality' to provide modern services. Moreover, it found that the hospitals of north Wales were largely dependent on general practitioners for their staffs, and concluded that in order to 'meet the hospital need not only are new buildings urgently required, but the need for settling a specialist team in the area is even more urgent'.[142] Hospital provision in south Wales was far more comprehensive, but here too there was a plethora of small hospitals and a deficiency in specialist services, and above all the survey team were struck by the lack of coordination of services. Overall, they concluded, the 'existing hospital service is characterised by difficulties, confusion and inadequacy'.[143]

In this volume Martin Powell sets out to consider the historiography of health and medicine in Wales in terms of theoretical debates concerning 'context and contingency'. To what extent, he asks, was Wales different? Did the differences simply reflect a different context, such as that produced by economic conditions or class formation, or were there factors unique to Wales, fused by culture or politics, for instance, which created a qualitatively different system in Wales? Powell demonstrates clearly that the pattern of hospital services in Wales was different. He indicates the inadequacy of hospital provision prior to the Second World War, and charts the different periodization and profile of development of both voluntary and municipal hospitals in Wales. With regard to the number of general practitioners he similarly demonstrates that Wales was relatively disadvantaged. Provision was therefore less comprehensive than in England, but was it different in nature? One argument, which has gained popular currency in Wales, is that the medical aid societies which developed before the First World War in Wales constituted an early form of communitarian provision. It has been suggested that the miners' medical services in South Wales 'at their best provided a universal and comprehensive medical service, unrivalled in the United Kingdom'.[144] Moreover, it has been held that the medical aid societies constituted an important part of an oppositional proletarian public sphere in south Wales, involving the 'rejection of professional control of medical services . . . the profit motive . . . and the very idea of individualism'.[145] However, Powell questions how representative these selected medical aid institutions were and whether they can be regarded as embryonic health centres. The strongest message of this informative and provocative chapter is the need for further research in order to identify what was unique in the Welsh situation.

Specifically, Powell identifies the need for a closer examination of the role of Welsh institutions, such as the Welsh Board of Health and the Welsh National Memorial Association (WNMA). The latter, although well described in an article by Linda Bryder, has never been the subject of a full-length history.[146] Established in 1910 as a Welsh national institution, its mission was to campaign to eradicate tuberculosis from Wales. The National Insurance Act of 1911 introduced the principle of free treatment in sanatoria for patients suffering from tuberculosis. The Act was amended to enable Welsh local authorities to delegate their obligation to provide services to the King Edward VII Welsh National Memorial Association. From 1912 onwards the association took responsibility for educational advice and treatment, providing a 'unified comprehensive anti-tuberculosis service with equal facilities throughout Wales'.[147] By 1928 the association was supporting 1,400 beds in four sanatoria and twelve hospitals, including the South Wales Sanatorium, Talgarth (304 beds) and the North Wales Sanatorium, Denbigh (234 beds).[148] However, despite this increase in the number of beds there was still less provision in Wales when measured in relation to the higher levels of mortality, for whereas England had an average of 69 beds per 100 deaths in 1929, Wales had only 52.[149]

The first Chair of Tuberculosis was established at Cardiff in 1920; new methods of diagnosis and treatment were introduced and evaluated, including ultra-violet light treatment for skin tuberculosis, surgical treatment of bone and joint and genito-urinary tuberculosis and various forms of collapsed lung therapy.[150] One of the world's leading thoracic surgeons, Hugh Morriston Davies, ran a small private establishment, Llanbedr Hall, near Ruthin, and acted as visiting surgeon to the WNMA.[151] Throughout Wales, many thousands of patients were treated for tuberculosis over a period of more than forty years, and it is a sad reflection on Welsh historiography that no major oral history project has been conducted. The intense experience of spending years in a sanatorium, and a patient's view of the extraordinary armoury of treatments, was captured by Herbert Williams in his autobiographical story *A Severe Case of Dandruff*.[152] His appeal for other surviving patients of the sanatoria led to a radio programme, where former inmates talked movingly of their experiences.[153] Despite many advances in treatment, the problem of tuberculosis in Wales remained serious throughout the inter-war years and especially so amongst the younger age groups. Death rates for tuberculosis amongst the age group 15–25 years, for instance, scarcely improved at all between 1921 and 1938.[154] By this time, local authorities were becoming vociferous in their complaints about the high cost of supporting tuberculosis treatment through the WMNA, with Flintshire protesting that expenditure on tuberculosis was swallowing up half of its gross expenditure on health services in the county.[155] There were concerns that the association was running a curative rather than a preventive service.

In 1938 a Committee of Inquiry was set up to investigate the anti-tuberculosis services in Wales, chaired by Clement Davies, MP for Montgomeryshire. Its revelations aroused the conscience of the nation.[156] The report publicly affirmed the close link between patterns of tuberculosis and social conditions. Detailed investigations in counties and districts with high rates of tuberculosis uncovered an astonishing level of poverty and public neglect of housing and sanitation. When the report was brought before the House of Commons, Jim Griffiths, MP for Llanelli, led the debate, giving an impassioned speech, later printed under the title *The Price Wales Pays for Poverty* (Llanelli, 1939). 'For that', he stated, 'is the fundamental fact which the report reveals. It reveals Wales as an impoverished nation. There are revelations of malnutrition, bad housing, poor schools, inadequate social services.' He referred to other recent reports on maternal mortality, on housing and on unemployment, and to a wealth of statistics that were testimony 'of the extent to which Wales is paying the penalty of its poverty in tuberculosis'.[157] During the debate, calls were made for a Cabinet Minister or a Cabinet Committee to deal with the problems affecting Wales.[158] The issue of health had once again provoked fundamental discussions concerning the government of Wales.

Health has been largely neglected in studies of devolution, which have tended to concentrate on political and constitutional change. The chapter by Charles Webster establishes the centrality of health in the devolution debates. Beginning with the establishment of the Welsh Insurance Commission in 1912, he dissects the various stages of evolution in the transfer of responsibilities for health to Wales and details the political tussles which preceded the transfer of executive responsibility to the Welsh Office in 1969. Political considerations weighed heavily, particularly concerns regarding the rising tide of nationalist sentiment, and this helps to explain what might appear as a sudden change of direction. Health was the largest portfolio to be transferred to the Welsh Office, and is now one of the major responsibilities of the new Assembly government.

Health and health services during the second half of the twentieth century

Meanwhile, how did the health of the people of Wales fare during the latter part of the twentieth century? During the Second World War the problem of tuberculosis in Wales was again highlighted when the medical examination of military recruits showed a high prevalence amongst applicants from Wales – 6 per cent of 1,869 men had been refused by the Welsh medical boards because they were found to have active tuberculosis.[159] However, during the war, the rates in Wales began to fall, and the gap narrowed between England and Wales. After the war, mass radiography schemes and improvements in treatment brought about rapid improvements.

Following publication of the Clement Davies Report, the dangers of slate dust were at last recognized and slate miners were included in the Silicosis Scheme of the Workmen's Compensation Act in 1940. However, few claims succeeded under this legislation and it was not until 1979 that a new Act was introduced, which enabled some 600 cases to receive compensation over the next eight years.[160]

The coal industry continued to cast a dark veil over the health of the Welsh people for decades after the Second World War. Older miners were still likely to develop lung and chest diseases, and other long-term limiting conditions such as heart and rheumatic complaints.[161] Such occupational diseases condemned many to a retirement of suffering. The legacy of unstable coal tips created anxiety amongst people dwelling in mining areas. In 1966 a sudden movement in a slag heap overshadowing one small Welsh community resulted in a calamity that exceeded the worst fears of all those who had warned against the dangers. On the morning of 21 October a coal tip suddenly moved, and within minutes had engulfed part of the village of Aberfan, killing 144 people, including 116 children attending Pantglas Junior School.[162] Whilst acknowledging this terrible blight on the lives of some families, most people enjoyed improvements in general health and life expectancy, and also in health services provision. As Jim Griffith had emphasized so clearly, the health problems in Wales were such that the remedies lay not in health measures alone, but in improvements in industrial and economic life. He believed that 'a greater diversity of industry and a better balance in its economic situation would itself lead to a healthier Wales'.[163] The broad measures adopted by the postwar Labour government, and especially those introduced by Jim Griffiths and Aneurin Bevan, 'the two outstanding figures in the Welsh Labour movement',[164] introduced new principles of social security, state-guaranteed welfare and universal health provision that transformed the living conditions of people in Wales during the 1950s. As R. Merfyn Jones has pointed out, post-war Wales was a very different place to Wales of the 1930s. The large expansion in social housing in the years following the Second World War contributed significantly to the improvements.[165] By 1965 out of the 225,000 new homes built in Wales, 144,000 had been constructed by local authorities.[166] The economy of south and south-west Wales was regenerated, with the growth of oil refineries, chemical works, new investment in steel and tin-plate works, and a rapid expansion in light industries, from crisps and clothing factories to washing-machine production and toy manufacturing. Women's economic activity rates increased significantly, bringing additional income to many households. Electrification revolutionized domestic life in rural areas and farming moved into a new phase of prosperity, with guaranteed subsidies on livestock production and on hill farming. The overall economic position and the welfare of urban and rural populations compared favourably with that of the 1930s. Infant mortality, one of the most sensitive indicators of social conditions, improved dramatically, and the high levels of maternal mortality began to fall, although they still remained higher in Wales than in England.

Health conditions therefore improved after the war. So too, did the health services, at last provided along more rational and comprehensive lines. Wales had stood testimony to Bevan's assertion that 'private charity and endowment' could not meet the costs of providing 'the best that medical skills can provide'. If the job of providing a modern health service is to be done, Bevan wrote in his brilliant exposition of socialized medicine, *In Place of Fear*, 'the state must accept financial responsibility'.[167]

Bevan's skilful negotiations and bold planning ensured that a nationalized health service providing treatment for all, free at the point of need, was brought into being after the Second World War.[168] This was of enormous importance to the people of Wales and particularly to women, the majority of whom had not been covered by National Health Insurance. All hospitals in Wales were nationalized and brought under the jurisdiction of a Welsh Regional Hospital Board, and for the first time there was an opportunity to plan an all-Wales hospital service. The inadequacies of the existing system were made clear by the war-time hospital surveys, previously mentioned. An enormous task of upgrading hospital facilities lay ahead. Many Welsh hospitals were in buildings which were totally unsuitable for the needs of modern medicine. A number of new hospitals had been erected during the Second World War, often as prefabricated structures for the US and Canadian military. Some, such as Glangwili in Carmarthen, continued to function as district hospitals for many years after, entirely unsuited to patient care. In the words of Dr Emyr Wyn Jones, the huts were 'anobeithiol o oer yn ystod y gaeaf ac yn annioddefol o boeth yn yr haf' (exceptionally hot in summer and extremely cold in winter).[169] Others occupied old workhouse sites, some dating back to the time of the New Poor Law. The money was not available to replace them, so a gradual process of upgrading took place. The Union Workhouse at St Asaph, for instance, was originally opened in 1840. An infirmary was joined to the workhouse in 1924 and a delivery ward, X-ray department and small theatre were opened. On the establishment of the National Health Service in 1948, a new phase of development commenced, 'and infirmary beds were utilised for medical, surgical, gynaecological, obstetrical, ophthalmic, dental and ENT patients'.[170] Between 1955 and 1957 rooms and outbuildings were adapted for use as a pathology laboratory, pharmacy, storerooms and works office. ENT facilities were further upgraded and in 1964–5 a new surgical suite was erected. Perhaps one of the most important developments was the appointment of specialist staff, in obstetrics, paediatrics, ENT, orthopaedics, rheumatology, geriatrics and so on. This process of adding to and upgrading buildings and appointing more full-time medical staff and specialists took place in many hospitals across Wales. St David's Hospital,

Bangor, for instance, saw improvements in facilities and staffing in the post-war years, including the opening of an Outpatients Department in 1959, followed by an operating theatre and a special baby-care unit, and in 1966 a new geriatric unit was opened.[171] This process of modernization and the careers of some of the specialists appointed in north Wales are beautifully captured in a series of personal portraits presented by retired anaesthetist, Buddug Owen.[172]

Pre-war patterns of popular belief regarding cures were not entirely abandoned, and the final vestiges of traditional practices were still occasionally encountered in the post-Second World War period. Dr Glyn Penrhyn Jones claimed that he witnessed a local *dyn hysbys* (medical magician; lit. a wise man) performing an elaborate healing ritual after consulting a 'secret book' at Llanllechid in the Ogwen valley in the 1950s.[173] During the 1960s teacher T. Llew Jones, fearing cancer, consulted an unqualified healer in Carmarthenshire after failing to obtain relief from orthodox medical provision at Glangwili Hospital and at the Royal Free Hospital, London. He described how following a feverish temperature his skin turned yellow and he began to feel weak and tired. The 'medicine' he received proved effective and he began to improve, at which point he was asked to return to the Royal Free as they had identified the cause of his illness. He had in fact contracted liver fluke from eating watercress brought to school by some of the farm children, a condition of which a rural herbalist might well have had expert knowledge.[174] On the whole, however, with the growth and development of the NHS in Wales, faith in modern biomedical solutions came to predominate and expectations shifted towards modern health provision.[175]

Progress in the early years of the NHS was slow. During the period 1948 to 1964 the health and particularly hospital services suffered resource starvation in relation to needs.[176] Planning for the health services in Wales was, and is, a hugely challenging task. Surveying the hospital services in Wales in 1969, G. Prys-Davies, chairman of the Welsh Hospital Board, spoke of the difficulty of calculating current need on the basis of past provision.[177] The low level of provision and the uneven distribution of population had created a long-standing problem. Bed-use statistics showed that there were long waiting lists for surgical specialties, and an imbalance in services, with uneven patterns between hospitals and regions. Generally the average duration of a hospital stay was longer in Wales than in England, and outpatient waiting lists were increasing. Needs in Wales were greater, reflecting poorer health. Wales had a higher proportion of skilled and unskilled workers than England. Ironically, whereas this meant higher levels of ill health (since there was a clear class gradient in health status), it had also meant lower expectations of the health services in the past, since the 'unskilled and semi-skilled did not make demands on the service to the same extent' as the more educated, professional classes. Therefore Wales had a higher level of unmet need that was now coming to the fore as socio-economic conditions were changing and expectations increasing apace.[178] The 1962 Hospital Plan for Wales identified the need for new district hospitals in towns such as Swansea, Bangor and Wrexham, and for the upgrading of smaller hospitals. There was massive investment in the new University Hospital of Wales at the Heath, Cardiff, complete with a new medical teaching centre.[179] Yet compared with the modernization of the hospital services in England, Wales still lagged behind. Within Wales there was an uneven distribution of services, with the most comprehensive and modern facilities being located in the most affluent areas, a phenomenon to which Julian Tudor Hart drew attention in his famous *Lancet* article, 'The Inverse Care Law'.[180] Central government began to recognize the uneven distribution of benefit accruing from investment in the health services across England and Wales and attempted to correct this by initiating a Resource Allocation Review, designed to divert resources to the more needy areas.[181] However, the introduction during the 1980s of new concepts of 'general management' and the creation of 'internal markets' represented 'an implicit rejection of past policies to correct such inequalities through planned resource allocations'.[182] The White Paper *Working for Patients* (1989) involved a rejection of central planning and the creation of a provider market. Targets, service frameworks and performance criteria became the crucial indicators of policy direction, during a unique epoch of change described in this volume by John Wyn Owen.

    The establishment of the Welsh Office in 1969 meant that it was possible for policies to develop in a slightly different direction, once administration was based in Cardiff rather than London. It is sometimes said that the Welsh Office did no more than reissue instructions emanating from the Department of Health, but the chapter by John Wyn Owen offers a different perspective. In 1984 he was appointed the first Director of the NHS in Wales, and this marked another stage in the process of devolution. In a first-hand account of his period as executive officer he describes the wide-ranging innovations that he piloted in Wales, and emphasizes the extent to which the health service in Wales at that time looked internationally for inspiration and models of good practice, especially in regard to public health. This chapter shows clearly that the health service in Wales was operating in the fast stream of change, adapting to new ideas and principles and pioneering innovative policy strategies, for instance the adoption of national service frameworks, benchmarking measures, employing health informatics. Wales was, in a sense, a testing ground during this period for many policies which have subsequently become hegemonic throughout the UK.

Since the 1960s there have been improvements in cardiac treatments and in cancer surgery and therapy, the introduction of facilities for kidney dialysis and body scanners that have revolutionized the practice of diagnosis. People working in the health services have witnessed rapid changes and innovation, and treatments and knowledge of the causes of disease have proceeded apace. However, despite investment in health promotion campaigns, such as Heartbeat Wales, rates of heart disease and diabetes in Wales have continued to rise, and so remain disproportionately high compared with England. There are areas in Wales which have the highest rates of low birth weights amongst infants, the highest rates of limiting long-term illness amongst the adult population and the highest rates of obesity amongst children of any areas in the UK – which perhaps correlates with the fact that Wales has the highest rates of child poverty.

Health inequalities

Illness, as Gareth Williams argues in the final chapter in this volume, is a lived historical experience that leaves its mark on how you live and how you die. Illness impacts on the lives of people, on their ability to perform tasks, on their relationships and on their memories. In Wales, as many other contributors have shown, we have a legacy of poor health and a history characterized by unequal life-chances. Ill health is inscribed in many of the autobiographical accounts of Welsh writers of the twentieth century. Health experiences relate to social patterns, and to material circumstances; in Wales, as elsewhere, they relate to structural changes in the economy.

Although, generally, health and life expectancy improved after the Second World War, the scale of inequalities remained stubbornly persistent. In the early 1930s Wales had a death rate eleven points above that of England and Wales combined. Forty years later 'that disparity was almost exactly the same'. Moreover, the 'massive and persistent difference between the death rates for the South East of England and those for Industrial South Wales' showed no signs of decreasing.[183] The death rates among particular age groups living in industrial areas diverged widely from those of the average for England and Wales. Male mortality from coronary heart disease for the age group 35–44 years in the valleys of Glamorgan was almost 75 per cent above the rate for England and Wales and three times the rate for East Anglia. Considerably higher death rates were experienced in parts of south Wales across a range of conditions, ranging from bronchitis to accidents.

Morbidity rates are harder to gauge precisely. Rates of limiting long-term illness, recorded by the Census of Population since 1991, indicate that Wales has some of the highest concentrations of sickness and ill health in the UK.[184] This also means higher consultation rates and higher general-practice workloads in these areas. A comparative morbidity survey carried out in 1970–2 showed that consultation rates in Tudor Hart's practice in Glyncorrwg were more than double the average of other practices participating in the study, and that hospital admission rates were 76 per cent higher.[185] In Wales, there was a 59 per cent increase in certified incapacity for work from illness between 1953–4 and 1972–3, compared with an increase of 30 per cent throughout the UK. High levels of claims for incapacity benefit were found in areas of high long-term male unemployment where there was little alternative employment following pit closures, and where they were 'particularly lacking protected light employment for those disabled by heavy industry'.[186] The Rhondda, Cynon Taf, the Rhymney valley and Blaenau Gwent continued to show rates of long-term illness considerably in excess of the average for England and Wales at the very end of the twentieth century.[187]

These higher rates of morbidity and mortality have implications both for the everyday lives of the people of Wales and for the costs of running the health service. In Wales as a whole the death rates from stomach cancer for men were 13 per cent higher and for women 21 per cent higher than the England and Wales average. Some of the highest rates of cancer are in the more rural areas of north and west Wales, where people still have to travel great distances to obtain treatment. The uneven distribution of illness and mortality, in terms of geography and social class, is a problem that presents a major challenge for health policymakers in Wales. The devolution of government to the Welsh Assembly offers new opportunities to tackle these problems.[188] Areas of Wales in which there are now, for example, higher than average infant mortality, premature death amongst adults and high rates of chronic illness are those very areas where there are concentrations of unemployment, low incomes, poor housing and limited access to transportation. These social conditions contribute to a lived and ongoing experience. In the final chapter of this book Williams describes how respondents to a study of the impact of the closure of Ebbw Vale steelworks described the effect on their lives and communities, their sense of loss and even heartbreak at the devastating consequences of economic decline. He places the Welsh experience within the broader context of debates on health inequalities and argues the need for a greater understanding of the human consequences of social inequality and economic exploitation.

This volume overall may be seen to tend towards a 'pessimistic' account of health, health services and social conditions in Wales. This should not lead to a fatalistic approach to the health of the Welsh people. Rather, the health conditions described in this book should alert people once again to the scale of the difficulties, both historically and in the present. As Jim Griffiths once declared 'we are not facing a predestined fate, we are facing a social problem'.[189] Health inequalities are the manifestation of social issues that confront Wales today. They represent a major challenge for the new Assembly government, but they can only be fully understood through an appreciation of the historical roots of ill health. Wales, more than most countries in the UK and indeed western Europe, has inherited both a huge backlog of health problems and a system of health care that has suffered from underinvestment and neglect. Unless the Assembly takes full account of the historical record, it is destined to repeat mistakes of the past and further deprive the people of their health rights for which Griffiths was making his impassioned plea in 1939.

Notes

[1] M. Hechter, *Internal Colonialism: The Celtic Fringe in British National Development, 1536–1966* (London, 1975); H. Kearney, *The British Isles: A History of Four Nations* (Cambridge, 1989); L. Colley, *Britons* (New Haven, CT, 1992); N. Davies, *The Isles: A History* (London, 1999); C. Kinealy,

A Disunited Kingdom?: England, Ireland, Scotland and Wales, 1880–1949 (Cambridge, 1999).

2   Jacqueline Jenkinson, *Scotland's Health, 1919–1948* (Oxford, 2002); John Stewart, 'The National Health Service in Scotland, 1947–1974: Scottish or British?', *Historical Research*, Vol. 76, no. 193 (2003), 389–410; Andrew Hull and Johanna Geyer-Kordesch, *The Shaping of the Medical Profession: The History of the Royal College of Physicians and Surgeons of Glasgow, 1858–1999* (London, 1999); C. Nottingham (ed.), *The NHS in Scotland: The Legacy of the Past and the Prospect for the Future* (Aldershot, 2000); M. Crowther, 'Poverty, health and welfare', in W. Hamish Fraser and R. Morris (eds), *People and Society in Scotland: Vol. II, 1830–1914* (Edinburgh, 1998), pp. 265–89; A. MacGregor, *Public Health in Glasgow, 1905–1914* (Edinburgh, 1967); Martin Gorsky, 'Threshold of a new era: the development of an integrated hospital system in north-east Scotland, 1900–1939', *Social History of Medicine*, Vol. 17, no. 2 (August 2004), 247–66; G. McLachlan (ed.), *Improving the Common Weal: Aspects of Scottish Health Services, 1900–1984* (Edinburgh, 1987); I. Levitt, *Poverty and Welfare in Scotland, 1890–1948* (Edinburgh, 1988); John Stewart, *Taking Stock: Scottish Social Welfare after Devolution* (Bristol, 2004); K. Woods and D. Carter (eds), *Scotland's Health and Health Service* (London, 2003).

3   Greta Jones and Elizabeth Malcolm, *Medicine, Disease and the State in Ireland, 1650–1940* (Cork, 1999); Greta Jones, *'Captain of all These Men of Death': The History of Tuberculosis in Nineteenth and Twentieth Century Ireland* (Amsterdam, 2001); Pauline Prior, *Mental Health and Politics in Northern Ireland: A History of Service Development* (Aldershot, 1993); R. D. Cassell, *Medical Charities, Medical Politics: The Irish Dispensary System and the Poor Law 1836–1872* (London, 1997).

4   R. Williams, 'West of Offa's Dyke', in D. Williams (ed.), *Who Speaks for Wales? Nation, Culture, Identity: Raymond Williams* (Cardiff, 2003), p. 35.

5   Tony Curtis, *Wales, The Imagined Nation: Studies in Cultural and National Identity* (Bridgend, 1986); Emyr Humphries, *The Taliesin Tradition: A Quest for the Welsh Identity* (Bridgend, 1989); Wynford Vaughan-Thomas, *Wales, a History* (London, 1985); Gwyn A. Williams, *When was Wales?* (Harmondsworth, 1985); Fiona Bowie, 'Wales from within: conflicting interpretations of Welsh identity', in Sharon MacDonald (ed.), *Inside European Identities: Ethnography in Western Europe* (Providence, RI, 1993), pp. 167–93.

6   H. Cushing, *The Life of Sir William Osler* (Oxford, 1940), p. 533. He made this remark in June/July 1916.

7   J. Cule, 'Sir William Osler and his Welsh connections', *Postgraduate Medical Journal*, Vol. 64 (1988), 568–74 (570). An eminent surgeon, and educator of world renown, Osler exerted an important influence over the development of medical education in Wales.

8   J. Aitchison and H. Carter, *A Geography of the Welsh Language* (Cardiff, 1994), p. 41; Mari A. Williams *'Yr Iaith Gymraeg yn ei Henbydrwydd': Y Gymraeg yn y 1950au* (Aberystwyth, 2001).

9   R. Merfyn Jones, *Cymru 2000: Hanes Cymru yn yr Ugeinfed Ganrif* (Caerdydd,

1999), pp. 176–7; Geraint H. Jenkins and Mari A. Williams, *'Let's do our Best for the Ancient Tongue': The Welsh Language in the Twentieth Century* (Cardiff, 2000); John Aitchison and Harold Carter, *Language, Economy and Society: The Changing Fortunes of the Welsh Language in the Twentieth Century* (Cardiff, 2000).

[10] For this paragraph and the next see Neil Evans, 'Two paths to economic development: Wales and the north-east of England', in Pat Hudson (ed.), *Regions and Industries: A Perspective on the Industrial Revolution in Britain* (Cambridge, 1989); idem, 'Gogs, Cardis and hwntws: region, nation and state in Wales, 1840–1940', in idem (ed.), *National Identity in the British Isles* (Coleg Harlech Occasional Papers in Welsh Studies, no. 3, 1989); idem, 'Regional Dynamics: North Wales, 1750–1914', in Edward Royle (ed.), *Issues in Regional Identity: Essays in Honour of John Marshall* (Manchester, 1998); idem, '"As rich as California": opening and closing the frontier, Wales 1780–1870', in Gareth Elwyn Jones and Dai Smith (eds), *The People of Wales: A Millennium History* (Llandysul, 1999).

[11] A. H. Dodd, *A Short History of Wales* (London, 1972), p. 147.

[12] See the map in R. A. Butlin, 'The historical geography of Britain', in *The Ordinance Survey Atlas of Great Britain* (London, 1982), p. 157.

[13] B. Jones, 'Banqueting at a moveable feast: Wales 1870–1914', in G. E. Jones and D. Smith (eds), *The People of Wales* (Llandysul, 1999), pp. 145–78 (150).

[14] Mining and quarrying employed 274,682 and metal manufacturing and engineering employed 98,558, totalling 373,240 out of a total occupied male workforce of 880,407. John Williams, *Digest of Welsh Historical Statistics*, Vol. I (Pontypool, 1985), p. 97.

[15] A. Borsay and D. Porter, 'Medicine and Health: Historical and Contemporary Perspectives',in A. Borsay, *Medicine in Wales c.1800–2000: Public Service or Private Commodity?* (Cardiff, 2003), pp. 1–20.

[16] J. Cule (ed.), *Wales and Medicine* (Llandysul, 1975).

[17] Colin Baber and John Lancaster (eds), *Healthcare in Wales: An Historical Miscellany* (Cardiff, 2000).

[18] John Cule, *Wales and Medicine: A Source-list for Printed Books and Papers Showing the History of Medicine in Relation to Wales and Welshmen* (Cardiff, 1980).

[19] J. Williams ab Ithel (ed.) and J. Pughe (trans.), *The Physicians of Myddfai* (Llandovery, 1861); H. E. F. Davies and M. E. Owen, 'Meddygon Myddfai', in J. Cule (ed.), *Wales and Medicine* (Llandysul, 1975), pp. 156–84; J. Pughe (trans.), *The Herbal Remedies of the Physicians of Myddfai* (Felinfach, 1987); J. Pughe (trans.), *The Physicians of Myddfai* (Felinfach, facsimile reprint, 1993); John Williams ab Ithel, *Meddygon Myddfai* (Felinfach, 1993); D. Hoffman, *Welsh Herbal Medicine* (Abercastle, Pembs, 1978).

[20] The Osler Library, McGill University, Montreal, Canada, Osler collection, item 3676, *The Physicians of Myddfai* – translated by John Pughe and edited by Revd John Williams ab Ithel, Llandovery, c.1861, with inserted letter from Sir John Rhŷs, 1908. For Sir John Rhŷs, see *The Dictionary of Welsh Biography down to 1940* (London, 1959), pp. 844–5.

[21] BMA Cymru Wales, The Voice of Doctors, 'Wales and Medicine – The Physicians of Myddfai', www.bma.org.uk/ap.nsf/content/the+physicians+of+myddfai, accessed 9 November 2003.

[22] F. Jones, *The Holy Wells of Wales* (Cardiff, 1954 and 1992); M. W. Annear, 'Some healing and holy wells of Wales' in Cule (ed.), *Wales and Medicine*, pp. 185–9.

[23] G. P. Jones, 'Folk medicine in eighteenth-century Wales', *Folk Life*, Vol. 7 (1969), 60–74 (66).

[24] K. Bosse Griffiths, *Byd y Dyn Hysbys: Swyngyfaredd yng Nghymru* (Talybont, 1977); R. C. Allen, 'Wizards or charlatans – doctors or herbalists?: an appraisal of the "Cunning Men" of Cwrt y Cadno, Camarthenshire', *North American Journal of Welsh Studies*, Vol. 1, no. 2 (Summer 2001), 68–85; Owen Davies, 'Charmers and charming in England and Wales from the eighteenth to the twentieth century', *Folklore*, Vol. 109 (1998), 41–52; Owen Davies, 'Cunning folk in England and Wales during the eighteenth and nineteenth centuries', *Rural History*, Vol. 8 (1997), 91–107.

[25] David LeVay, *The Life of Hugh Owen Thomas* (Edinburgh and London, 1956); Emyr Wyn Jones, 'Hugh Owen Thomas – Gŵr o Dras', in *Ar Ffiniau Meddygaeth* (Denbigh, 1971), pp. 21–35; F. Watson, *The Life of Sir Robert Jones* (London, 1934); for obituaries of Robert Jones, see *British Medical Journal* (January 28 1933 and January 21 1933), p. 170 and p. 123; Emyr Wyn Jones, 'Canmlwyddiant geni syr Robert Jones', in *Ar Ffiniau Meddygaeth*, pp. 36–45; N. Hywel Jones 'The bone-setters of Anglesey', *Transactions of the Anglesey Antiquarian Society* (1981), 57–8; Roger Cooter, *Surgery and Society in Peace and War: Orthopaedics and the Organisation of Modern Medicine, 1880–1948* (Basingstoke, 1993).

[26] The Roberts family of Merioneth offer a good example of a medical dynasty who sent their sons to gain formal qualifications, see Edward Davies, 'Meddygon Stiniog', *Rhamant Bro, Cylchgrawn Cymdeithas Hanes Bro Ffestiniog*, rhif 17 (Haf, 1999), pp. 20–8.

[27] H. Hughes-Roberts, *Meddygon Esgyrn Môn* (Liverpool, 1935), p. 78.

[28] James Patterson Ross and W. R. LeFanu, *Lives of the Royal College of Surgeons of England, 1965–1973* (London, 1981), p. 186.

[29] I. G. Jones, '1848 and 1868: "Brad y llyfrau Gleision" and Welsh politics', in *Mid-Victorian Wales: The Observers and the Observed* (Cardiff, 1992), p. 173, n. 20.

[30] T. G. Davies, 'And where shall she find a doctor? Incidents in the history of medicine in Gower during the nineteenth century', *Morgannwg*, Vol. 45 (2001), 29–54.

[31] H. Glyn Davies, *Edrych yn Ôl: Hen Atgofion am Geredigion* (Liverpool, 1958), 60–5.

[32] A. E. Williams, *Meddyginiaethau Llafar Gwlad* (Cardiff, 1983).

[33] T. Llew Jones and Dafydd Wyn Jones, *Cyfrinach Wncwl Daniel* (Llandysul, 1992); T. Llew Jones and Dafydd Wyn Jones, *Cancer Curers – or Quacks? The Story of a Secret Herbal Remedy* (Llandysul, 1993); Cyril Scott, *Victory over Cancer* (London, 1939).

34 H. Parri, *Meddygon y Ddafad Wyllt* (Denbigh, 1984).
35 Anne E. Jones, 'Folk medicine in living memory in Wales', *Folk Life*, Vol. 18 (1980), pp. 58–68; P. S. Brown, 'The vicissitudes of herbalism in late nineteenth and early twentieth century Britain', *Medical History*, Vol. 29, no. 1 (1985), 71–92; H. Bowles, 'Cure for all ills?', *Gwent Local History*, Vol. 58 (1985), 30–6.
36 A. Digby, *The Evolution of British General Practice, 1850–1948* (Oxford, 1999), p. 34.
37 Information from my father F. R. Williams, Ivy Cottage, Cadoxton, Neath, Glamorgan.
38 Emyr Wyn Jones, *Lloffa yn Llŷn – Trem yn Ôl* (Denbigh, 1994); T. G. Davies, 'Dau iachawr o Abertawe: y Baron Spolasco a James Rogers', *National Library of Wales Journal*, Vol. 25 (1987), 98–113.
39 Emyr Wyn Jones, 'Sir John Williams: his background and achievement (1840–1926)', in Cule (ed.), *Wales and Medicine*, pp. 86–95; Ruth Evans, *John Williams, 1840–1926* (Cardiff, 1952); Iorwerth Hughes Jones, 'The medical aspects of the life of Sir John Williams, Bart', *National Library of Wales Journal*, Vol. 9, no. 2 (Winter, 1955), 235–8.
40 Emyr Wyn Jones, 'Sir John Williams', 93–4.
41 D. Geraint James, 'Dr Isambard Owen (1850–1927)', in Cule (ed.), *Wales and Medicine*, pp. 96–106; G. A. Jones, 'The life and work of Sir Isambard Owen, 1850–1927' (unpublished MA thesis, University of Wales, 1967).
42 J. Gwynn Williams, *The University of North Wales: Foundations 1884–1927* (Cardiff, 1985).
43 Peter H. Thomas, 'Medical men of Glamorgan: Dr Donald Rose Paterson (1862–1939)', in Stewart Williams (ed.), *Glamorgan Historian*, Vol. 5 (Cowbridge, 1968), 38–60; P. H. Thomas, 'Medical men of Glamorgan: William Thomas Edwards, 1821–1915', in Stuart Williams (ed.), *Glamorgan Historian*, Vol. 8 (Barry, 1972), 121–45.
44 W. A. Evans, 'Dr Evan Pierce of Denbigh', *Transactions of the Denbighshire Historical Society*, Vol. 15 (1966), 158–68; Buddug Owen, *Meeting Pioneers* (Denbigh, 1994), 'Not on the Denbigh Column', pp. 18–26. See also Robert Hughes Parry's account of Dr O. Wynne Roberts and Dr Jones Evans of Pwllheli, in his autobiography *Within Life's Span* (Ilfracombe, 1973), pp. 110–12. A good example from south-west Wales is provided by E. Vernon Jones, 'A Saint and his Progeny', *Carmarthen Historian*, Vol. 8 (1971), 46–68 (48–53). Dr John Hughes (1817–97) played a leading role in the town of Carmarthen for over fifty years, holding many public offices, including that of coroner, chairman of the Board of Guardians, chairman of the School Board, surgeon to the artillery militia stationed in the town, factory surgeon, police surgeon, income tax commissioner, and so on.
45 As Hettie Glyn Davies, like many others, remarked: 'Ni fyddai neb yn 'mofyn doctor os na fyddai'r salwch yn ddrwg iawn' (nobody would call the doctor unless the illness was extremely serious), H. Glyn Davies, *Edrych Yn Ôl*, p. 60.
46 *Mesur Yswiriant Cenedlaethol: Eileb o gofnodeb yn egluro y mesur ar ôl bod drwy dŷ y cyffredin cyn belled ag y mae a fynno ag yswiriant iechyd cenedlaethol (cyfieithiedig o Cd. 5995)* (Cardiff, 1912).

[47] William George, *Yswiriant Cenedlaethol Iechyd neu Ddeddf Yswiriol 1911: Esboniad a Rhydd Gyfieithiad gan William George Criccieth* (Caernarfon, 1912), p. 5. 'The Insurance Act of 1911 is a revolutionary Bill – that is, it involves important transformations in the machinery of society, the wheels of which when this Bill is operating will turn in a very different way from that which they did before. Indeed, if we may be allowed to follow the metaphor further we might say that there is good reason to believe that this New Great Wheel will be of enormous help in raising the lower ranks from the depths of ill health and poverty and bringing them within reach of healthy air and the fullness of life.'

[48] Ibid., pp. 107–10.

[49] I. G. Jones, 'The people's health in mid-Victorian Wales', in *Mid-Victorian Wales: The Observers and the Observed* (Cardiff, 1992), pp. 24–53; D. C. James, 'The genesis of sanitary reform', *Welsh History Review*, Vol. 11 (1982), 50–66; A. Croll, 'Writing the insanitary town: G. T. Clark, slums and sanitary reform', in B. Ll. James (ed.), *G. T. Clark: Scholar Ironmaster in the Victorian Age* (Cardiff, 1998), pp. 24–47; A. H. Williams, 'Public health and local history', *The Local Historian*, Vol. 14, no. 4 (1980), 202–10.

[50] Raymond K. J. Grant, 'Merthyr Tydfil in the mid nineteenth-century: the struggle for public health', *Welsh History Review*, Vol. 14 (1989), 574–94; Raymond K. J. Grant, *Water and Sanitation: The Struggle for Public Health in Merthyr Tydfil* (Cowbridge, 1993); J. Gross, 'Water supply and sewerage in Merthyr Tydfil, 1850–1914', *Merthyr Historian*, Vol. 2 (1978), 67–78; J. Gross, 'Dr T. J. Dyke, 1816–1900', *Merthyr Historian*, Vol. 12 (2001), 21–6; I. G. Jones, 'Health and sanitary engineering in mid-nineteenth century Merthyr Tydfil', *Journal of the South East Wales Industrial Archaeology Society*, Vol. 2, no. 2 (1976), 27–48; I. Gwynedd Jones, 'The politics of survival', *Llafur*, Vol. 2, no. 1 (1976), 18–31 and reprinted in idem, *Communities: Essays in the Social History of Victorian Wales* (Llandysul, 1992), pp. 24–53.

[51] Huw Williams, 'Pontypridd: public health', in H. Williams (ed.), *Pontypridd: Essays on the History of an Industrial Community* (Cardiff, 1981), 33–41; H. Richards, 'Investment in public health provision in the mining valleys of south Wales, 1860–1914', in C. Baber and J. Williams (eds), *Modern South Wales: Essays in Economic History* (Cardiff, 1986), pp. 128–39.

[52] D. C. James, 'Public health in nineteenth century Cardiff' (unpublished MA thesis, University of Wales, 1974); D. C. James, 'The genesis of sanitary reform in Cardiff', *Welsh History Review*, Vol. 11 (1982), 50–66.

[53] R. D. Till, 'Public health and community in the borough of Neath, 1835–60', *Welsh History Review*, Vol. 5 (1971), 377–92; Colin James, *Study Based on the Clerk's Report Book of the Swansea Local Board of Health, 1855–66* (Lampeter, 2000); T. G. Davies, 'Health and hospitals', in Ralph A. Griffiths (ed.), *The City of Swansea: Challenges and Changes* (Stroud, 1990), pp. 165–78.

[54] Stephen Roberts, '"Necessary precaution": public health in Wrexham, 1830–1848', *Trafodion Cymdeithas Hanes Sir Dinbych*, Vol. 45 (1996), 59–88. David Lee Williams, 'A healthy place to be? The Wrexham coalfield in the interwar period', *Llafur*, Vol. 7, no. 1 (1996), 87–95.

55 *Public Health in Mid-Victorian Wales: Correspondence from the Principality to the General Board of Health and the Local Government Act Office, 1848–71*, transcribed and edited with an introduction by A. H. Williams (Cardiff, 1983). A copy of this typescript, running to over 1,750 pages in four volumes, is deposited in the university libraries of Wales, as well as at the National Library of Wales, other copyright libraries, the Institute of Historical Research and the Wellcome Unit for the History of Medicine in Oxford.
56 G. Roberts, 'Iechyd cyhoeddus yn Sir Caernarfon, 1870–1939' (unpublished Ph.D. thesis, University of Wales, 1993); Steven D. Thompson, 'A social history of health in interwar south Wales' (unpublished Ph.D. thesis, University of Wales, 2001); see also Owen Gruffydd Roberts, 'Sanitary reform, civic politics and ideas of health in Wales, 1870–1900. With special reference to Swansea' (unpublished Ph.D. thesis, University of Wales, 2003).
57 A. Fletcher, 'Cholera in north-east Wales, 1832', *Denbighshire Historical Society Transactions*, Vol. 44 (1995), 25–44; D. C. James, 'The cholera epidemic of 1849 in Cardiff: a case study', *Morgannwg*, Vol. 25 (1981), 164–79; G. Penrhyn Jones, 'Cholera in Wales', *National Library of Wales Journal*, Vol. 10 (1957–8), 281–300; E. G. Parry, 'A poor man's plague – the cholera epidemic', *Brycheiniog*, Vol. 22 (1986–7), 42–56; G. Owen, 'The Bangor typhoid epidemic of 1882', *Transactions of the Caernarfonshire Historical Society*, Vol. 26 (1965), 157–68; G. Robert, 'Closing the stable door after the horse has bolted: preventing the spread of smallpox and cholera in Caernarfonshire, 1870–1910', *Transactions of the Caernarfonshire Historical Society*, Vol. 55 (1994), 109–28; T. Meirion Hughes, *Caernarfon Ddoe: Y Colera a'r Gronfa Ddŵr Newydd* (Caernarfon, 1996).
58 I. G. Jones, 'The people's health in mid-Victorian Wales', 52.
59 N. Evans, 'The Welsh Victorian city: the middle class and civic and national consciousness in Cardiff, 1850–1914', *Welsh History Review*, Vol. 12, no. 3 (1985), 350–87; P. E. Jones, 'Bangor local board of health, 1850–83', *Transactions of the Caernarfonshire Historical Society*, Vol. 37 (1976), 87–132; H. Richards, 'Investment in public health provision'.
60 J. H. L. Mabbitt, *The Health Services of Glamorgan* (Cowbridge, 1973), p. 37.
61 W. Williams, *A Sanitary Survey of Glamorganshire* (Cardiff, 1895); J. Gross, 'Water supply and sewerage in Merthyr Tydfil, 1850–1974', in *Merthyr Historian*, Vol. 11 (1978), 67–78; O. Roberts, 'The politics of health and the origin of Liverpool's Lake Vyrnwy water scheme, 1871–92', *Welsh History Review*, Vol. 20, no. 2 (2000), 308–35; R. Coopey and O. Roberts, 'Public utility or private enterprise? Water and health in the nineteenth and twentieth centuries', in Borsay (ed.), *Medicine in Wales*, pp. 21–39.
62 G. Roberts and A. Evans, *The Centenary of Minffordd Hospital, 1895–1995* (Bangor, 1996), p. 34.
63 J. Gross, 'Hospitals in Merthyr Tydfil, 1850–1974', *Merthyr Historian*, Vol. 2 (1978), 79–92.
64 Roberts and Evans, *The Centenary of Minffordd Hospital*; G. Roberts, 'Closing the stable door after the horse has bolted'.
65 For a brief account of this vessel, see John Mayberry, *I Saw Three Ships: The Story of HMS Hamadryad, Cardiff's Hospital Ship, 1866–1905, and Gospel and*

Educational Ships, HMS Thisbe and HMS Havannah (St Michaels on Wyre, Lancs, 1987).
[66] Sea air was often regarded as having beneficial effects on health, see John Hassan, The Seaside, Health and Environment in England and Wales since 1800 (Aldershot, 2003).
[67] J. Brownlee, An Investigation into the Epidemiology of Phthisis in Great Britain and Ireland, Special Report Series, Great Britain, Medical Research Committee, no. 18 (London, 1918); J. Brownlee, An investigation into the epidemiology of phthisis in Great Britain and Ireland, part 3, Special Report Series, Great Britain, Medical Research Committee, no. 46 (London, 1920). (London); E. G. Bowen, 'The incidence of phthisis in relation to race-type and environment in south and south-west Wales', Journal of the Royal Anthropological Institute, Vol. 58 (1928); idem, 'A clinical study of miners' phthisis in relation to the geography and racial features of the Cardiganshire lead mining area', first published in 1930, reprinted in Harold Carter and Wayne K. Davies, Geography, Culture and Habitat, Selected Essays (1925–1975) of E. G. Bowen (Llandysul, 1976), pp. 86–99.
[68] C. J. Williams, 'The lead miners of Flintshire and Denbighshire', Llafur, Vol. 3, no. 1 (Spring 1980), 87–96 (92).
[69] C. Jones, Calon Blwm (Llandysul, 1994).
[70] J. Gwynne Morgan, 'The place of nickel in the history of industrial disease', in Cule (ed.), Wales and Medicine, pp. 68–74.
[71] E. Davies, The North Wales Quarry Hospitals and the Health and Welfare of the Quarrymen (Caernarfon, 2003).
[72] L. Bryder, 'Tuberculosis, silicosis, and the slate industry in north Wales, 1927–1939', in P. Weindling (ed.), The Social History of Occupational Health (London, 1985), pp. 108–26.
[73] Ibid., p. 112.
[74] H. D. Chalke, An Investigation into the Causes of the Continued High Death Rate from Tuberculosis in Certain Parts of North Wales (Cardiff, 1933).
[75] Bryder, 'Tuberculosis, silicosis, and the slate industry in north Wales', pp. 117–8.
[76] M. Lieven, Senghennydd: The Universal Pit Village, 1890–1930 (Llandysul, 1994); N. Williams, 'The Senghennydd Colliery disaster', in Stewart Williams (ed.), Glamorgan Historian, Vol. 6 (Cowbridge, 1969), 148–59; John Brown, The Valley of the Shadow: An Account of Britain's Worst Mining Disaster, the Senghennydd Explosion (Port Talbot, 1981); T. Boyns, 'Work and death in the south Wales coalfield', Welsh History Review, Vol. 12 (1985), 514–37; T. Boyns, 'Technical change and colliery explosions in the south Wales Coalfield, 1870–1914', Welsh History Review, Vol. 14 (1986–7), 115–77; Parry Davies, 'Gresford Colliery explosion', Transactions of the Denbighshire Historical Society, Vol. 22 (1973), 272–328; Stanley Williamson, Gresford: The Anatomy of a Disaster (Liverpool, 1999).
[77] B. L. Coombes, These Poor Hands: The Autobiography of a Miner Working in South Wales (London, 1939; repr. Cardiff, 2004), see for examples, pp. 105, 160–1, 168–9.

[78] G. Howells and C. Rees, 'Pneumoconiosis: a study of its effects on miners' health in south Wales 1900–1980', *Nursing Standard*, Vol. 13, no. 26 (17 March 1999), 39–41; Kim Howells, 'Victimisation, accidents and disease', in D. Smith (ed.), *A People and a Proletariat: Essays in the History of Wales 1780–1980* (London, 1980), pp. 181–98; Enid M. Williams, *The Health of Old and Retired Miners in South Wales* (Cardiff, 1933); Keith Strange, 'Accidents at work in Merthyr Tydfil c.1840–1850', *Merthyr Historian*, Vol. 3 (1980), 54–64.

[79] A. Meiklejohn, 'The development of compensation for occupational diseases of the lungs in Great Britain', *British Journal of Industrial Medicine*, Vol. 11 (1954), 198–212; N. Woodward, 'Why did south Wales miners have high mortality? Evidence from the mid-twentieth century', *Welsh History Review*, Vol. 20, no. 1 (June 2000), 117–42; J. S. Haldane, 'Silicosis and coal-mining', *Transactions, Institution of Mining Engineers*, Vol. 80 (1930–1), 415–51; Mark Bufton and Joseph Melling, 'Coming up for air: experts, employers, and workers in campaigns to compensate silicosis sufferers in Britain, 1918–1939', *Social History of Medicine*, Vol. 18, no. 1 (2005), 63–86.

[80] E. L. Collis and J. C. Gilchrist, 'Effects of dust upon coal trimmers', *Journal of Industrial Hygiene*, Vol. 10 (1928), 101–110 (101).

[81] S. L. Cummins and A. F. Sladden, 'Coal-miner's lung: an investigation into the anthracitic lungs of coal-miners in south Wales', *Journal of Pathological Bacteria*, Vol. 33 (1930), 1095; E. Posner, 'Milestones in the history of mineral dust pneumoconioses', in Cule (ed.), *Wales and Medicine*.

[82] D. J. Davies, *Silicosis and the Welsh Miner* (Caernarfon and Cardiff, 1931); H. Francis and D. Smith, *The Fed: A History of the South Wales Miners in the Twentieth Century* (London, 1980; Cardiff, 1998); Mick Bloor, 'The South Wales Miners Federation, miners' lung and the instrumental use of expertise, 1900–1950', *Social Studies of Science*, Vol. 30, no. 1 (2000), 125–40.

[83] E. Posner, 'Milestones in the history of mineral dust pneumoconiosis', in Cule (ed.), *Wales and Medicine*.

[84] J. C. McVittie, 'Pneumoconiosis in coal miners', *Postgraduate Medical Journal*, Vol. 25 (1949), 186; Morris Greenberg, 'A battle for compensation for Welsh coal miners: J. S. Haldane v "Sericite" Jones, 1932–1934', *American Journal of Industrial Medicine*, Vol. 32 (1977), 309–14.

[85] James Griffiths, *Pages from Memory* (London, 1969), p. 55.

[86] D'Arcy Hart recalled that the MRC were asked to 'sort things, make recommendations, and do it urgently', P. D'Arcy Hart, 'Chronic pulmonary disease in south Wales coal mines: an eye-witness account of the MRC surveys (1937–1942), edited and annotated by E. M. Tansey', *Social History of Medicine*, Vol. 11, no. 3 (December 1998), 459–68 (462).

[87] P. D'Arcy Hart and E. A. Aslett, *Chronic Pulmonary Disease in South Wales Coalminers*: Vol. 1. *Medical Studies*, Medical Research Council, Special Report Series, 243 (London, 1942), Vol. 2, *Environmental Studies*, 244 (London, 1943) and Vol. 3, *Experimental Studies*, 250 (London, 1945).

[88] A. L. Cochrane, 'Pulmonary tuberculosis in the Rhondda Fach: a survey of a mining community', *British Medical Journal*, Vol. 2 (1952), 843–53.

[89] D'Arcy Hart, 'Chronic pulmonary disease', 467.

90 George Davey Smith, introduction to A. R. Ness, L. A. Reynolds, E. M. Tansey (eds), *Population-based Research in South Wales: The MRC Pneumoconiosis Research Unit and the MRC Epidemiology Unit*, The Wellcome Witnesses to Twentieth Century Medicine, Vol. 13 (November 2002), xvii.
91 A. L. Cochrane, *Effectiveness and Efficiency: Random Reflections on Health Services*, The Rock Carling Fellowship (London, 1971); A. Maynard, I. Chalmers (eds), *Non-random Reflections on Health Services Research: On the 25th Anniversary of Archie Cochrane's 'Effectiveness and Efficiency'* (London, 1972).
92 Ness et al., *Population-based Research in South Wales*.
93 Lynn Davies, 'Aspects of mining folklore in Wales', *Folk Life*, Vol. 9 (1971), 79–107; 98–102 relate to folk medicine.
94 Ibid., also oral recollections gathered by Julian Tudor Hart, and shared with members of the History of Medicine in Wales Society at a meeting in Swansea on 8 September 2003.
95 Deirdre Beddoe, 'Towards a Welsh women's history', *Llafur*, Vol. 3, no. 2 (Spring 1981), 32–8. Her own subsequent publications have gone a long way to rectifying this deficit.
96 Dot Jones, 'Counting the cost of coal: women's lives in the Rhondda, 1881–1911', in Angela John (ed.), *Our Mothers' Land: Essays in Welsh Women's History* (Cardiff, 1991).
97 Neil Evans and Dot Jones, '"A blessing for the miner's wife": the campaign for pit-head baths in the south Wales coalfield, 1908–1950', *Llafur*, Vol. 6, no. 3 (1994), 5–28.
98 Borsay (ed.), *Medicine in Wales*; Buddug Owen, *Meeting Pioneers*, pp. 63–72; 86–98; 99–105.
99 *Report of the Labour Committee of Inquiry*, issued by the Parliamentary Labour Party, 1928.
100 Susan A. Williams, 'Relief and research: the nutrition work of the National Birthday Trust Fund, 1935–9', in David F. Smith, *Nutrition in Britain: Science, Scientists, and Politics in the Twentieth Century* (London, 1997), pp. 99–122; Susan A. Williams, *Women and Childbirth in the Twentieth Century: A History of the National Birthday Trust Fund, 1928–93* (Stroud, 1997).
101 Williams, 'Relief and research', 111–15.
102 Elizabeth Peretz, 'The cost of modern motherhood to low income families in interwar Britain', in V. Fildes, L. Marks and H. Marland (eds), *Women and Children First: International Maternal and Infant Welfare, 1870–1945* (London, 1992), pp. 257–80.
103 Jane Williams (Ysgafell) (ed.), *The Autobiography of Elizabeth Davis: Betsy Cadwaladr: A Balaclava Nurse*, with a new introduction by Deirdre Beddoe (Cardiff, 1987).
104 Zillah Jones, *A Sister's Log: A Nurse's Reminiscences* (Llandysul, 1964), p. 9.
105 Fflorens Roberts, *Mae Bod yn Fyw yn Fawr Ryfeddod* (Dinbych, 1996); 'Memories of a Young Nurse', in John Gruffydd Jones et al. (eds), *A History of Abergele Hospital: Confronting the White Plague* (Denbigh, 1999), pp. 79–109.

[106] Sara Brady, 'Public service and private ambitions: nursing at the King Edward VII Hospital, Cardiff during the First World War', in Borsay (ed.), *Medicine in Wales*, pp. 108–27.

[107] Maggie Furness, 'Welsh Voices: fifty years of oral orthopaedic history', *International History of Nursing Journal*, Vol. 7, no. 3 (2003), 83–93.

[108] David Mills Evans, *A District Nurse in Rural Wales before the National Health Service*, edited and prepared for publication by Dr W. T. R. Pryce (Llanrwst, 2003).

[109] Anthea Symonds, '"It's a funny job really": the contradictions of health visiting', in Borsay (ed.), *Medicine in Wales*, pp. 171–94.

[110] Susan J. Pitt, 'Private lives and public bodies: childbirth in post-war Swansea', in Borsay (ed.), *Medicine in Wales*, pp. 154–70.

[111] J. Stewart, 'A Welsh life, a medical life: Dr Emyr Wyn Jones (1907–1999) Interviewed', *The National Library of Wales Journal*, Vol. 32, no. 1 (Summer 2001), 107–19 (109).

[112] Ibid., p. 112; Emyr Wyn Jones, 'Y Bysedd Cochion: Ei rhin a'i Rhawd', in idem, *Bysedd Cochion a'r Wladfa Gyntaf* (Denbigh, 1997), pp. 13–38; idem, 'Y Bysedd Cochion' in Baber and Lancaster (eds), *Healthcare in Wales*, pp. 25–54; Dr J. H. Thomas recalled that 'digitalis' was used by an old woman herbalist as a treatment for dropsy; J. H. Thomas, *Yng Nghwmni'r Meddyg* (Swansea, 1990), pp. 69–79.

[113] J. Stewart, 'A Welsh life', pp. 111–12.

[114] N. Jewson, 'The disappearance of the sick-man from medical cosmology, 1770–1870', *Sociology*, Vol. 10 (1976), 225–44.

[115] J. Thomas, *Y Doctor Tomos* (Y Bala, 1968), p. 16.

[116] Ibid., p. 5.

[117] Gwyn Thomas, *A Country Doctor's Diary* (Denbigh, 2001), p. 24.

[118] Trevor Hughes, *Eighty Years on Call* (Bala, 1971).

[119] N. Naunton Davies, 'Two and a half centuries of medical practice: a Welsh medical dynasty', in Cule (ed.), *Wales and Medicine*, pp. 216–21; another renowned member of this medical dynasty was Henry Naunton Davies, see S. Roberts, 'Henry Naunton Davies (1927–1899): A devoted family doctor and a brave rescuer', *Journal of Medical Biography*, Vol. 11 (2003), 163–6; E. Pride, *Rhondda My Valley Brave* (Risca, Newport, 1975), p. 174.

[120] A. Digby, *Making a Medical Living* (Cambridge, 1994), p. 77.

[121] R. H. O. B. Robinson and W. R. LeFanu, *Lives of the Fellows of the Royal College of Surgeons of England, 1952–64* (London, 1970), p. 173.

[122] Robert Hughes Parry, *Within Life's Span*, pp. 99–112; see also his *Under the Cherry Tree* (Llandysul, 1969).

[123] Ministry of Health, *First Report of the Welsh Consultative Council of Medical and Allied Services in Wales* (London, Cmd. 708, 1920), p. 6.

[124] A. W. Sheen, 'The Welsh National School of Medicine' in *The Book of Cardiff, Ninety-Sixth Annual Meeting of the British Medical Association held at Cardiff in July, 1928* (Cardiff, 1928), pp. 38–41; A. Trevor Jones, 'The new medical centre and the development of medical education in Wales', in Cule (ed.), *Wales and Medicine*, pp. 23–9.

[125] Ivor Davies, *Memoirs of a Welsh Physician* (Aberystwyth, 1959) for personal recollections of the founding of the medical school in Cardiff. On medical education in this formative period see Abraham Flexner, *Medical Education in Europe* (New York, Carnegie Foundation for the advancement of Teaching, Bulletin No. 6, 1912); Thomas Neville Bonner, 'Abraham Flexner as critic of British and Continental medical education', *Medical History*, Vol. 33 (1989): 472–9.

[126] T. I. Ellis, *The Development of Higher Education in Wales* (Wrexham, 1935), pp. 187–8.

[127] Frances Collingwood, 'The Welsh National School of Medicine', *History of Medicine*, Vol. 2, no. 2 (Summer 1970).

[128] See, for instance, Thomas Mullin, *The Story of a Toiler's Life* (Cardiff, 1921; reprinted by University College Dublin Press, 2000, edited by Patrick Maume), the story of an Irish doctor who trained in Galway and practised in Cardiff, where he described how, during the 1880s, he consulted a medical directory to discover the areas with the lowest rates of doctors per head of population, and identified half a dozen centres including Preston, Barrow, Oldham and Wolverhampton, but Cardiff was first on the list so he settled on Cardiff; A. D. Morris, 'Two colliery doctors . . . the brothers Armstrong of Treorchy', in Cule (ed.), *Wales and Medicine*, pp. 208–15 – their father migrated from Scotland to north Wales, and they grew up in Wales; Francis Maylett Smith, *The Surgery at Aberffrwd: Some Encounters of a Colliery Doctor Seventy Years Ago*, edited by Denis Hayes Crofton (Hythe, Kent, 1981); F. M. Smith came from Yorkshire, the son of a Nonconformist minister, and towards the end of his medical training suffered a severe loss of hearing resulting in his having difficulty finding a post, but after a fortnight's locum in a neighbouring valley he was appointed to a practice in Aberffrwd, where he spent nearly seven years as an 'overworked colliery doctor'.

[129] Neil Evans, 'Through the prism of ethnic violence: riots and racial attacks in Wales, 1826–2002', in Charlotte Williams, Neil Evans and Paul O'Leary, *A Tolerant Nation? Exploring Ethnic Diversity in Wales* (Cardiff, 2003), pp. 93–108 (102–5).

[130] 'From the Raj to the Rhondda', BBC Four documentary, broadcast on 26 November 2003; 'Raj to Rhondda: how Asian doctors saved the NHS', broadcast on BBC 2, 12 October 2004.

[131] J. T. Hart, *Going for Gold: A New Approach to Primary Medical Care in the South Wales Valleys* (London, 1997).

[132] Martin Powell, 'Wales and the National Health Service', *Llafur*, Vol. 8, no. 1 (2000), 33–43 (33).

[133] See for instance Digby, *The Evolution of British General Practice*. It should be noted that Anne Digby provides a genuinely British account of the history of general practice, drawing on a rich array of sources from Wales. Two chapters in this volume cite Cronin as an authority.

[134] John Howie, 'Research in general practice', in Irvine Loudon, John Horder and Charles Webster (eds), *General Practice under the National Health Service 1948–1997* (London, 1998), pp. 146–64 (155); R. C. Humphreys, *A History of*

Research in General Practice in Wales: 1950–1992 (Swansea, 1994); 'The Good Doctor', videotape, BBC Television (1996), *Pioneers*, Part 6; Dr Julian Tudor Hart, videotape (30 minutes) deposited at the Wellcome Library, Video and Audio Collection, 882V.

135 Martin Powell, 'How Adequate was hospital provision before the NHS? An examination of the 1945 South Wales Hospital Survey', *Local Population Studies*, Vol. 48 (1992), 22–32; idem, 'Wales and the National Health Service'.

136 A. S. Aldis, *Cardiff Royal Infirmary, 1883–1983* (Cardiff, 1984); D. L. Baker-Jones, '"To supply the sick poor"', *Carmarthenshire Historian*, Vol. 15 (1978), 3–28; William E. Beer, *A Portrait of the C & A Hospital, Bangor: The People and the Place* (Mold, 2000); John Coles, *Beside the Seaside: Health Care in Tenby* (Tenby, 1995); idem, *A Brief History of the Hospitals of Pembroke and Pembroke Dock* (Pembroke Dock, 1995); Gwen Davies, *Builth Cottage Hospital: A Centenary History 1897–1997* (Llandrindod Wells, 1997); T. G. Davies, *Deeds Not Words: A History of the Swansea General and Eye Hospital, 1817–1948* (Cardiff, 1988); idem, 'Health and Hospitals', in Ralph Griffiths (ed.), *The City of Swansea: Challenges and Change* (Stroud: 1990), pp. 165–78; D. I. Evans, 'Hospital services in Aberystwyth before 1948', *Ceredigion*, Vol. 5, no. 2 (1965), 168–208; Neil Evans, '"The First Charity in Wales": Cardiff Infirmary and South Wales Society, 1837–1914', *Welsh History Review*, Vol. 9, no. 3 (1979), 319–46; J. Gross, 'Hospitals in Merthyr Tydfil, 1850–1974'; John Ingham, 'The early days of the Caernarvonshire and Anglesey Hospital', *Transactions of the Caernarfonshire Historical Society*, Vol. 11 (1950), 61–72; Gareth Jones, *The Aneurin Bevan Inheritance: The Story of the Nevill Hall and District NHS Trust* (Abertillery, 1998); O. V. Jones, *The Progress of Medicine: A History of the Caernarfon and Anglesey Infirmary, 1809–1948* (Llandysul, 1984); T. B. Jones and W. J. T. Collins, *History of the Royal Gwent Hospital* (Newport, 1948); Ann Lewis, 'The story of Merthyr General Hospital', *Merthyr Historian*, Vol. 4 (1989), 114–30; A. Lewis and M. Lloyd, 'The story of St Tydfil's Hospital', ibid., Vol. 6 (1992), 1–21; Gwenda M. Matthews, *Colwyn Bay Community Hospital: History and Development (1898–1993)* (Colwyn Bay, 1993); R. C. B. Oliver, 'Llandrindod Wells Hospital: its beginnings and early years', *Transactions of the Radnorshire Society*, Vol. 51 (1981), 7–15; Brian Owen, *The History of the War Memorial Hospital, Llanidloes, 1920–1948* (Llanidloes, 1998); Robert Owen, *The History of Abergele Hospital: Confronting the White Plague: 'Ymladd y Pla Gwyn'* (Denbigh, 1999); Robert Phelps, *Ysbyty Dewi Sant, Bangor, 1913–1994* (Llangefni, 1994); R. R. Powell, *A Miners' Hospital: An Illustrated History of Mountain Ash General Hospital* (Mountain Ash, 1997); Glynne Roberts, *Canmlwyddiant Ysbyty Minffordd/The Centenary of Minffordd Hospital, Bangor, 1895–1995* (Bangor, 1996); J. K. Roberts and I. Lancefield, 'The early history of the Stanley Sailor's Hospital, Holyhead, 1871–1926', *Transactions of the Anglesey Antiquarian Society and Field Club* (1997), 69–86; Steven Thompson, '"To relieve the sufferings of humanity, irrespective of party, politics or creed"? Conflict, consensus and hospital provision in Edwardian south Wales', *Social History of Medicine*, Vol. 16, no. 2, 247–62; idem, 'Hospital provision, charity and public responsibility in Edwardian

Pontypridd', *Llafur*, Vol. 8, no. 3 (2002), 53–65; idem, '"Without any distinction of sect, or creed, or politics"'?: Charity and hospital provision in nineteenth-century Aberystwyth', *Ceredigion*, Vol. 14, no. 2 (2002), 38–56.

[137] Ministry of Health, *Second Report of the Welsh Consultative Council on Medical and Allied Services in Wales* (London, Cmd. 1448, 1921), p. 10.

[138] Ibid., p. 11.

[139] Ibid., p. 11.

[140] J. L. Williams, *Digest of Welsh Historical Statistics: Volume II* (Cardiff, 1985), p. 152.

[141] Ernest Rock Carling and T. S. McIntosh, *Hospital Survey: The Hospital Services of the North-Western Area* (London, 1944).

[142] Ibid., 104.

[143] A. Trevor Jones, J. A. Nixon and R. M. F. Picken, *Hospital Survey: The Hospital Services of South Wales and Monmouthshire* (London, 1945), pp. 12, 83.

[144] Ray Earwicker, 'Miners' medical services before the First World War: the south Wales coalfield', *Llafur*, Vol. 3, no. 2 (Spring 1981), 39–52.

[145] Steven Thompson, 'A proletarian public sphere: working-class provision of medical services and care in south Wales, *c*.1900–1948', in Borsay (ed.), *Medicine in Wales*, pp. 86–107 (100).

[146] Linda Bryder, 'The King Edward VII Welsh National Memorial Association and its policy towards tuberculosis 1910–1948', *Welsh History Review*, Vol. 13 (1986), 194–216.

[147] Glynne R. Jones, 'The King Edward VII Welsh National Memorial Association, 1912–1948', in Cule (ed.), *Wales and Medicine*, pp. 30–41 (31).

[148] D. A. Powell, 'The King Edward VII Welsh National Memorial Association', in *The Book of Cardiff*, pp. 42–44 (42).

[149] Linda Bryder, *Below the Magic Mountain: A Social History of Tuberculosis in Twentieth-Century Britain* (Oxford, 1988), p. 82.

[150] Glynne R. Jones, 'The King Edward VII Welsh National Memorial Association', p. 33.

[151] Kathleen Jones, *Hugh Morriston Davies: Pioneer Thoracic Surgeon, 1879–1965* (Ruthin, 1998); Glyn Penrhyn Jones, 'Portread o Lawfeddyg', in *Newyn a Haint yng Nghymru* (Caernarfon, 1983), pp. 175–80; Buddug Owen, *Meeting Pioneers*, pp. 37–44.

[152] Herbert Williams, *A Severe Case of Dandruff* (Llandysul, 1999).

[153] Idem, '*A Little Like Being a Leper*', broadcast on BBC Radio Wales, 5 April.

[154] Anne Hardy, 'Reframing disease: changing perceptions of tuberculosis in England and Wales, 1938–70, *Institute of Historical Research*, Vol. 76, no. 194 (November 2003).

[155] Linda Bryder, *Below the Magic Mountain*, p. 93.

[156] John Davies, 'Y gydwybod gymdeithasol yng Nghymru rhwng y ddau ryfel byd', in Geraint H. Jenkins (ed.), *Cof Cenedl IV: Ysgrifau ar Hanes Cymru*, Vol. 4 (Llandysul, 1989), pp. 153–78; John Davies, 'The communal conscience of Wales in the inter-war years', *Transactions of the Honourable Society of the Cymmrodorion* (1998), 145–60.

[157] *House of Commons Debates*, 'Anti-Tuberculosis Service, Wales and Monmouthshire', Hansard HC (Series 5), Vol. 345, cols 1330–1421 (22 March 1939), col. 1331.
[158] Ibid., Sir W. Jenkins, col. 1374.
[159] Anne Hardy, 'Reframing disease', p. 539.
[160] E. Davies, *The North Wales Quarry Hospitals*, pp. 221–4.
[161] A. L. Cochrane, R. G. Carpenter and F. Moore, 'The mortality of miners and ex-miners in the Rhondda Fach', *British Journal of Industrial Medicine*, Vol. 21 (1964), 38–45; J. E. Cotes, P. D. Oldham and A. J. Thomas, 'The prevalence of coronary heart disease in a mining valley', *Proceedings of the Royal Society of Medicine*, Vol. 48 (1955), 673–4; J. E. Cotes, T. T. Higgins and A. J. Thomas, 'Relationship of coronary heart disease to respiratory disability: investigation of a random sample of coal-workers aged 55–64 from a mining valley in south Wales', *British Medical Journal*, Vol. 1 (1956), 601–603.
[162] Tony Austin, *Aberfan: The Story of a Disaster* (London, 1967); J. Miller, *Aberfan: A Disaster and its Aftermath* (London, 1974); Martin Johnes, 'Uneasy relationships: the Aberfan disaster 1966, Merthyr Tydfil Borough Council and local politics', *Welsh History Review*, Vol. 20 (June 2000), 143–66; Iain McLean and Martin Johnes, *Aberfan: Government and Disasters* (Cardiff, 2000).
[163] J. Beverley Smith, 'James Griffiths: an appreciation', in *James Griffiths and His Times* (a volume commissioned by Labour Party Wales, printed by Maddock and Co., Ferndale, Rhondda, 1976), pp. 58–118 (89).
[164] Kenneth O. Morgan, 'The red dragon and the red flag: the case of James Griffiths and Aneurin Bevan', Welsh Political Archive Lecture, 1988, National Library of Wales; reprinted in Kenneth O. Morgan, *Modern Wales: Politics, Places and People* (Cardiff, 1995), pp. 443–53. They were leading architects of the National Insurance, National Health Service and Housing Acts of 1946 and of the National Assistance Act of 1948.
[165] The house building programme owed much to the efforts of Aneurin Bevan, who had responsibility for housing as well as health, and despite the shortage of resources after the war, over a million permanent homes were built in England and Wales in the six years 1945–1951; Morgan, 'Aneurin Bevan and the Welfare State', in Morgan, *Modern Wales*, pp. 454–62; Claire Beckett and Francis Beckett, *Bevan* (London, 2004).
[166] R. Merfyn Jones, *Cymru 2000*, pp. 127–8 (117).
[167] Aneurin Bevan, *In Place of Fear* (London, 1952), p. 79.
[168] Charles Webster (ed.), *Aneurin Bevan and the National Health Service* (Oxford, 1991).
[169] Interview with Beti George, 'O'r Crud i'r Bedd', S4C (1998).
[170] E. Parry-Jones, *From Workhouse to Hospital: A Story of H. M. Stanley Hospital, St Asaph* (Denbigh, 1981), p. 14.
[171] Joan Povey and Jasmine Hughes, *Ysbyty Dewi Sant, Bangor, 1913–1994/St David's Hospital, Bangor, 1913–1994* (Llangefni, 1994).
[172] Buddug Owen, *Meeting Pioneers*. For further insights into the work of consultant surgeons in north Wales during the post-war period, the extent to which they were integrated into Welsh culture, and the close medical links

which continued between Liverpool and north Wales, see J. Howell Hughes, *A Surgeon's Journey* (Denbigh, 1989) and Guto Roberts, *Doctor Pen-y-Bryn: Atgofion Owen E. Owen* (Penygroes, 1985).
[173] G. P. Jones, 'Folk medicine in eighteenth century Wales', p. 74.
[174] T. Llew Jones, *Fy Mhobol i* (Llandysul, 2002), pp. 80–3.
[175] However, during the latter years of the twentieth century, biomedicine was increasingly challenged and there was a resurgence of interest in 'alternative medicine'.
[176] Charles Webster, *A Political History of the NHS* (Oxford, 1998), p. 35.
[177] G. Prys-Davies, *Survey of the Hospital Service in Wales* (Cardiff, 1969), p. 1.
[178] Ibid., p. 2.
[179] Trevor Jones and John Surtees, *The Medical Teaching Centre, Cardiff: An Account of the Clinical and Academic Facilities Provided for the University Hospital of Wales and the Welsh National School of Medicine at Heath Park, Cardiff* (Cardiff, 1971).
[180] Julian Tudor Hart, 'The Inverse Care Law', *The Lancet*, 27 February, 1971, pp. 405–12.
[181] Charles Webster, *The Health Services since the War, Vol. II* (London, 1996), pp. 609–12. Appointed in May 1975, the Resource Allocation Working Party reported in September 1976. Some of the earliest complaints about the inequity of resource allocation apparently emanated from the Welsh Regional Hospital Board, see Charles Webster, 'Investigating inequalities before Black' in Virginia Berridge and Stuart Blume (eds), *Poor Health: Social Inequality before and after the Black Report* (London, 2003), pp. 81–103, 95.
[182] Richard Prentice, 'Health care and housing policies', in idem, *Change and Policy in Wales: Wales in the Era of Privatism* (Llandysul, 1993), pp. 205–28 (207).
[183] Gareth Rees, 'Health, the distribution of health services and poverty in Wales', in Gareth Rees and Teresa Rees (eds), *Poverty and Social Inequality in Wales* (London, 1980), pp. 93–115 (95, see table 5.1).
[184] Martyn Senior, 'Area variations in self-perceived limiting long term illness in Britain, 1991: Is the Welsh experience exceptional?', *Regional Studies*, Vol. 32, no. 3 (1998), 265–80; Paul Boyle, Anthony Gatrell and Oliver Duke-Williams, 'Do area-level population change, deprivation and variations in deprivation affect individual-level self-reported limiting long-term illness?', *Social Science and Medicine*, Vol. 53 (2001), 795–9.
[185] J. Tudor Hart, 'General-practice workload, needs, and resources in the National Health Service', *Journal of the Royal College of General Practitioners*, Vol. 26 (1976), 885–92 (885).
[186] Ibid., 888. The medical and social conditions described by Hart were graphically depicted in a documentary film made by Karl Francis entitled *Above us the Earth* (1977), which traced the closure of the Ogilvie colliery in the Rhymney valley, and the effects this had on the local community. At the same time it documented the painful drawing to a close of the life of an individual miner, who had worked in the colliery for most of his working life, and during his final days was suffering the painful effects of emphysema.

[187] S. Monaghan, *An Atlas of Health Inequalities between Welsh Local Authorities* (Cardiff, 1998).

[188] S. Monaghan, J. Davidson and D. Bainton, *Freeing the Dragon: New Opportunities to Improve the Health of the Welsh People* (London, 1999).

[189] Jim Griffiths, *House of Commons Debates* (March 1939), col. 1334.

1

Sickness and Health in Caernarfonshire, 1870–1939

GLYNNE ROBERTS

There are houses with roses round the door, but inside they are not fit for people to die in, never mind live in.[1]

The period under review highlights some of the most spectacular changes in health status ever seen, with the main achievements in the seventy years following 1870 being more intimately linked to social reform than medical advancements. The conquest of infectious diseases was not so much the mastering of the unknown by medical science, but the culmination of a prolonged process that resulted in the improvement of health standards at an unprecedented rate. The main threads of this chapter, therefore, consider the preventative 'upstream' influences on health,[2] and the uneven path trodden by local authorities in attempting to meet higher expectations and improve the well-being of their local populations.

The social influences on health can generally be periodized into two phases, bridged by the First World War. In the initial period, legislation and the most vocal and vehement efforts focused on sanitary improvements and the battle to secure uncontaminated drinking water. State intervention increased expectations on local authorities to engineer a world of pure water supplies and effective sewerage removal; to provide regular refuse collection and, ultimately, better living conditions. An acute awareness of the need for such 'upstream' preventative endeavours is demonstrated in comments made by Dr Hugh Rees in 1892: 'Measures of cleanliness before hand are of more importance for the protection of a district . . . than the removal or disinfection of filth after the disease has actually made its appearance.'[3] Between 1919 and 1939, having generally secured the primary objective, housing developments became the main plank of public health reform. However, the onerous and unrealistic expectations placed on local authorities to initiate reform prolonged the agony of poverty for many communities, particularly in areas where the starting point was so miserably low.

During the second half of the nineteenth century, medical science shifted gradually from the miasmatic theory that disease emanated from bad smells and noxious effluvia. The overall health improvements were not the culmination of a carefully planned strategy, but a haphazard conclusion to a number of fortuitous circumstances. Tackling many of the main causes of miasma, however, with the primary emphasis on cleanliness and the avoidance of dirt, led to substantial investments in sanitary improvements, which in turn provided many of the desired outcomes. Public health linked to social reform often resembled a moral crusade.[4] While influential individuals may have been thin on the ground in Caernarfonshire, the ripple effect from the endeavours of nineteenth-century reformists had a significant impact on the manner, if not the pace, of local reform.

The decline in the overall death rate between 1870 and the mid-twentieth century was extraordinary. Over three generations, crude death rates fell by 50 per cent, and deaths from infectious diseases by some 90 per cent. Overall general mortality rates declined from 20.5 per cent in 1861 to 16.9 per cent in 1901; correspondingly, life expectancy increased at birth from 40.2 per cent in 1841 to 51.5 per cent in 1911.[5] One of the main indicators of poverty was the infant death rate, which was wholly unacceptable in parts of Caernarfonshire. Speaking in 1907, Dr Peter Fraser, the Medical Officer of Health (MoH), complained that: 'It has been over 50% above this standard in . . . the quarrying districts of Ogwen and Gwyrfai and in the crowded towns of Llanrwst, Bethesda and Caernarvon.'[6]

In many ways, the impact of three diseases – smallpox, typhoid and tuberculosis – encapsulated the nature of local efforts to effect health improvements. Smallpox emphasized the medical contribution to combating infectious diseases but, for all the effectiveness of inoculation, accounted for only one-twentieth of the total decline in death rates throughout England and Wales.[7] Conversely, mortality rates for typhoid, scarlet fever and whooping cough declined long before the introduction of effective immunization procedures.

Caernarfonshire incorporated three diverse communities. The county's towns demonstrated significant differences in the pace of progress: in Bangor, reforms were evident, with confident strides taken to enact substantial improvements. Conversely, there were also towns such as Caernarfon, where advancements were much more gradual. Secondly, rural communities were subject to the vagaries of the fragile agricultural economy, and were areas where health improvements permeated more slowly than in the towns. The very rurality of these areas often masked the true extent of potential public health risks that would have wreaked so much more devastation in an urban environment. Straddling the first two communities were the slate-quarrying communities of Bethesda, Llanberis and the Nantlle valley, demonstrating both the problems of industrial towns and also the inherent deficiencies of rural environments.

The evolving health responsibilities of local government in Caernarfonshire were crucial. Some local authorities within the county, even during the 1930s, stood accused of being wholly ineffectual; the magnitude of the expected transformation was beyond their grasp and vision. Central edicts might have provided the tools that led to widespread housing, hospital and sanitary reform in Bangor, but in the hands of local authorities such as Gwyrfai these tools were often blunt and ineffective.

What came to be regarded as mainstream health-service provisions – the employment of medical personnel and the provision of hospitals – developed mostly in an ad hoc and irregular manner across the county. Developments aimed at improving health services and social conditions were not necessarily based on the health needs but on the drive of key individuals, spontaneous reactions to temporary crises and financial considerations. There were numerous examples of how failings in public awareness led to avoidable outbreaks of infectious disease, and how responding to crises dictated the direction of health policy at a localized level, even when the full impact and devastation of the infectious diseases had passed.[8]

Although Caernarfonshire was on the western fringes of the British Isles, there was fear of infection coming from over the sea as well as the land. Dr Hunter Hughes, MoH for the Pwllheli Poor Law Union, devised a scheme whereby the local constabulary would keep a watch on shipping and sailors, and designated medical practitioners were appointed to enforce procedures aimed at preventing infectious cases from reaching dry land. In 1871, complaints were received that ships coming to Porthmadog could have smallpox cases aboard, and as part of the same concerns, a ship was set aside offshore by the Beaumaris

Port Sanitary Authority to accommodate any smallpox cases from dry land or from ships.[9]

Smallpox was a disease that attacked with no respect for age or social status. During 1871–80, 42,000 people died from smallpox in England; during this epidemic 28 deaths occurred in the Caernarfon Union. Between 1891 and 1900, there were only 27 recorded cases across the whole of Caernarfonshire, and less than half of these died.[10] However, stark memories of the devastation caused by smallpox remained within communities long after the disease itself had ceased to pose a threat. As much as 96 per cent of the decline in smallpox death rates occurred before the turn of the century,[11] so that many of the protracted discussions about the provision of appropriate facilities overestimated the real need.[12]

The authorities' responses to smallpox were two-pronged: taking an aggressive stance in aiming to vaccinate the whole population, whilst also developing effective defensive mechanisms through providing isolation facilities. With the latter option particularly, it often proved to be too little too late, as the disease had all but been eradicated before the small network of hospitals was completed. Within the Deiniolen area, up to 120 people were said to have suffered from smallpox as part of the 1871–2 epidemic,[13] and one of the main preventive options was to engage the local constabulary and to isolate cases within their own homes. Gwyrfai Council did not discover a more functional solution until land on the Faenol Estate was offered to them in 1901 to build an isolation hospital.[14] Although significantly underutilized, the completed hospital proved useful in dealing with the few cases that occurred.

In 1903, the county MoH, Dr Fraser, outlined a plan whereby the whole of the Caernarfonshire population would have a smallpox isolation facility within ten miles of their homes.[15] By 1907, four such hospitals had been built, with metal buildings erected in Gwyrfai and Llandudno, a small hospital in Llysfaen and a house near Colwyn Bay. For the rest of the 100,000 population, there was no hospital isolation provision, so it was fortuitous that the disease no longer posed a major public health threat.[16]

It was often beyond the scope of most local authorities to contemplate working collaboratively with neighbouring authorities. Consequently, when it came to establishing isolation hospitals, one local authority area invariably shouldered the responsibility and the recurring financial burden, whereas adjoining areas would either remain without adequate provisions, or would undertake to develop similar facilities. Such needless duplication was seen when Caernarfon and Bangor both opened isolation hospitals within six years of each other,[17] so that there were two hospitals, fulfilling the same purpose, less than ten miles apart.

Typhoid was a disease that emanated from insanitary environments,[18] with the declining death rate substantiating the successful attempts to provide clean water supplies. Between 1871 and 1910, across the four Poor Law Unions in Caernarfonshire, a total of 835 typhoid deaths were recorded, with the endemic nature of the disease leading to it being known as *clefyd Stiniog* (Ffestiniog sickness) in Blaenau Ffestiniog.[19]

Typhoid figures recorded for Caernarfonshire increased during 1881–90 compared to the previous decade, primarily because of the horrendous effects of the epidemic that struck Bangor in 1882. In many ways, the responses to the Bangor typhoid epidemic emphasize the watershed in medical science. Dr E. O. Price's assertion that in both human and monetary costs the 'epidemic was thrice as expensive as it need have been'[20] indicates the reluctance with which the local Sanitary Authority was able to work in harmony with the MoH. Dr Rees, the MoH, identified the source of the infection in a farmhouse located above the city in May 1882; three months later, the authorities were still floundering in their attempts to prevent further contagion. Reporting mechanisms did not assist communication between local medical practitioners, so that the full extent of the outbreak was not immediately evident. While individual doctors dealt with isolated cases, they were unaware that they had an epidemic on their hands until the end of June when 25 cases were recorded in one week.[21]

The management of typhoid patients emphasized the inherent problems with existing health structures. Paupers were catered for under the Poor Law, and the more affluent sections of society were able to secure their own nursing and medical support. For those who fell between these two categories – a substantial proportion of the population – local authorities had to ensure suitable isolation facilities.

Most developments – such as building Minffordd Hospital in Bangor or Gallt-y-Sil in Caernarfon – came about as a direct response to devastating outbreaks of infectious disease. Bangor had neither the population density nor the ability realistically to meet the onerous financial obligations of exclusive use, but local pressures brought about by the recollections of the 1882 typhoid epidemic[22] were reinforced in 1889 when contagious scarlet fever patients had to be removed from crowded communities. One household in the Hirael area of Bangor suffered five deaths from scarlet fever,[23] ensuring that efforts to establish an infectious diseases hospital remained at the forefront of public opinion, and dovetailed with other municipal aspirations such as the pier and ferry developments.[24]

The process whereby Bangor City Council built Minffordd Hospital provides a useful insight into the achievements of a forceful local authority.[25] This may have been a conventional 'downstream' activity, but it was a key component in the overall responses to counter infectious diseases. The Poor Law Infirmary and the Caernarfon and Anglesey (C & A) voluntary hospital (serving the counties of Caernarfonshire and Anglesey) were the cornerstones of health provisions in the city,[26] with the development at Minffordd seen as a practical response to the reluctance of the other hospitals to accommodate infectious cases. The allied 'upstream' improvements to water and sewerage supplies and a later extensive housing-development programme put the City Council at the forefront of developments within the county. The whole programme highlighted the civic ethos of the Council, with its proactive municipal management and reflected glory when developments came to fruition. Such action led to justifiable self-congratulation by the city's councillors and, with the advent of higher education establishments, coupled with a strong commercial base, Bangor's councillors proved much more active, able and forward thinking than their counterparts in adjoining areas.

The decline in death rates from tuberculosis – the disease that most clearly singles out the delayed responsiveness of Caernarfonshire – provides the best measure of the intrinsic link between living conditions and ill health. The reduction in tuberculosis death rates accounted for almost half the total reduction in all death rates across England and Wales between 1850 and 1900,[27] and the efforts to eradicate its hold over communities provide a clear gauge of the success of social legislation over medical advancement.

Of all the infectious diseases, the history of tuberculosis is the most tragic, as this disease, above all others, was so intimately associated with poverty and adversity. Known locally as *y dicáu* (decay), tuberculosis or 'consumption' was an endemic disease in Caernarfonshire. Until the middle of the 1940s, prevention, control and treatment of tuberculosis depended ultimately on the provision of good quality and wholesome food, access to sunshine, fresh air and plentiful rest.[28] The conditions in many parts of Caernarfonshire were perfect for the spread of the disease: ill-ventilated and overcrowded houses; low-paid employment leading to significant pockets of poverty; higher than average rainfall, and working conditions that at best hindered progress but mainly maintained the devastating impact of the disease.

The synergistic effects of poor working and living conditions meant that the local MoHs in Caernarfonshire were still deeply troubled by tuberculosis long after other areas had delivered radical programmes to eradicate the disease. Moves to improve the public's health had been underpinned by the Public Health Acts of 1848 and 1875, backed up crucially by social legislation to introduce medical inspections in schools (1907), old age pensions (1909) and National Insurance (1911). The NAPT (National Association of the Prevention of Consumption and other forms of Tuberculosis) had been formed in England in 1898, whereas in Wales the driving force became the Welsh National Memorial Association (WNMA). Through these measures, central government both accepted a greater responsibility for the health of the population, but also abdicated ultimate authority by devolving to these organizations the main tasks of producing comprehensive interventional programmes.

In Wales, much of the treatment available was provided via a network of sanatoria, encouraged and sustained by the fund-raising activities of the WNMA. The success of their campaign is borne out in the provision of hospital beds, increasing from 23 in 1912 to over 1,000 in 1926.[29] Between 1926 and 1935, 1,915 patients from Caernarfonshire received care in sanatoria or other specialist provisions, with Gwyrfai contributing almost 20 per cent of this total.[30] This 'downstream' activity by the WNMA entailed a focusing of resources on the wider infrastructure of pharmacies, institutional provisions and establishing departments for propaganda and research. The real task of tackling the underlying causes of tuberculosis fell on the shakier foundations offered by the emerging local authorities.

Where tasks were ill defined and not enforced, inertia reigned. The battle against tuberculosis was ultimately won through better housing than in the provision of hospital beds. However beneficial the stay in a sanatorium may have been, sufferers still had to return to their ill-ventilated and overcrowded homes at the end of their period of respite. Dr Thomas Evans, MoH for Swansea, criticized the WNMA focus on treatment 'as to hinder it from devoting itself to the real task of prevention'.[31] If the ultimate objective was to impact on prevalence and mortality, Wales did not fare particularly well compared with other areas in the UK. Between 1901 and 1905, death rates from tuberculosis were significantly higher in Scotland than in Wales; by 1925, the rates in the two countries were running in parallel, while by 1936, Scottish rates had decreased to a level comparable to England, leaving Wales lagging behind.[32] Considering that the tuberculosis death rates in parts of Caernarfonshire were significantly higher than the all-Wales average, the magnitude of the task facing local authorities was daunting. The Caernarfonshire MoH added his own vilification of the efforts of the WNMA, claiming that 'the decrease in the death-rate does not come up to expectation'.[33] Fully occupied sanatoria were a visible testimony to the failure of all other attempts to eradicate the disease.

Under the 1875 Public Health Act, local authorities were tasked with developing a broad range of public health measures. The Caernarfonshire Combined Sanitary Authority (consisting originally of nine urban and six rural councils) was established in 1876, primarily to share the cost of employing a full-time MoH. The first incumbent was Dr Hugh Rees, but he eventually relinquished his duties in 1890 due to ill health, reinforcing the concerns about the excessive workload expressed by one of the authority's members at the time of his appointment: 'I don't think this man will have time to sleep. And giving him five years' trial; why the man will give it up in twelve months.'[34] By 1908, because of the geographical area served and the magnitude of the tasks ahead, the area was split into three, each with its own MoH. There was little opportunity for the MoHs to develop long-term objectives, and while they reported a range of nuisances and circumstances detrimental to the health of local communities, their recommendations and findings often fell on the deaf ears of local councillors.[35] Invariably, individual MoHs found themselves working in isolation, with powers of observation but no power of implementation, highlighting extensive social problems, all the while knowing that there was little that could be achieved to demonstrate even short-term gains and improvements to health status.

The impact of tuberculosis had a dramatic, negative effect upon the spirit of communities. So endemic was the disease that the battle to eradicate it had as much to do with winning hearts and minds as with the scientific and social advances. The WNMA publication *The Crusade against Consumption* sounded the battle-cry for 'a persistent warfare against the prevailing ignorance and fatalism'.[36] Numerous planned activities were arranged through mobile exhibitions, slide lectures and the production of appropriately targeted literature.[37] To overcome the innate pessimism, more tangible achievements at a community level were required, of which there was little discernible evidence in many areas of Caernarfonshire.

Regardless of the unfavourable living conditions, there were certain preventive actions that could have been taken to improve the chances of avoiding the spread of tuberculosis. Dr Parry, in his 1906 report to the Caernarfonshire Sanitary Committee, complained that people were not keen on fresh air and that they held the belief that the root of all illness was to be found in cold air. Consequently, by keeping windows closed – even nailed down – there was a conviction that diseases were prevented from entering the home.[38] These were the very conditions that helped spread the tubercle bacillus, frustrating the efforts to eradicate the disease in a part of the country where 'consumption should be all but unknown in a district where we need never lack for fresh air'.[39]

By the first decade of the twentieth century, when many of the other infectious diseases had all but been eradicated, tuberculosis accounted for one death in every eight in the UK; for one-third of all deaths in men aged 25–44 and a quarter of all deaths in women aged 25–44.[40] There was a need to cut through the prejudice and the long-standing, melancholic beliefs of generations if prevention campaigns were to be successful. The inherent fatalism of the local population is evident throughout this period as staunchly Calvinistic communities put their faith in higher authorities than the local MoH, as evidenced in the 1933 Chalke inquiry: 'The population is poor, ill-housed, and full of the fatalistic and poetical uplift which gives such fervour to religious movements in Wales, and it puts up patiently with material conditions which might be thought intolerable elsewhere.'[41] The innate pessimism was related to the fact that this disease hit people in the prime of their lives, whereas the visitations of other infectious diseases were more dramatic, intermittent and short-lived. Tuberculosis did not have the same immediacy. The onset was often gradual and painful, and, unlike diseases such as smallpox, there was no quick-fix medication available to raise expectations.

The harmful effects of the slate industry exacerbated the endemic nature of tuberculosis in Caernarfonshire through a combination of weakening the chest through the inhalation of slate dust and the permanent presence of tuberculosis within quarrying communities. Dr Mills Roberts, a surgeon employed at Dinorwig Quarry Hospital in Llanberis, attributed the prevalence of ill health within these communities to nutritional deficiencies, unsuitable clothing, insufficient sanitary arrangements, the dampness of the atmosphere and, most controversially of all, to early marriage and intermarriage.[42] Notwithstanding Dr Roberts's allegiance to his employers, he identified the key components that contributed to the seemingly insurmountable problems associated with eradicating tuberculosis.

In his inaugural lecture, Professor Lyle Cummins, the first incumbent of the David Davies Chair in Tuberculosis, developed the argument that people living in cramped, overcrowded conditions in the major urban centres were able to develop a level of immunity that was not present in the more rural communities of Caernarfonshire. He claimed it was more dangerous for the inhabitants to leave their home environments to seek work in the large industrial centres than to remain in their own communities.[43] Such comments are borne out throughout this whole period, with numerous accounts of seemingly fit and healthy young people seeking employment in cities such as Liverpool, and returning home within a few years suffering from the disease.[44]

Underpinning the overall improvements in health and well-being were the protracted efforts to enact housing legislation. At the end of the period under review, it was felt that 'a number of local authorities in Wales have not taken advantage of their statutory powers',[45] particularly in relation to housing programmes. Across Caernarfonshire, a total of 8,152 houses were built between 1919 and 1940,[46] but the process was often painful and fraught with accusations of intransigence. Dr E. O. Price complained in 1914 that the lack of progress with housing reform was 'the weak spot of the tuberculosis campaign'.[47] The enormity of the tasks facing each type of community in Caernarfonshire was clearly demonstrated in the comments made by Dr R. Bruce Lowe in 1895, who demonstrated that in housing provisions alone, there was tremendous variance across Caernarfonshire:

> In the older towns some of the better class or artisan dwellings are fairly satisfactory, but back-to-back houses, and dwellings that are damp, dilapidated, insufficiently lighted and ventilated, were met with. In the industrial, or quarrymen's villages, the houses were, on the whole, of a good sort. The worst samples of dwellings were to be found in the purely rural parts.[48]

As early as 1899, councillors in Caernarfon were drawing up proposals for four major housing projects.[49] A quarter of a century later, local newspaper editorials were outspoken in their condemnation of the lack of progress: 'There is not a Council in the country that has talked more about houses than Caernarvon Town Council. Neither is there a Council that has done less . . . They have accomplished nothing.'[50] A tuberculosis exhibition in 1911 used models of houses based on examples found in Caernarfon to demonstrate what to avoid when designing and building new houses![51] It was felt that while 'improvement is impossible while the people live under such depressing conditions',[52] there was an additional imperative to respond when considering the extent of the problem. Early in 1908, the County MoH visited over 150 houses around Caernarfon and found that their condition was invariably beyond superficial repair.[53] Caernarfon Town Council embarked on a strategy of 'levelling up', where the lower social classes would move to housing vacated by those slightly higher up the social scale, who themselves would take a step up to better quality houses.[54] There is little evidence that this policy was successful, as shown in the frustration of Robert Roberts, the town's Sanitary Inspector, that 'no relief has reached those where the pressure is greatest'.[55] Councillors floundered with the magnitude of the task with which they were faced, and failed miserably to demonstrate tangible achievements.

To meet the demand for new housing successfully local authorities had to accept their responsibilities as landlords, rather than the previous, and easier, reliance on private enterprise. Housing was a local problem that required national solutions. Interventions by Ministry of Health officials,[56] and national condemnation when it was shown that 10 per cent of the 1,641 houses inspected in Caernarfon were overcrowded and unsuitable,[57] finally led to the Town Council taking full advantage of the 1935 Housing Act. A five-year plan was prepared to build 130 houses on the town's Ysgubor Goch site,[58] thereby alleviating many of the most acute housing problems.

The watershed for housing reform came in the post-war period. Addison's Housing Act (1919) led to a number of attempts during the 1920s and 1930s to implement ambitious housing projects. It was estimated in 1923 that 2,326 additional houses were required in Caernarfonshire, of which 75 per cent would be provided by local authorities. The gap between expectation and reality was highlighted when it was reported in 1923 that four of the seventeen local authorities within Caernarfonshire had hitherto failed to build any houses. By 1926, Bangor had built a credible 127 houses towards its target of 405.[59] In contrast, Gwyrfai – more rural, less municipal, demonstrating less drive and determination – was condemned for only providing 6 of the expected 326 homes.[60] The damning evidence led to the conclusion that 'the conditions in Gwyrfai are appalling'.[61] Obvious comparisons can be drawn between the approaches adopted in Bangor and Caernarfon. Bangor had established itself as the county's centre for health and learning, whereas Caernarfon was the traditional centre of commerce. Positive moves were seen in Bangor in the pre-1914 period to alleviate many of the more profound overcrowding and insanitary conditions. The borough surveyor, J. Gill, noted that in newly built houses in the city, the death rate was 8 per 1,000 population, whereas for Bangor as a whole, the rate was 14 per 1,000.[62] However subjective such an assessment may have been, it nevertheless established housing as a major public health issue that was seen to have an immediate impact on improving health status.

Many of the comments associated with the state of housing were linked to the moral implications of the overcrowded surroundings. This was evident in the COPEC (Christian Order in Politics, Economics and Citizenship) housing survey of Bangor in 1924,[63] where unsatisfactory housing conditions were seen as the precursor to moral weakness and spiritual degeneration. Although there were notable examples of unacceptable housing conditions – such as a house with one living room and one bedroom where three families (five adults and nine children) resided – the overall COPEC findings in Bangor were favourable.

COPEC followed up the study by ensuring that funding was provided for twenty three-bedroomed houses in Bangor, with priority being given to young families who previously lived in unsuitable accommodation.[64] Good quality housing at affordable rents was provided – meeting a demand that had been largely unachievable in Caernarfon through the prevarications of the 'levelling up' debate. Over a ten-year period from 1928, a further 816 houses were built in Bangor, placing the Council's house-building and slum-clearance programme alongside the most progressive in the UK.[65] As a result of this ambitious programme, many of the housing problems in Bangor were alleviated. By 1936, it was reported that only 3.7 per cent of houses were classified as overcrowded, compared with 22.1 per cent in Pwllheli.[66] The view that Bangor had dealt competently with housing was also reflected in the Clement Davies inquiry: 'When they [Bangor City Council] have completed their present schemes, they will not only have done away with their slum houses, but also have got rid of their overcrowding.'[67] The available evidence suggests that in the rural areas there was very limited progress, by authorities who rarely exhibited the same sense of urgency as their more urban counterparts. The perilous state of rural housing was well chronicled, from the observation in the 1860s that 'on the whole I have never seen in England as many bad cottages as I saw in North Wales',[68] to the laments of D. Lleufer Thomas almost a half-century later that 'in quality, as well as in quantity, the housing accommodation of most rural districts in Wales is deficient'.[69] The Royal Commission on Labour (1893) reported that the overall standard of agricultural cottage improved as you moved eastwards across north Wales, so that the cottages of Arfon and Eifionydd were generally of a better quality than in the Llŷn Peninsula.[70]

The main problems lay not in the availability but in the condition of the houses. Wages for agricultural labourers were generally lower than for quarrymen and town workers,[71] so that offering new houses at an affordable rent would not have been a viable proposition to rural councils and it would have been difficult for them to recoup their initial outlay. To the extent that an 'aristocracy of labour' existed,[72] the agricultural labourer was placed lower down the scale than industrial workers from quarries, ports and towns, so that economic factors had a greater bearing on housing conditions in rural areas than in the nearby towns.

People in rural areas had neither the economic means to access better quality housing, nor the ability to move because of the scarcity of good quality housing within their localities. Damning reports were published, linking the prevalence of infectious disease to the condition of local housing, listing a catalogue of unacceptable living conditions: walls built of mud, not stone; windows that were too small, leaving houses ill ventilated; floors of soil, not easily cleaned; pigsties adjacent to kitchens and cowsheds next to bedrooms.[73] The Welsh Housing Association reported in 1912 that it was no coincidence that Anglesey and parts of Caernarfonshire experienced the highest cancer rates in Europe.[74]

There were claims that housing legislation at the end of the nineteenth century was geared more to dealing with the slums of London and other large cities than with the problems of rural housing.[75] As a consequence, people living in industrial towns were experiencing better health outcomes by the end of the century. A report to the Llŷn Sanitary Committee in 1916 noted that although unsuitable houses had been found in Nefyn, Abersoch and Mynytho, the only available housing locally, in Pwllheli, was in a worse condition.[76] Twenty years later, the local MoH, Dr Lloyd Owen, complained that there remained a serious shortage of houses for the working classes in Llŷn, and that the local authority had not submitted any proposals to resolve the situation. The inability to finance ambitious projects was often at the heart of the lethargy, although it could be argued that public-health problems were more visible and ominous in the more densely populated areas.

Housing conditions, allied to more stable employment opportunities, provided the main reasons for the attraction of the slate-quarrying areas over more traditional agricultural districts. Even within the slate-quarrying communities, there is a need to differentiate between the situation in the larger communities of Llanberis and Bethesda, where conditions were 'far above the average',[77] and the Nantlle valley in Gwyrfai, which encompassed rural and urban elements, 'displaying most of the disadvantages of both and few of the advantages of either'.[78] Whereas Bethesda and Llanberis came under the stewardship of two of the largest quarry-owners in the world, Penrhyn and Assheton-Smith, the Nantlle valley quarries were smaller and therefore more prone to the effects of even minor economic fluctuations. As a result of the questionable economic viability of the quarries, the depression that hit the slate industry by the end of the 1920s meant that there were a number of empty houses available within these communities.[79]

There is an abundance of evidence regarding the Gwyrfai housing crisis. Regardless of previous inactivity, Councillor Jones Parry of Clynnog stated in 1926 that the proposals to build four houses in each parish in Gwyrfai were far too ambitious,[80] at a time when the death rate from tuberculosis was 44 per cent higher in Gwyrfai than in Bangor, and the cancer death rates twice as high.[81] The local council was accused of ignoring Local Government Board recommendations, of ignoring public opinion and of purposely failing to fulfil their responsibilities.[82] Not surprisingly, Gwyrfai was referred to as the 'black spot in the darkest county',[83] and on seeing the condition of some houses in the district, Clement Davies commented that he had to remind himself that he was living in the twentieth century.[84]

The need for housing reform in Gwyrfai was greater than in any other district in Caernarfonshire, but it was not a decline in living conditions that was seen, but rather an unwillingness to meet the increased expectations of the times. Following the 1933 Chalke report, the *British Medical Journal* referred to the living conditions in Gwyrfai as a 'sombre tragedy',[85] a situation that had hardly improved by 1936 when it was reported that 8.3 per cent of houses in the district were overcrowded. When compared with the other slate-quarrying districts of Ogwen (4.4 per cent) and Bethesda (3 per cent), it can be seen that serious problems remained in Gwyrfai. The effects of the Clement Davies inquiry reverberated through the British press, with headlines such as 'Homes worse than slums of Shanghai' and 'Ten live in 2-roomed hovel'[86] giving a full flavour to the indictment in the report. By the end of the 1930s, however, over 650 new houses had been built by the council and private builders, leading W. Hughes Jones to claim that a 'revolution' had occurred:

> A wizard has been to the Gwyrfai district. Gone are the old rags, and the holes and the walls, and the leaking roofs and the sunless lethal bedchambers. Gone are the overcrowded houses. In their place are neat, widely scattered stone bungalows with wide open windows.[87]

That the health status of the local population was so greatly improved by the late 1930s compared with the 1870s is due mainly to the eradication of the infectious diseases and the vastly improved living conditions. Certainly, the overall reduction in the prevalence of infectious diseases mirrors corresponding improvements in sanitary provisions, uncontaminated water supplies, better housing and an improved standard of living. Many of the improvements were down to the component parts mentioned by the chairman of the North Wales Medical Committee in his annual speech in 1902. While a growing proportion of the population was putting its faith in the medical profession, the doctors themselves were emphasizing that it was only through fighting for social, educational and sanitary reform that real health improvements were to be found:

> Whatever might be done through the investigations of science and preventive measures, they would have to rely pre-eminently upon the observation of the laws of health, such as the encouragement of manly exercises, which tended to improve the physical stamina; seeing that the food supplies were not adulterated, and that as far as possible the air and water supplies were pure, and more particularly that the question of proper housing among the

labouring population became a prominent plank in the platform of social legislation.'[88]

Notes

[1] Ministry of Health, *Report of the Committee of Inquiry into the Anti-Tuberculosis Service in Wales and Monmouth* (1938), evidence, Vol. 7, pp. 27–8 (National Library of Wales MS 15357), D. Thomas Jones, Chair of the Gwyrfai Council Housing Committee, giving evidence to the enquiry.

[2] 'Upstream' activity would focus on the causes of poor health and inequalities in health (the factors that push people into the river of ill health). 'Downstream' activities look at individual behavioural or other risk factors (pulling drowning people out of the river). Upstream activities would include preventative measures such as housing policy, nutritional interventions and public education, whereas the downstream approaches would encompass hospital and medical provisions. Consequently, most of the factors that improve the public's health lie outside the domain of mainstream health services. (G. Davey Smith, S. Macintyre, I. Chalmers, R. Horton, R. Smith, 'Using evidence to inform health policy: case study,' *British Medical Journal*, Vol. 322 (2001), 222–5.

[3] *Caernarvon and Denbigh Herald*, 9 September 1892.

[4] A. S. Wohl, *Endangered Lives: Public Health in Victorian Britain* (London, 1983).

[5] Ibid., p. 329.

[6] *Caernarvon and Denbigh Herald*, 20 September 1907.

[7] T. McKeown and C. R. Lowe, *An Introduction to Social Medicine* (Oxford, 1966), p. 13.

[8] G. Roberts, 'Closing the stable door after the horse has bolted: preventing the spread of smallpox and cholera in Caernarfonshire, 1870–1910', *Caernarfonshire Historical Society Transactions*, Vol. 55 (1994), 109–28.

[9] *Caernarvon and Denbigh Herald*, 2 September 1892.

[10] Ibid., 25 July 1902.

[11] T. McKeown, *The Modern Rise of Population* (London, 1976), p. 59.

[12] F. B. Smith, *The People's Health 1830–1910* (London, 1979), p. 156.

[13] *Caernarvon and Denbigh Herald*, 12 October 1872.

[14] *North Wales Chronicle*, 19 January 1901.

[15] Ibid., 13 June 1903.

[16] *Caernarvon and Denbigh Herald*, 25 July 1902.

[17] Roberts, 'Closing the stable door'.

[18] W. A. R. Thomson (ed.), *Black's Medical Dictionary* (1978), p. 303.

[19] E. Jones, *Stiniog* (Caernarfon, 1988), p. 41.

[20] E. O. Price, *The Bangor Typhoid Epidemic of 1882* (Bangor MS 15595), p. 24.

[21] Ibid., p. 11.

[22] Ibid., p. 11.

[23] *Caernarvon and Denbigh Herald*, 1 November 1889.

[24] P. E. Jones, *Bangor: A Study in Municipal Government* (Cardiff, 1986).

25 G. Roberts and A. Evans, *The Centenary of Minffordd Hospital 1895–1995*, (Bangor, 1996).
26 P. E. Jones, *Bangor: A Study in Municipal Government*, pp. 33–54.
27 Wohl, *Endangered Lives*, p. 130.
28 F. F Cartwright, *A Social History of Medicine* (London, 1977).
29 *North Wales Chronicle*, 5 May 1917.
30 Annual Reports of the Registrar General 1926–35.
31 *Welsh Outlook* (February 1919), Appendix, p. 8.
32 Ministry of Health, *Report of the Committee of Inquiry into the Anti-Tuberculosis Service in Wales and Monmouth* (1938), p. 20.
33 Medical Officer of Health, Caernarvon County Council, *Annual Report* 1925, p. 10.
34 R. Bruce Lowe, *Report to the Local Government Board on Sanitary Progress and Administration in the Caernarvonshire Combined District* (1895), PRO MH12/16073, p. 1.
35 Roberts (1994), 'Closing the stable door'.
36 Welsh National Memorial Association, *The Crusade against Consumption*, (Newtown, 1910).
37 Ibid.
38 *North Wales Chronicle*, 15 June 1906.
39 *Caernarvon and Denbigh Herald*, 23 July 1909, editorial.
40 Linda Bryder, *Below the Magic Mountain: A Social History of Tuberculosis in Twentieth-Century Britain* (Oxford, 1988), p. 1.
41 'Tuberculosis in north Wales', *British Medical Journal*, editorial (30 September 1933), p. 613.
42 Report on Open Quarries (1894), *Minutes of Evidence given before the Committee appointed to Inquire into the Dangers to Health, Life and Limb*. Appendix 3, p. 24, evidence of Dr Mills Roberts, 29 June 1893.
43 *North Wales Chronicle*, 4 November 1921.
44 G. Roberts, *Iechyd Cyhoeddus yn Sir Gaernarfon, 1870–1939*, unpublished Ph.D. thesis, Aberystwyth, 1993).
45 Ministry of Health, *Report of the Committee of Inquiry into the Anti-Tuberculosis Service in Wales and Monmouth* (London, 1939), p. 93.
46 J. Williams, *Digest of Welsh Historical Statistics*, Vol. 2, (Cardiff, 1985), p. 88.
47 *North Wales Chronicle*, 1 May 1914.
48 R. Bruce Lowe, *Report to the Local Government Board on Sanitary Progress and Administration*, p. 5.
49 *North Wales Chronicle*, 24 February 1900.
50 *Caernarvon and Denbigh Herald*, 16 February 1923.
51 Ibid., 3 March 1911.
52 Ibid., 21 February 1908.
53 P. Fraser, *Report on the Dwellings in the Courts and Poorest Parts of the Town*, Gwynedd Archives Service, XDI/ 626.
54 *Caernarvon and Denbigh Herald*, 5 February 1926.
55 Ibid., 8 February 1929.
56 *North Wales Chronicle*, 6 July 1934.

57 Housing Act 1935, *Report on the Overcrowding Survey in England and Wales, 1936*, p. 144.
58 *North Wales Chronicle*, 15 November 1935.
59 P. E. Jones, *Bangor: A Study in Municipal Government*, p. 269.
60 *Caernarvon and Denbigh Herald*, 3 August 1923.
61 Ministry of Health, *Report of the Committee of Inquiry into the Anti-Tuberculosis Service in Wales and Monmouth* (1938), evidence, Vol. VII, pp. 27-8.
62 *North Wales Chronicle*, 31 January 1913.
63 Christian Order in Politics, Economics and Citizenship, University of Wales, Bangor MS 19232.
64 *Caernarvon and Denbigh Herald*, 17 February 1928.
65 P. E. Jones, *Bangor: A Study in Municipal Government*, p. 269.
66 Housing Act 1935, *Report on the Overcrowding Survey*.
67 Ministry of Health, *Report of the Committee of Inquiry into the Anti-Tuberculosis Service in Wales and Monmouth* (London, 1939), p. 154.
68 Commission on the Employment of Children, Young Persons and Women in Agriculture, (1867), pp. 34-5.
69 D. Lleufer Thomas, 'The Housing Problem in Wales', *Welsh Housing and Development Association Yearbook* (1916), p. 24.
70 Royal Commission on Labour, *The Agricultural Labourers*, Vol. 2, *Wales* (1893), p. 149.
71 Cartwright *A Social History of Medicine*, pp. 95-6.
72 E. J. Hobsbawm, 'The aristocracy of labour reconsidered', in idem, *Worlds of Labour* (London, 1984), p. 227.
73 Dr Parsons, *Report to the Local Government Board on the Sanitary Circumstances of the Pwllheli Rural District and on Diphtheria There* (10 October 1887), Harvester Microform 387, p. 1.
74 *Caernarvon and Denbigh Herald*, 14 June 1912.
75 Ibid., 20 December 1912.
76 *North Wales Chronicle*, 21 January 1916.
77 Ibid., 18 July 1913.
78 H. D. Chalke, *An Investigation into the Causes of the Continued High Death Rate from Tuberculosis in Certain Parts of North Wales* (Bangor, 1933), p. 14.
79 Roberts, 'Closing the stable door'.
80 *Caernarvon and Denbigh Herald*, 19 February 1926.
81 *North Wales Chronicle*, 31 January 1913.
82 Ibid., 10 October 1913.
83 *Caernarvon and Denbigh Herald*, 11 March 1938.
84 Ministry of Health, *Report of the Committee of Inquiry into the Anti-Tuberculosis Service in Wales and Monmouth* (1938), evidence, Vol. VII, p. 19.
85 'Tuberculosis in North Wales', *British Medical Journal*, editorial (30 September 1933), p. 614.
86 *Daily Sketch*, 14 March 1939.
87 W. Hughes Jones, *A Challenge to Wales* (Liverpool, 1938) p. 38.
88 *Caernarvon and Denbigh Herald*, 18 July 1902.

2

'Sea Wall against Disease':[1] Port Health in Cardiff, 1850–1950

NEIL EVANS

The importance of attention to the hygienic condition both of our merchant vessels and our seaports is clearly seen; for a foul ship, instead of merchandise, carries from land to sea the seeds of depopulating diseases, and a foul seaport supplies the soil in which they rankly germinate.[2]

Introduction

Ports are particular kinds of towns and this gives them particular health problems. The novelist Linda Grant, drawing on her (or rather her character's) own experience of Liverpool and sundry other ports, observes: 'Ports don't inhabit the country they are in. Our backs are turned against the land, looking out for the stranger. Traders, traders all.'[3] Urban and labour historians are currently trying to specify the distinctiveness of ports. Essentially they are being seen as interfaces between nations and global trade, a position which gives them peculiar social characteristics. Their workforces are dominated by casual labour, and close relationships develop between sailors, dockers and the engineering trades which keep the ships functioning. These workers are semi-detached from the wider labour movement.[4]

Issues of health were an important aspect of this distinctiveness once Britain's filthy towns were cleaned up in the mid-Victorian period. The conditions in which epidemics could really flourish were ended. Keeping further infection out by the sanitary inspection of shipping became a viable option. The approach to this problem which had evolved over much of Europe was to use physical barriers to the transmission of disease. In cholera epidemics in Europe it was common to use police measures and even troops in attempts to resist the spread of cholera. The maritime equivalent was quarantine under which infected ships were detained for long periods and kept in isolation. Both the ill and the healthy were held together. Such policies were increasingly challenged in the nineteenth century, on a number of grounds. For one thing, they notably failed to work and disease tended to spread faster in countries which adopted draconian measures than in those which did not. A ready explanation was available for this in the anti-contagionist ideas which were developed in the period. Epidemics were seen as being the result of polluted air rather than of direct transmission through contagion. This suggested that public health reform was an alternative and more effective policy. So the lack of success of physical barrier methods was underpinned by medical theory. Furthermore such an approach chimed in with the emergent ideology of laissez-faire, and was particularly attractive in Britain where international trade was such a central economic activity.[5]

Port sanitary matters were generally a concern of the later nineteenth century after the more basic public health problems of rapidly growing towns had been addressed.[6] The exponential growth of trade in the late nineteenth century created a global system which in many ways paralleled the globalized world of the early twenty-first century. The potential for spreading disease was greatly increased.[7] The coming of steamships magnified the problem because of the speed with which they moved between ports.[8]

The policies which evolved became known as the 'English system' and were rooted in anti-contagionist theory. They focused on inspecting ships from infected ports and isolating only those who were ill rather than whole crews and complements of passengers. Interruptions to trade were minimized, though it was not possible to end quarantine entirely until the 1890s because of the measures which other countries would take against British commerce unless this was retained for bubonic plague and yellow fever. The English system dealt with non-quarantine diseases like smallpox, cholera, scarlet fever and measles.[9]

These issues were fully discussed in the 1869 Commission on Sanitation and, as a result, port sanitary authorities were introduced in the Public Health Act of 1872 to implement the English system. Such action was seen not simply as a measure for the protection of the ports themselves but as part of a national defence system against disease.

The measures which are carried out in our ports and littoral districts with a view of preventing the introduction of cholera from foreign countries are intended not only for the benefit of places receiving the infection, but also for the protection of the country at large ... The sanitary arrangements of the districts which form as it were our first line of defence, and upon which our security from invasion must greatly depend, are matters, therefore, which concern the whole nation.[10]

Effective port sanitation depended on the cooperation of the port sanitary authority with the general sanitary authority for the port as well as with inland authorities so that contacts of infected people could be traced and these in turn inspected or isolated.[11]

Public health in Cardiff

Cardiff was no exception to this chronological pattern and as one of the UK's major ports it was a vital link in the chain of defence. By 1914 it was the largest tramp shipping port in the world as well as the greatest coal-exporting port and its growth had been astronomic. In 1801 it had contained under 2,000 people which rose to just over 18,000 in 1851 but to a massive 182,000 in 1911.[12] Concern with port sanitary matters came only late in the day when more fundamental issues of shore hygiene had been addressed. If there was any issue of sanitation which involved the port in the early 1850s it concerned the Irish immigrants who were seen as an imported health risk and one which H. J. Paine, the Medical Officer of Health (MoH), was keen to exclude. Appropriately enough when port health issues first appear in the MoH's report it is in regard to cholera which was imported by visiting sailors in 1853–4 and ultimately spread to the rest of the town. In all, there were 171 deaths, of whom 30 were seamen and a total of 44 having some connection with shipping. But there were no efforts made to try to limit this importation, despite the clear recognition of the source. In 1857 an epidemic of smallpox spread from the shipping into the Irish area of Newtown. In all there were 161 deaths.[13]

By the early 1860s the town's death rate had fallen from over 30 per 1,000 before the adoption of the Public Health Act in 1849 to around 20 per 1,000 by 1862. It was in this context that there seemed to be a possibility of containing disease by some port sanitary measures. In that year the MoH reported 22 deaths from fever, 3 of which were cases of seamen removed from vessels. Residents in George Street and in Loudon Square complained of the risks to them. This was especially the case because of the prevalence of the highly contagious typhoid on board ship. Yet to leave cases on board ship made them hard to treat and gave the stricken seamen the dubious comforts of a hammock. This led Paine to make the first case for a seamen's hospital of some kind: 'The rapidity of transport now renders it a matter of serious consideration, as fever from foreign ports may be here, and has in some ports been introduced with serious results.'[14] But the local Board of Health made no response until the next appearance of cholera in 1866. The warning was repeated:

> The importation of yellow fever into Swansea by the *Hecla*, from Cuba, laden with copper ore, whereby 13 deaths from that disease occurred in the harbour, another on board the *Eleanor*, and one in Llanelly, directed public attention to the circumstances, that the rapid transit now affected through the employment of steam power in our commercial trades exposed us to the dangers of disease from which this country was before exempt; and that such diseases when imported spread, not merely by actual contagion, but by miasma among our people. The necessity of a provision to meet this danger I have frequently impressed upon your board.[15]

The outbreak of yellow fever mentioned in Swansea was the only one which ever occurred in Britain. On all other occasions it was kept within the port but this outbreak spread to the shore adding to the fears engendered by cholera.[16] Cholera had been advancing since the spring of 1865 from Egypt and concern was naturally felt because of the constant communication between Egypt and Britain. By early 1866 France, Belgium and Holland all had outbreaks while a few cases had been recorded at Southampton the previous autumn. The dangers of cholera led to some action being taken, and Mr Boyle, the agent to the Marquess of Bute, used his influence with the government to procure an old ship, *HMS Hamadryad*, for use as a seamen's hospital. This was to obviate the need for sending cholera cases to the workhouse or to scattered seamen's lodging-houses, both of which would have increased the risk of spreading infection through the town. In July cholera finally reached Cardiff in a ship coming from London docks. The body was buried at sea and the ship fumigated but other vessels subsequently introduced further cases and the epidemic ultimately spread to the town. A cholera hospital was established in Tyndall Street which was close both to the docks and to the likely areas of high incidence of the disease in the town.[17]

This third cholera epidemic to strike Cardiff was the least serious and showed that the public-health measures taken in the 1850s had done much to control death rates. It now became feasible to try to prevent an epidemic by means of rigorous attention to the medical inspection of vessels. The declining impact of cholera in Cardiff is indicated in table 2.1.

Table 2.1: Deaths from Cholera in Cardiff

Year	Deaths	Rate per 1000
1849	350	21.80
1854	175	6.36
1866	47	1.25

Source: Cardiff Medical Officer of Health, Annual Report, 1866.

The formalization of port sanitary authorities in the early 1870s was also prompted by the issue of cholera. The danger of cholera in 1873 led to a provisional order being made to create a port sanitary authority in Cardiff. In fact this led to the detection of seven cases of smallpox rather than of cholera. Under powers given by an Order in Council a steam vessel was used to visit all foreign ships on arrival in the Roads.[18] Questions about the health of the crew and the port from which the vessel had sailed then had to be answered. Captains faced severe penalties if they gave false information. Ships were detained in quarantine if the answers were unsatisfactory. Logbooks were also examined for evidence of disease on the voyage. This system was maintained from 9 September 1873 until 25 March 1874 when the danger was deemed to have passed.[19] The virtues of this system in containing smallpox were commented upon by Paine:

> The great number of seamen who suffered from the disease, and the length of time which elapsed before the disease spread among the inhabitants – namely one year and three months – proves the great advantage accruing from the sanitary supervision of which was exercised over the shipping . . .[20]

By then, the *Hamadryad* had been fitted up to take up to sixty-five patients and had become self-supporting by means of a voluntary levy on shipping of two shillings per hundred tons' register which in turn gave the right to free treatment to the crews of ships paying the levy.

'SEA WALL AGAINST DISEASE' 83

This worked well and quickly provided a surplus of income over expenditure of £400.[21] The main practical problem of inspection at Cardiff was the circumstance that the dock gates opened directly into the Bristol Channel and therefore no real opportunity was provided for inspection of vessels before they entered the port. This problem was circumnavigated by enlisting the aid of pilots who boarded vessels in the channel and asked the standard questions about sickness on the voyage. These were:

1) From what port have you come?
2) Have you had any communication with another vessel during this voyage?
3) Is every person on board in good health?
4) Has anyone died on board during the voyage?
5) Has anyone been ill, and if so from what disease has he suffered?[22]

The nature of medical problems at sea can be indicated from the kind of cases which were admitted to the *Hamadryad* for a single year as in table 2.2.

Table 2.2: Admissions to *HMS Hamadryad*, 1882

Disease	Admitted	Death	Recovery
Smallpox	5	1	4
Measles	3	–	3
Scarlet fever	2	–	2
Fever	19	3	16
Ague	10	–	10
Rheumatic fever	45	–	45
Erysipelas	5	3	2
Phthisis	8	6	2 (relieved)
Bronchitis, Pleurisy and Pneumonia	43	5	38
Heart disease	12	3	9
Other diseases	318	1	317
Injuries	109	7	102

Source: Cardiff MoH Report, 1882.

Cholera again prompted the next major shift in port health policy in Cardiff in 1883 when arrangements were made to secure a temporary isolation hospital on Flat Holm in the Bristol Channel and a mooring station was provided near the island where vessels from inspected ports could be visited by the port sanitary inspector. The site was in the middle of the channel and six miles from land. The inhabitants of the island totalled twenty-five. Initially a tent was provided as accommodation and it was erected on an elevated location but in a depression which gave some protection from the elements.[23] In addition to the inspection of vessels the MoH made an arrangement with the Medical Superintendent of the *Hamadryad* to report all special cases of sickness to him. In 1886, when there was an outbreak of cholera at Bilbao, a quarantine boat operated in the Roads to intercept all vessels entering with a foul bill of health. But no cases of cholera came to light as a result of this.[24]

The methods of port health

Port sanitary measures, as we have seen, became part of a distinctive British strategy for dealing with public health which had evolved by the last decade of the nineteenth century. The MoH who succeeded Paine in Cardiff, Edward Walford, explained to the public the essence of the arrangements in some detail:

> Although the old term 'quarantine' is still used by some as applied to the protective measures used in our ports, it has long ceased to imply any routine detention. The system in force is that known as 'Medical Inspection' and consists in the medical inspection of all infected vessels, the removal, where possible, of any infected persons, the disinfection or destruction of any infected articles, and the thorough disinfection and cleansing of the vessel. At the same time the names and addresses of persons leaving the vessel are taken and forwarded to the place of destination of such persons, in order that they may be kept for a time under medical supervision. No undue interference with the shipping takes place (the whole process occupying only a matter of a few hours) as in the old form of quarantine where all vessels, infected or not infected, coming from any country in which there was at the time of leaving a case of cholera, were subjected to a useless and prolonged detention.[25]

A commercial nation certainly welcomed any system which assisted the free flow of shipping. Walford also thought it had the virtue of removing the false security provided by quarantine and directing attention towards measures which would prevent diseases like cholera from taking hold:

> In the place of resisting disease by military cordons by land and by unjustifiable detentions by sea, we rely on internal sanitation, on the provision of pure water, and efficient drainage. And on the removal of all decomposing

and harmful impurities from the neighbourhood of habitations ... by further efforts in the same direction we shall, in time, be able to exclude Asiatic Cholera from our country ... No such results can be shewn to have followed the adoption of the most stringent system of quarantine; on the contrary, the quarantining countries are essentially those which cholera invades, and for the most part they are those where sanitation makes but slow progress. The system has apparently, by engendering a false sense of security, retarded the execution of works of sanitary improvement, whereas the abandonment of it in England has probably been one of the most powerful of the many stimulants which the cause of sanitary reform has ever received.[26]

In the mid 1890s the provision for dealing with infectious diseases was improved by the construction of a permanent hospital on the island of Flat Holm to replace the weather-battered tents. This included a crematorium for the disposal of the bodies of the infected. This facility was also used by the adjoining Barry Port Sanitary Authority for the isolation of its infectious cases. These comprehensive arrangements engendered a sense of confidence: 'It is highly improbable, therefore, with all these precautions, that any such case could be brought ashore from vessels coming into any of the docks at Cardiff or at Barry.'[27]

The Port Sanitary Authority had been permanently constituted in 1882 and took in an area which included parts of Glamorgan as well as the Cardiff waterfront. The work was nothing if not methodical. The Port Sanitary Inspector was aided by an inspector of nuisances who inspected all vessels for defects – to check whether they were well ventilated, clean and lighted. The main problems were constantly found to be defective ventilation, impure water, overcrowding, defective bulkhead drainage and leaks in water closets. In such cases the owner was informed and formal notice usually issued. Much of the restitution seems to have been achieved amicably without recourse to legal proceedings.[28] It was soon claimed that this work had produced tangible results in that the numbers of defective vessels failed to grow at the same rate as the growth of shipping using the port.[29] The figures for inspections and defective vessels in appendix 2 (p. 94) broadly bear out this analysis. But this did not stop conditions on board ships occasionally becoming issues of public discussion. In the sparring which preceded and ran through the national seamen's strike of 1911, the conditions of ships' forecastles was one of the insults which was traded between owners and sailors in a replay of the common Victorian 'pig or the sty' debate on housing. The MoH at Newport complained of the state of things. A Cardiff shipowner knew where to place the blame:

> one of the most successful owners, spoke in strong terms of the British seaman, who, he said, was dirtier in his language and his manners than foreigners. It was useless attempting to train them into cleanliness, for whatever was provided they spoilt by their carelessness and dirty habits.[30]

The union's view, by contrast, was that quarters were too cramped and off-duty time too short for men to be able to keep them clean: in this restricted space sweat-sodden clothes had to be dried near their food. It was an indication of the general lack of care that the shipowners showed for the welfare of their crews.[31]

But there was to be no break in the routine of this work until the late 1930s when a sudden deterioration in conditions on board ship was revealed. Of course after the massive confrontation of the international strike of 1911 the National Sailors' and Firemen's Union had generally settled into a cosy relationship with the Shipping Federation and was hardly a campaigning body. When combined with the apparently cosy relationship between the MoH's staff and the shipowners there was little leverage which could be exerted to try to improve seamen's conditions. When the deterioration in conditions became an issue in the mid-1930s it was soon resolved by recourse to the corporate structure of relations between the union and the shipowners and an agreement was reached through the National Maritime Board.[33]

New developments in port health

By the end of the 1890s new duties began to devolve upon the port sanitary officials. By 1897 frozen meat was being imported from a variety of locations mainly from the River Plate and Buenos Aires, sometimes via London and Liverpool. The officials were required to inspect such cargoes. This could have more serious consequences. When, in 1911, Beggs's warehouse was burned down in the docks during the seamen's and dockers' strike the inspectors had to spend some weeks with the salvage men deciding what had to go to the corporation destructor and what could be sold at auction.[33]

As the century drew to a close, the central concern of the Port Sanitary Authority shifted away from cholera towards the control of bubonic plague. A new bubonic plague epidemic had been gathering force in central Asia from the 1850s but in 1894 it attracted international attention when it swept through the filthy and unregulated streets of Hong Kong. Its impact was greatest within the British Empire which served as a conduit for the disease but it had a much more severe impact in the East than in the West. In Hong Kong the black rat was isolated as the vector of the disease and this meant that preventative measures could be taken.[34] In August 1899 the Local Government Board issued a circular warning of this danger and an inspector was despatched to Cardiff to discuss the issue. He was pleased with the preparations which had been made but it proved to be the start of a new area of work. Very soon rats found on vessels which came from infected ports (Bilbao from whence came the iron ore for south Wales works was one of them) were killed and burned.[36] Rats would become one of the key issues to face port sanitary authorities in the first part of the twentieth century. In 1901, for the first time, a tally of rats caught – 1,868 – was included in the Annual Report. These tallies would recur each year and become much enhanced as efforts were made to eliminate as far as possible the rats which were the carriers of disease. By 1908 around twice the number of rats were destroyed – 3,112. The next year measures to destroy mosquitoes were added to this, given the realization of their role in the spreading of yellow fever. By 1910 the number of rats destroyed each year had averaged over 5,000 for three years – with 8,720 accounted for in the last year. The fears were based on small outbreaks of plague in Glasgow, Liverpool, Cardiff and Leith in the previous decade. But it was never a fundamental issue in Cardiff – like so much of port health work it was routine preventive work, necessary, but not leading to dramatic events or much controversy. Nor did bubonic plague raise issues in many other Western ports, though it may have contributed something to anti-Chinese feeling. Only in the East did it arouse major public issues and provide the raw material for Marriott's sensational bestseller.[36]

Cholera, of course, still remained a concern but it was treated along the existing procedures rather than with innovations in policy as was the case with plague. Apart from this there was little in the way of new work until the outbreak of the First World War. The major innovation was a concern for the treatment of venereal disease which led to the establishment of a clinic for seamen. This was the result of regulations issued by the Local Government Board on 12 July 1916 and further regulations on sailors which followed. The clinic – exclusively for sailors – at the Hamadryad was opened on 16 April 1917 and soon was well frequented. Ever since 1905 this hospital had been a permanent building on shore but it retained the name of the vessel which had been its first home until it closed.

Venereal disease remained a regular concern of the Port Sanitary Authority but it was clearly – again – unspectacular work which produced no major new developments until the Second World War. In 1935 there was some public controversy over the issue in Cardiff, when the British Social Hygiene Council and the British Council for the Welfare of the Mercantile Marine published a report on social conditions in docklands. Cardiff naturally figured amongst these. Much of the report was unexceptionable but when it was finally published its author, Captain F. A. Richardson, chose to use it to launch an attack on the port's black population. It claimed that 88 per cent of the venereal disease cases in the Hamadryad originated abroad and that 50 per cent of the cases in Cardiff and district were traceable to Bute Street cafes. It simply said that the blame was placed on Cardiff's black and mixed-race population, which was seen as living in idleness and vice. 'Half-caste' girls had for some time been seen as having no future other than prostitution; they spread the disease far and wide – at least as far as up the south Wales valleys, transmitted through rugby crowds which came into Cardiff on international match days and ended their festivities with a tour of Bute Street's night life. The *Western Mail* drew the moral:

> In considering the numbers of black seamen in Cardiff it is interesting to note that the expenditure on the treatment of venereal disease in that city is the second largest of any city in the United Kingdom, and that the total population is barely a quarter of a million.[37]

Perhaps we need to retrace the steps in this argument to make it clearer. Foreign sailors brought it in; these are then equated with black sailors resident in Cardiff. Their offspring are the prostitutes who spread venereal disease to the Valleys and doubtless beyond. It is entirely to the credit of the professionalism of Cardiff's public health officials that this tendentious mélange is entirely absent from the MoH's Annual Report for the year. It was a matter for credit to refuse to be concerned with such racist accusation which went far beyond the eugenicist position common amongst medical professionals in the period and reached the outer limits of right-wing extremism.

The normal position of medical professionals was evident in the attitudes displayed towards tuberculosis. In 1934 the MoH announced with some delight that he had nailed the myth of Cardiff's exceptionally high incidence of tuberculosis. It was true that the rate was above that of the towns with which it was usually compared. But it was not above that for ports, and particular attention was given to the incidence of the disease amongst seamen – especially Arab seamen who were seen to be particularly susceptible to it. South Shields which also had a large proportion of Arab seamen was also shown to have an above average incidence of the disease. Of course racial explanations of tuberculosis and of other diseases were common in the inter-war period.[38] In this case it gave the MoH an opportunity to relieve what was clearly felt to be some public pressure upon him over the disease.[39] In fact, racial explanations were usually symptoms of other matters – disproportionate exposure to poor housing conditions and nutrition, and the length of time in which the group had lived in such conditions. Those recently arrived had not had time to develop such immunities. On Tyneside in the 1930s this included the Irish who were two generations behind the rest in 'urban industrial selection'.[40] When the Cardiff Medical Officer of Health was writing for the professional audience in the *Lancet* rather than for local political consumption he chose to stress the sanitary conditions in which sailors worked; indeed he did not mention racial factors.[41]

The end of the First World War brought new problems with the impact of the influenza pandemic.[42] It was present on board ships in the docks from 15–31 March 1918 and 19 September 1918 until 30 April 1919. Patients were treated on board ship or conveyed to hospital as appropriate.[43] The end of the war also saw the introduction of more stringent requirements for the destruction of rats by the Rat and Mice (Destruction) Act of 1919 which required occupiers of premises to take steps periodically to destroy the rat and mouse population, on pain of severe penalties. This was particularly enforced in 1926 when the impact of the coal strike drastically reduced the volume of shipping to be inspected (as well as the amount of infectious diseases imported) and advantage could be taken of the respite from inspection to concentrate on vermin control.[44]

The fact that port sanitary matters were a national issue as well as one which particularly concerned the particular port was recognized by government in 1920 by the payment of half the costs by the Ministry of Health. This produced requirements about the amount of time devoted to port sanitary matters by some of the MoH staff. These were met at Cardiff with some modifications of the requirements of the Ministry. Such changes came in the context of the threat of plague from Europe and of typhus in the aftermath of the war. Influenza continued to be a problem on board ship too.[45]

By the 1920s port sanitary administration – never the subject of high drama – had become routine and plodding: 'The preventative organization at the Port leaves little to be desired,' the MoH reported rather languidly in 1922.[46] But there is no reason to think that this work was other than highly competently done. Professionalism had matched itself to the problems and there seemed to be little of consequence to report. But there was never room for complacency as a shock experienced in 1924 illustrated. As we have seen, protection against plague and rat infestation was a major concern of the Port Sanitary Authority from the turn of the century onwards. Plague was still prevalent in the world at large but no case had been known at Cardiff for many years. A ship which had been moored at the port and twice given a clean bill of health experienced two cases of plague two weeks after leaving the port. As it had called nowhere else in the meantime, it followed that the infection must have been present when at Cardiff. Ten rats (the low figure being compatible with the master's statement that the ship was rat-free) were destroyed when the vessel was fumigated at Suez and these almost certainly carried the bacilli. A lesson was drawn:

> there is also the possibility that the rats passed over from some other vessel against which she was lying at the docks.
>
> The important point is that, if this vessel or any other vessel which brought these rats had been lying at the quayside, the warehouses and the town might have become infested with plague infected rats, and an extensive outbreak might have started.
>
> These facts reveal the loop-holes which necessarily exist in any reasonably limited scheme for controlling the entry of infectious diseases by sea. ... the supervision of vessels lying at the buoys presents a problem which has not yet been solved.[47]

But this was a rare breach in the sea wall. Generally it was well maintained and, where some water crept through, a finger was speedily applied to the hole.

Conclusion

One of the great problems in historical studies of public health is that of evidence. The most readily available sources – and sometimes almost the only ones – are the official records of the agencies charged with enforcing public health regulations and preventing outbreaks of disease. The historian can feel like the Medical Officer of Health's public relations consultant rather than an independent investigator. The main sources deployed here are of these official kinds – so does this mean that the conclusions drawn are inherently favourable to the medical professionals?

In the course of this discussion perhaps four independent ways of checking the conclusions have emerged. One is the public health record. The lack of any major epidemic of cholera or bubonic plague in a world where they were endemic and where Cardiff had close trading links with many infected areas must say something about the efficacy of port health measures. Major epidemics were possible in ports where health provision was less effective, as the devastation of both Hamburg and St Petersburg in 1892 demonstrates. It has been suggested that this was luck as much as anything and that there were serious gaps in the defences in the late nineteenth century. But this applies only to the smaller ports of Wales and it is difficult to believe that luck alone kept Britain free from major epidemics of killer diseases which ravaged many of its trading partners – though Cardiff was clearly not the most vulnerable of ports as its trade was heavily skewed to exports and many ships entered the port with only skeleton crews.[48] Part of the inequality in the imperial world was in health care and the machinery of administration.[49] The second control is the investigation conducted by Parliament in the 1890s into port health, which generally gave all the south Wales ports a gold star. Cardiff was placed in a group of ports (which included the other major south Wales ports) of which it was said:

> the arrangements were not only highly satisfactory in themselves but they were carried out with a devotion to duty on the part of many of the Medical Officers of Health, such as must be regarded as having largely contributed to the marked success with which imported cholera was controlled at nearly all English [sic] ports during 1892 and 1893.

The procedures enforced embodied the best practice known in Britain and generally the quality of administration was rated as 'good'.[50]

The last two ways of auditing the MoH come from separate incidents in the Edwardian period. Both were, at first sight, episodes which questioned the professional competence of port health. However, closer inspection of the incidents in their full context qualifies the criticisms made. In 1908, Edward Nicholl exposed the appalling nature of conditions in seamen's boarding houses in Cardiff, places which had consistently been given a clean bill of health by the Medical Officer of Health for decades.[51] Then in the strike of 1911 one of the major issues which the seamen's union stressed was the poor state of the forecastles in which the seamen lived. Again these had been regularly inspected and generally acquitted by the MoH. Do these examples make his perspective a tendentious one? Of course, both of the Edwardian investigations had political purposes: Nicholl was campaigning for his Council seat and offering vigorous opposition to the dominant Liberal-Nonconformist view of Cardiff's docklands, that the problems were rooted in the drink trade and vice. Reform would come from controlling these forces. Nicholl by contrast offered a public health approach and stressed the racial composition of the boarding houses. It was a polarization which would have a deep and enduring impact on politics and race relations in the city.[52] Similarly the National Sailors' and Firemen's union was trying to win recognition from the owners and its campaign was part of a protracted struggle and perhaps any hand was welcome at the pumps.

With both these campaigns, perhaps the underlying issue was that of expectation. Sailors – and dockers – worked in casual trades and these were associated with expectations of low standards of living and conditions. The MoH's inspection process most probably endorsed such low standards, while eradicating the worst conditions. This meant there was plenty for a disaffected Tory or for a trade union to agitate about without inventing anything – but also that medical inspection was enforcing what were seen as acceptable standards for a group of workers for whom little was expected. Dockland areas had acquired unsavoury reputations and sailors were widely seen as unruly and unreflective. By-laws were enforced within a context of such apprehensions. Ports were, after all, distinctive places and they had cognate images.[53] The standards of accommodation required by law were lower both at sea and ashore for sailors as compared with the shore-based working class.[54] Undoubtedly the medical officers swayed towards the shipowners rather than the workers but they had some degree of independence. They contributed many important analyses which greatly aid our understanding of the nature of urban society in the nineteenth and twentieth centuries. In the mid 1850s H. J. Paine produced the first sophisticated analysis of social areas in Cardiff; in the early 1930s one of his successors produced a detailed anatomy of

'SEA WALL AGAINST DISEASE' 93

the continuing growth of the city. They shared many of the prejudices of their times. Paine was notably hostile to the Irish – yet he also managed to explain their lower infant mortality rate in the 1880s effectively, even though his predilection was to consider them as irredeemably dirty and uncouth. Similarly in the 1930s there was a rush to explain away the city's high incidence of tuberculosis in racial terms. But to his credit the MoH gave no support to the lurid stories about venereal disease which emanated from a retired sea captain in 1935. Overall one can have a high regard for their professional integrity and intelligence. Yet we always need to be on guard against their self-presentation of their successes and to scour the crevices of the archives for those fleeting pieces of evidence which show them in different and less flattering lights. This will hardly change our general favourable image. But it will produce real people with limitations rather than impossibly proficient professionals.

Appendix 1:
Infectious Diseases Notified to Port Sanitary Authority at Cardiff, 1888–1909

Year	Notified	Died	Year	Notified	Died
1888	31	–	1899	11	3
1889	33	3	1900	16	6
1890	28	1	1901	9	2
1891	25	2	1902	3	0
1892	15	6	1903	18	1
1893	17	5	1904	9	0
1894	13	1	1905	5	2
1895	17	0	1906	25	3
1896	9	1	1907	10	0
1897	16	1	1908	18	–
1898	6	3	1909	22	–

Source: Cardiff MoH reports, 1888–1909.

Appendix 2:
Vessels Inspected by Port Sanitary Authority at Cardiff, 1890–1950

Year	Inspected	Defective	Year	Inspected	Defective
1890	1740	409	1921	5147	453
1891	1864	340	1922	6712	591
1892	4,608	813	1923	7405	566
1893	5494	780	1924	7265	609
1894	6424	1249	1925	6574	875
1895	5825	928	1926	4451	600
1896	6222	951	1927	6569	847
1897	6257	866	1928	5984	723
1898	5627	1101	1929	6249	486
1899	7170	1597	1930	5889	735
1900	6711	1026	1931	5045	357
1901	8227	1421	1932	4699	332
1902	8179	1404	1933	4506	419
1903	8072	1228	1934	4414	514
1904	8171	1408	1935	4115	505
1905	8116	1269	1936	3884	418
1906	8332	1167	1937	4068	512
1907	8129	1304	1938	3826	816
1908	8241	986	1939	–	–
1909	8477	933	1940	1288	553
1910	8377	809	1941	1009	433
1911	7720	950	1942	1030	405
1912	8188	1501	1943	661	246
1913	8671	964	1944	694	195
1914	8325	1402	1945	2342	128
1915	8203	1118	1946	2329	284
1916	8067	1040	1947	2263	352
1917	6590	635	1948	2559	328
1918*	6764	643	1949	2200	283
1919*	7583	1163	1950	2711	335
1920	7870	880			

Source: Cardiff MoH reports, 1890–1950.

Appendix 3:
Patients Treated at Hamadryad VD Clinic, Cardiff, 1917–1933

Year	First Time	Total	Patient in Days
1917 (from 16/4)	572	7191	2692
1918	790	4361	5297
1919	972	17040	6281
1920	1234	12872	4679
1921	868	12242	3352
1922	786	12856	3775
1923	821	13704	3722
1924	615	16212	2697
1925	616	16008	3104
1926	565	12702	2536
1927	640	13995	2426
1928	646	15347	3195
1929	704	15027	2093
1930	731	12670	1639
1931	487	9853	1372
1932	606	10004	1707
1933	519	9918	2220

Source: Cardiff MoH reports, 1917–1933.

Notes

[1] J. Greenwood Wilson, 'Sea wall against disease', *Doctor* (February 1944). Wilson was the Medical Officer of Health (MoH) of Cardiff.

[2] Registrar General's Report for the December Quarter, 1865, cited in the Cardiff MoH Report, 1866, 25–6.

[3] Linda Grant, *The Cast Iron Shore* (London, 1996, paperback edn. 1997) p. 3.

[4] Frank Boeze, ' Militancy and pragmatism: an international perspective on maritime labour, 1870–1914', *International Review of Social History*, Vol. 36 (1991), 165–200; Josef W. Konwitz, 'Port cities and urban history', *Journal of Urban History*, Vol. 19 (1993), 115–20; Robert Lee, 'The socio-economic and demographic characteristics of port cities: a typology for comparative analysis', *Urban History*, Vol. 25 (1998), 147–172; Sarah Palmer, 'Ports', in Martin Daunton (ed.), *The Cambridge Urban History of Britain Vol. III, 1840–1950* (Cambridge, 2000), pp. 133–50.

[5] Krista Maglen, '"The first line of defence": British quarantine and the port sanitary authorities in the nineteenth century', *Social History of Medicine*, Vol. 15 (2002), 413–28.

[6] Anne Hardy, 'Cholera, quarantine and the English preventive system, 1850–1895', *Medical History*, Vol. 37 (1993).

[7] Karl Polanyi, *The Origins of Our Time: The Great Transformation* (London 1945) is the classic discussion of the international system and the parallels with

the present are brought out in Beverley J. Silver and Giovanni Arrighi, 'Polanyi's "double movement": the belle epoque of British and American hegemony compared', *Politics and Society*, Vol. 31 (2003), 325–55.
[8] John R. Guy, 'Wales, the Baltic Trade and cholera in the late nineteenth century', in John H. Cule and John Lancaster (eds), *Russia and Wales: Essays on the History of State Involvement in Health Care* (History of Medicine Society of Wales, 1994), pp. 87–100; Myron Echenberg, 'Pestis Redux: the initial years of the third bubonic plague pandemic, 1894–1901', *Journal of World History*, Vol. 13 (2002), 429–49.
[9] Maglen, '"The first line of defence"'.
[10] Edward Walford, *Notes on the Effect of the Improved Sanitation on the Public Health of Seaport Towns*, (np; nd [Cardiff? 1890?]), p. 3.
[11] Maglen, '"The first line of defence"'.
[12] M. J. Daunton, *Coal Metropolis: Cardiff, 1870–1914* (Leicester, 1977), chapters 1 and 2.
[13] Cardiff MoH Reports, 1853, 1854, 1857.
[14] Ibid., 1862, p. 16.
[15] Ibid., 1866, p. 25.
[16] C. E. Gordon Smith and Mary E. Gibson, 'Yellow fever in south Wales, 1865', *Medical History*, Vol. 30 (1986), 322–40; P. D. Meers, 'Yellow fever in Swansea, 1865', *Journal of Hygiene*, Vol. 97 (1986), 185–91.
[17] Cardiff MoH Report, 1866, p. 25.
[18] A stretch of the Bristol Channel which formed the route into Cardiff and where ships waited in order to get into the port.
[19] Cardiff MoH Report, 1873, pp. 4–6.
[20] Ibid., pp. 24–5.
[21] Ibid., 1878, pp. 33–4.
[22] Ibid., 1879, p. 33
[23] Ibid., 1883, p. 58; 1884, p. 63.
[24] Cardiff Port Sanitary Authority Annual Report, 1886, p. 8.
[25] Dr Walford, 'Sanitation in Cardiff', in John Ballinger (ed.), *Cardiff: An Illustrated Handbook* (Cardiff, 1896), pp. 93–4.
[26] Walford, *Notes on the Effect of the Improved Sanitation*, pp. 3–4.
[27] Walford, 'Sanitation in Cardiff', p. 94.
[28] Cardiff Port Sanitary Authority Annual Reports, 1889; 1890.
[29] Ibid., 1914, p. 45.
[30] *South Wales Daily News*, 16 May 1911.
[31] Neil Evans, '"A tidal wave of impatience": the Cardiff General Strike of 1911', in Geraint H. Jenkins and J. Beverley Smith (eds), *Politics and Society in Wales, 1840–1922: Essays in Honour of Ieuan Gwynedd Jones* (Cardiff, 1988), pp. 135–59; pp. 142–3.
[32] Cardiff MoH Annual Reports, 1936; 1937.
[33] Cardiff Port Sanitary Authority Annual Reports, 1897, 1898, 1911, p. 51; Evans, '"A tidal wave of impatience"'.
[34] Echenberg, 'Pestis Redux'; Edward Marriott, *The Plague Race: A Tale of Fear, Science and Heroism* (London, 2002).

35 M. W. Flinn, 'British steel and Spanish ore, 1871–1914', *Economic History Review*, 2nd Series, Vol. 8 (1955), 84–90.
36 Echenberg, 'Pestis Redux'; Marriott, *Plague Race*.
37 Neil Evans, 'Regulating the Reserve Army: Arabs, Blacks and the local state in Cardiff, 1919–1945', in Kenneth Lunn (ed.), *Race and Labour in Twentieth-Century Britain* (London, 1985), pp. 92–6.
38 Michael Worboys, 'Tuberculosis and race in Britain and its Empire, 1900–1950', in Waltraud Ernst and Bernard Harris (eds), *Race, Science and Medicine, 1700–1960* (London, 1999), pp. 144–66; Greta Jones, *Social Hygiene in Twentieth-Century Britain* (London, 1986); John Welshman, *Municipal Medicine* (Oxford, 2000).
39 Cardiff MoH Annual Report, 1934.
40 David Byrne, *Complexity Theory and the Social Sciences: An Introduction* (London, 1998), pp. 38–9; 110–11 (179). Byrne's discussion is based on a report on tuberculosis on Tyneside in the 1930s – F. C. S. Bradshaw, *Causal Factors in Tuberculosis* (London, 1933).
41 J. Greenwood Wilson, 'Slum clearance at sea', *The Lancet*, 12 September 1936, pp. 646–9. I am grateful to Pam Michael for this reference.
42 For some of the context see Howard Phillips and David Killingray (eds), *The Spanish Influenza Pandemic of 1918–19: New Perspectives* (London and New York, 2003); also, Alfred W. Crosby, *America's Forgotten Pandemic: The Influenza of 1918* (Cambridge, 1989).
43 Cardiff Port Sanitary Authority Annual Reports, 1918, p. 8; 1919, p. 11.
44 Ibid., 1919, p. 28; 1926.
45 Ibid., 1920, pp. 12–13.
46 Ibid., 1922.
47 Ibid., 1924.
48 Daunton, *Coal Metropolis*, chapter 3.
49 See Richard Evans, *Death in Hamburg*, (Oxford, 1988).
50 *Port and Riperian Sanitary Survey*, PP 1895 (VII, C (2nd series) 52), pp. 504–10.
51 This issue will be discussed fully in terms of its impact on racial issues in Neil Evans, *Darker Cardiff: The Underside of the City, 1840–1960*, in progress.
52 Ibid.
53 Boeze, 'Militancy and pragmatism'; Ross Cameron, '"The most colourful extravaganza in the world": Images of Tiger Bay, 1845–1970', *Patterns of Prejudice*, Vol. 31 (1997), 59–90; Valerie Burton, 'Boundaries and identities in the nineteenth-century English port: Sailortown narratives and urban space', in Simon Gunn and Robert J. Morris (eds), *Identities in Space: Contested Terrains in the Western City since 1850* (London, 2001), pp. 137–51; eadem, '"As I wuz a-rolling down the highway one morn": Fictions of the nineteenth-century English Sailortown', in Bernhard Klien (ed.), *Fictions of the Sea: Critical Perspectives on the Ocean in British Literature and Culture* (London, 2002), pp. 141–56.
54 Greenwood Wilson, 'Slum clearance at sea', pp. 645–6.

3

Unemployment, Poverty and Women's Health in Inter-war South Wales

STEVEN THOMPSON

Health and mortality were extremely controversial issues during the inter-war period and became politicized to a greater degree than ever before. Evidence relating to the health of the population was utilized by critics of the government in their denunciations of official economic, unemployment and welfare policies, and even used to question the very nature of capitalist development in Britain. Similarly, inter-war governments employed a great deal of data relating to health and mortality in their defence of official economic and welfare policies. These issues have continued to provide a focus for disagreement ever since, most noticeably in the so-called 'optimistic' and 'pessimistic' interpretations formulated during the 1970s and, more especially, the 1980s.[1] Disagreements centre on the precise effects of unemployment on the standards of health of the population and whether or not the period should be characterized as a time of marked improvement or significant deterioration in standards of health and levels of mortality.[2] The health and welfare of 'vulnerable' groups of the population, notably women and children, occupy an important place in these contemporary and historiographical disagreements. It is believed that the supposed vulnerability of such groups left them more susceptible to subtle social and economic changes and, as such, that their standards of health can serve as a sensitive indicator of the effects of economic depression and unemployment on human health. This study is partly conceived in these terms and considers the effects of economic depression on the health and mortality experiences of women in inter-war south Wales.

The Welsh historiography relating to women's health in the inter-war period is much less controversial than the work written in a British context, and the conclusions are more 'pessimistic' in character. Comments that various forms of mortality were higher in south Wales than in the rest of Britain are common, while it is often asserted that certain mortality indicators, most notably maternal and tuberculosis mortality, increased during the inter-war period. Such inequalities and changes in levels of mortality are explicitly or implicitly attributed to the economic depression. In the same way, comments are made that working-class women suffered anaemia, headaches, constipation, rheumatism, gynaecological problems and a host of other ailments and illnesses, and again, such epidemiological phenomena are associated with unemployment and poverty, and often in a relatively simplistic cause-and-effect manner.[3]

However, nowhere in the Welsh historiography is it satisfactorily established that mortality increased as a direct result of economic depression, unemployment and poverty. Too often, the specific effects of the inter-war depression are confused with the more general consequences of women's lives in industrial communities, while assertions about the precise influence of unemployment on standards of health are vague in character. In addition, the extent to which the health problems of the inter-war period also characterized other periods of Welsh history is insufficiently considered. In the British historiography, levels of unemployment and mortality rates are wrenched from particular social and economic contexts and insufficient attention is given to the specificities of local circumstances. Biological phenomena and social determinants are considered on a general level but, on the whole, demographic studies are not integrated into an understanding of the wider epidemiological and ecological framework. As Winter recognizes, it is misleading to treat unemployment as an independent variable and mortality as a dependent variable. 'To make sense of the immediate consequences of unemployment,' Winter argues, 'it must be seen as part of a network of economic relations, support systems and social attitudes that are deeply embedded in the class structure.'[4]

Therefore, it is necessary to place our understanding of health in inter-war south Wales on a surer empirical footing and to distinguish more closely between the specific effects of economic depression and the structural factors that were characteristic of industrial communities. We need to follow Landers's example and conceptualize the relationship between mortality and its social determinants as a 'vital regime', which he defines 'not as a loosely related collection of vital rates, but as an unbounded network of relationships between the demography of human populations and the structures of their social, economic and political life, as well as their biology and ecology'.[5] This study of women's health, and the wider project of which it is a part,[6] goes some way to meeting Anne Crowther's call for detailed local studies which relate mortality data in the inter-war period to specific local circumstances.[7]

Women's lives in inter-war south Wales

A fundamental factor in the health and mortality of women in south Wales was the nature of their everyday lives in industrial communities.[8] South Wales was one of the most important regions of British industrial development during the modern period. By the late nineteenth and early twentieth centuries the metallurgical districts along the rims of the coalfield, initially developed in the first half of the nineteenth century, were superseded in importance by the massive expansion of the coal industry in the central valleys of south Wales. During the late Victorian and Edwardian periods people poured into the valleys of south Wales so that the region was inhabited by over a million and a half individuals by 1911. This relatively late industrial development meant that, since the majority of houses were built according to the more stringent building by-laws of the late nineteenth century, housing conditions were better than in other industrial or urban areas of Britain that experienced industrialization and urbanization in the early nineteenth century. Nevertheless, the very large number of terraced houses built in close proximity in the narrow valleys, and the generally unwholesome character of such a heavily industrialized region, meant that south Wales was a relatively unhealthy environment for its inhabitants.

More relevant to women, the working environment formed by the home was often dirty and damp, while domestic work was labour-intensive and onerous. Cleaning, washing clothes, preparing food and raising children were time-consuming and tiring tasks. In a sense, women worked longer 'shifts' than their husbands, invariably working anything up to seventeen or eighteen hours a day, and were often required to draw baths and prepare meals at various times of the day as male members of the household finished their different shifts at the local colliery. The preparation of these baths took its toll on women's health as the daily toil of lifting and carrying large pans of water caused women to strain themselves. Miscarriages and stillbirths were common consequences of such activities.[9]

Women in mining districts, and in particular south Wales, married early and raised large families. Fertility rates were high and many working-class women faced a large number of pregnancies in quick succession during their adult lives. The large number of pregnancies placed an onerous burden on women's bodies and predisposed women to a series of ailments and illnesses, and occasionally permanent injuries and disabilities. Dot Jones has commented that 'The unremitting toil of childbirth and domestic labour killed and debilitated Rhondda women as much as accident and conditions in the mining industry killed and maimed Rhondda men.'[10]

This, broadly, was the nature of women's lives in the industrial districts of south Wales at the start of the inter-war period. The economic depression of the 1920s and 1930s served further to intensify the pressures that acted upon women. They were forced to manage their household budgets on smaller incomes and the strain of doing so often resulted in mental health problems. Perhaps the most important way in which unemployment and poverty affected women's health, however, was through the deterioration that occurred in dietary standards. Unemployment often served to lessen the food resources available to a family and it is clear that the dietary standards of 'unemployed families' were inferior to those of 'employed families'.[11] However, while differences *between* families were highly significant, the divisions *within* families also conditioned experiences and determined living standards. While it is useful to utilize 'households' or 'families' as the unit of analysis, it also needs to be remembered that resources were not allocated equally among the members of those units but were competed for by individuals within them.[12]

Most importantly, gender relations influenced the allocation of food resources within families. There was a cultural ideal that the earning capacity of the family needed to be maintained and that this was best achieved by maximizing the food consumption of the (usually male) breadwinner(s).[13] This assumed a greater relevance during the inter-war period as the threat of unemployment, or short spells of joblessness, led women to place the earning capacity of their husbands or the nutrition of their children before their own dietary needs to an even greater extent than previously.[14] Many contemporary investigators noted that it was the women of unemployed families who were bearing the brunt of the deterioration in dietary standards that unemployment occasioned.[15] Maggie Pryce Jones of Trelewis, remembering the allocation of food resources in her family and her mother's place in this hierarchy, stated how it was: 'The best for Dad, the next best for the children; for her, I suspect now, nothing.'[16]

Children below a certain age were protected from the worst effects of poverty by the sacrifices of their parents and, most especially, their mothers, but when girls reached a certain age they too experienced shortages in their food intake. This was borne out by the findings of the Rhondda school medical officer and his staff during the mid to late 1930s when medical inspection was extended to children attending secondary and continuation schools in the district. They found that the girls attending these schools were 'physically inferior' to the boys and asserted that this was because of the lack of opportunities for girls to enjoy open-air exercise, to the employment of girls in domestic duties and, most importantly, to diets deficient in 'the constituents which serve to maintain physical fitness, such as milk and other dairy products, eggs, and green vegetables'. Girls paid the price for these dietary disadvantages and experienced more 'defects' such as anaemia, blepharitis, defective vision and postural 'deformities' such as curvature of the spine and flat feet.[17]

These various factors helped determine the levels of mortality experienced by girls and women. It might be argued that mortality is a rather blunt tool with which to measure the impact of unemployment and poverty on standards of health and that the true costs of the depression are more likely to be revealed by data relating to morbidity.[18] And yet historians have recognized mortality rates as sensitive indicators of the social and economic well-being of a population.[19] They have been used in the 'standard of living' debate,[20] in disagreements over the impact of the First World War on civilian health[21] and, of course, in the controversy over the 'healthy or hungry thirties'. Mortality rates are also more easily obtainable and suffer fewer methodological problems than data relating to morbidity. Therefore, this study utilizes mortality rates in an attempt to ascertain female standards of health during the Depression. General death rates are disaggregated so as to determine subtle patterns and changes in mortality. As Webster points out in relation to infant mortality, official, optimistic interpretations were based upon aggregate death rates, but a different perspective is offered by a finer analysis of the mortality data.[22]

Patterns of female mortality

The demographic experiences of men and women differed in important respects during the inter-war period. Certainly, men and women experienced many of the same determinants of health in similar ways but, equally important, men and women also experienced various social and economic factors differently which, in turn, produced differing demographic experiences. Men and women had different working environments, inhabited different public environments, varied in the success with which they satisfied the demands they made on the food resources of the household, made differing demands on the health services utilized by a family, and, of course, differed biologically. Occupational factors, for example, played some part in male standards of health, while housing conditions exerted a greater influence on women's health.

The first thing to note about female mortality in inter-war south Wales is that it was exceeded by male mortality. In most societies in the modern, developed world male mortality exceeds female mortality and in all age groups. Various social and biological factors determine this phenomenon.[23] Throughout the inter-war period, crude male mortality rates for England and Wales varied between 112 per cent and 116 per cent of the corresponding female rates but the experience in south Wales differed to some extent from this pattern.[24] In the administrative county of Glamorgan the crude male death rate remained in excess of the female rate until the early 1930s to the same extent as the England and Wales rates but from the mid to late 1930s the male rate diverged even more markedly from the female rate, so that in the period 1935–9 the male rate was 122.5 per cent of the female rate. The male excess in Monmouthshire and Merthyr was generally less than the England and Wales excess, while in Cardiff and Swansea the male excess was relatively high. The male rate in Cardiff varied from about 115 per cent to 135 per cent of the female rate.

If the focus is altered so as to examine smaller administrative units within south Wales then it becomes clear that the districts where the male excess mortality was at its lowest were typically the most industrialized districts of the coalfield that experienced the highest levels of unemployment in the inter-war period. But was this due to higher female mortality in these districts and lower male death rates or was it due to differences in the sex-specific age-structure? Standardized sex-specific mortality rates reveal that male mortality in industrial districts of south Wales was in excess of male mortality in England and Wales as a whole but that female mortality was in excess of the corresponding England and Wales rates to a greater degree. Table 3.1 illustrates this point. Therefore, despite the fact that overall male mortality was greater than female mortality, it was the girls and women of the industrial districts of south Wales who suffered the penalty for living in these areas to a greater degree than the boys and men. This contrasts with male and female mortality in the more prosperous towns of Cardiff, Swansea and Newport, all of which exceeded the corresponding male and female England and Wales averages to the same degree.

Table 3.1: Standardized sex-specific death rates in selected areas of south Wales, 1920–39[25]

		Standardized sex-specific death rates (England and Wales male rate = 100 and England and Wales female rate = 100)			
		1920–4	1925–9	1930–4	1935–9
Aberdare UD	Male	103.3	112.0	116.3	132.9
	Female	121.1	121.5	132.4	140.1
Bedwellty UD	Male	112.7	108.4	123.9	125.9
	Female	118.8	110.0	137.9	135.8
Blaenavon UD	Male	116.2	104.7	113.9	133.2
	Female	132.5	119.0	135.9	144.2
Gelligaer UD	Male	99.3	111.0	119.1	130.3
	Female	119.1	122.3	127.6	140.3
Merthyr Tydfil CB	Male	114.9	116.5	120.4	130.3
	Female	122.4	127.0	141.7	144.4
Mountain Ash UD	Male	109.9	111.4	119.5	129.4
	Female	113.8	121.1	126.3	138.6
Rhondda UD	Male	110.9	114.4	118.4	131.3
	Female	119.8	125.8	134.1	140.5

Clearly, there was something about the coal-mining communities that had a more deleterious effect on female mortality than male mortality. Excess female mortality in south Wales was marked in certain age groups. Unfortunately, age-specific death rates cannot be calculated for the smaller administrative units in south Wales but those for the larger units are sufficient for the purposes of this study.[26] Significantly, female mortality in the 15–24 age group increased in the administrative counties of Glamorgan and Monmouthshire and in Merthyr Tydfil in the period 1921–5 to 1931–5. In the case of Merthyr, the increase was substantial and the death rate increased from 4.14 deaths per 1,000 females in 1921–5 to 5.26 in 1931–5. Furthermore, the England and Wales rates in this age group demonstrate the tendency for male mortality to exceed female mortality. A male rate of 3.14 deaths per 1,000 males in 1921–5 corresponded with a female rate of 2.84, while in the period 1931–5 the male rate stood at 2.70 and the female rate at 2.38. In south Wales, male mortality exceeded female mortality by much less and was even exceeded by female mortality in some districts. In the two administrative counties, in Newport in the period 1921–5 and in Merthyr in the period 1931–5, female mortality exceeded male mortality, whereas the more prosperous boroughs of Cardiff and Swansea experienced excess male mortality, a pattern more closely approximating that of England and Wales as a whole.

Moreover, the two administrative counties and Merthyr County Borough experienced female mortality equal to, or exceeding, male mortality in the 25–44 age group whereas Cardiff, Newport and Swansea more closely resembled the England and Wales pattern of excess male mortality. In the 45–65 age group, excess male mortality was often quite significant in the more prosperous areas but was limited in the more depressed areas. The area with the smallest differential in male and female mortality in this age-group was Merthyr. Here, male mortality approximated to male mortality in other areas, while female mortality was much higher than elsewhere and almost approximated the level of male mortality.

If these age- and sex-specific death rates for south Wales are expressed as a percentage of the equivalent rates for England and Wales then it is evident that not only did south Wales experience higher levels of mortality than the England and Wales average but that in many cases the excess mortality in south Wales was considerable. The level of excess mortality was greatest in the 15–24 age group and for females in particular. The excess mortality of women in south

Wales over women in England and Wales as a whole in this age group rose during the inter-war years and, in the case of Merthyr, was a staggering 221 per cent of the England and Wales rate in 1931–5, having experienced female mortality at 145.8 per cent of the England and Wales rate for the same age group in the period 1921–5. Therefore, the point made above regarding higher than expected female mortality in the industrial areas of south Wales can be further refined to demonstrate that the high female mortality was the result of significantly higher mortality in the 15–24 and 25–44 age groups. High adult female mortality was a noted mortality pattern of other depressed areas during the inter-war period. An article published in the *New Statesman and Nation* in 1935 commented that female mortality in the 'depressed areas' exceeded female mortality in the 'rest of the country' to a greater extent than male mortality in the 'depressed areas' exceeded male mortality in the 'rest of the country'.

Table 3.2: Excess male and female mortality in 'depressed areas' over 'rest of the country', 1934[27]

Age group	Percentage excess of deaths in 'depressed areas' over 'rest of the country', 1934	
	Male	Female
0–14	30	30
15–44	16	24
45–64	16	21
65 and over	16	21
Total	18	23

The article maintained that this pattern of mortality was a result of the economic depression. However, it is not enough to show that death rates in the depressed areas were higher than elsewhere, rather that they were higher in the depressed areas in the inter-war period than they had been before the First World War.[28] As far as south Wales is concerned, Dot Jones has shown how female mortality at ages between about 15 and 45 years was relatively high in the Rhondda for many decades before the First World War, during a time of relative prosperity, and maintains that this was a consequence of the everyday nature of women's lives in industrial communities.[29] This evidence seems to suggest that the high female mortality in these age groups during the inter-war period was not solely a consequence of economic depression but a characteristic feature of the mortality landscapes of these industrial communities during the late nineteenth and early twentieth centuries. The cause of excess female mortality in the young adult age groups in south Wales can primarily be attributed to high tuberculosis mortality. Figure 3.1 illustrates the rates for the county borough of Merthyr Tydfil and Rhondda Urban District, two very depressed communities, and compares them with England and Wales as a whole.

Figure 3.1: Sex- and age-specific mortality from pulmonary tuberculosis, Merthyr County Borough, Rhondda Urban District and England and Wales, 1931–3.[30]

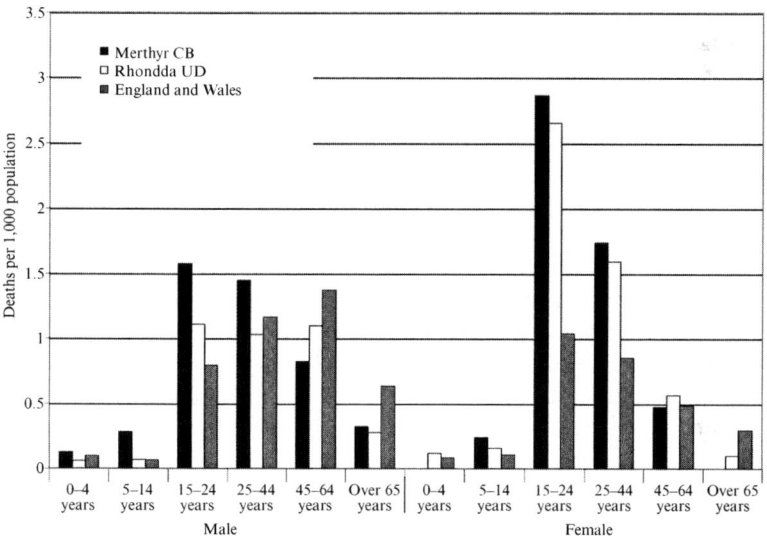

The usual tendency was for female tuberculosis mortality to exceed male mortality during childhood and early adulthood but for male mortality to exceed female mortality after about the age of 30.[31] In Merthyr and the Rhondda, on the other hand, female mortality consistently exceeded male mortality in the age groups between 15 and 44 years of age. In the 15–24 age-group, female mortality from pulmonary mortality in Merthyr in 1931–2 was 275 per cent of the England and Wales rate and only slightly less in the Rhondda. Furthermore, the Registrar-General's Decennial Supplement for the period 1930–2 found that while miners continued to experience low levels of pulmonary tuberculosis relative to other workers, their wives experienced relatively high levels of mortality from this cause in comparison with the wives of other workers.[32] The causes of excess female tuberculosis mortality in Merthyr and the Rhondda in the 15–44 age group were many and varied. Firstly, the strain of constant childbearing imposed intolerable strains on women's bodies that made them more susceptible to the effects of the disease, and this was of significance in the mining districts characterized by high fertility rates and low ages at which women married.[33] However, teenage girls experienced higher levels of tuberculosis mortality than their male counterparts and this was not due to the effects of pregnancy. Rather, the onset of puberty contributed to the peak in female mortality at this age since metabolic changes in the bodies of teenage girls increased the need for protein and when protein is unavailable, resistance to infection decreases.[34] The effects of menstruation would also have depleted the nutritional status of teenage girls and it is significant that high levels of anaemia, another possible consequence of menstruation, were found among girls attending secondary and continuation schools in the Rhondda in the 1930s.[35]

These biological factors were exacerbated by a cultural practice that favoured the nutrition of boys and young men of this age over girls and young women. The earning power of boys of this age needed to be safeguarded and boys who contributed to the household income were able more successfully to satisfy their demands on the food resources of the household.[36] It is also possible that girls and young women from the valley communities contracted tuberculosis while in service and returned home to die, thereby inflating the death rate. Lastly, girls and women were more likely to nurse sick members of the family and this increased the likelihood of contracting tuberculosis.

The precise consequences of the economic depression are harder to discern but it is significant that mortality from pulmonary tuberculosis for females aged 15–24 and 25–44 was greater in Merthyr in 1931–3 than in 1921–3.[37] While death rates from this cause were increasing for adult males in Merthyr, the increases for females were even greater. Female mortality in the 15–24 age group increased from 1.94 deaths per 1,000 females in 1921–3 to 2.86 in 1931–3, while the death rate for the 25–44 age group increased from 1.6 to 1.74 deaths per 1,000 females. These increases were confirmed by an official analysis of the mortality statistics that was specifically intended to refute suggestions that unemployment had caused an increase in ill health and mortality. Despite its overwhelmingly optimistic conclusions, E. Lewis-Faning's report was forced to concede that female mortality in the 15–24 age group had increased in Merthyr Tydfil in the period 1920–2 to 1930–2, and that this was because of increases in heart disease and tuberculosis mortality.[38]

Therefore, despite the influence of structural factors that contributed to the high female mortality levels in south Wales, the economic conditions of the inter-war depression caused increases in age-specific female mortality and, in particular, tuberculosis mortality in Merthyr Tydfil, one of the most depressed towns in depressed south Wales. A confidential investigation carried out by senior Ministry of Health officials in 1934 described the increasing mortality among young adults in south Wales as 'striking' and, while failing adequately to explain this increase, concluded that unemployment could not be ruled out as a factor.[39] Public statements, however, were confined to observations that unemployment could not be causing premature death because tuberculosis mortality in England and Wales as a whole was declining, or that overall death rates in certain districts of south Wales were decreasing.[40] Certain medical officers in south Wales opposed this interpretation and posited a causal link between unemployment and poverty on the one hand and tuberculosis mortality on the other.[41]

Maternal mortality

Even more controversial than tuberculosis mortality during the inter-war period was the issue of various types of 'reproductive mortality', including maternal mortality, stillbirth mortality and various forms of infant mortality. These demographic indicators can be used to ascertain the health status of women. Of these forms of mortality, it was the issue of maternal mortality that received most attention during the inter-war period and has figured most prominently in the historiographical debates over unemployment and standards of health. In the first place, it is important to note that various investigations into maternal mortality carried out before the First World War found that mortality rates were significantly higher in Wales than in other parts of Britain.[42] This was as true of the rural areas of Wales as it was of the industrial valleys of south Wales. Therefore, the fact that maternal mortality was high in inter-war south Wales relative to other parts of Britain is insufficient as evidence of the demographic impact of the Depression.

However, the more 'pessimistic' interpretations of health in interwar Britain argue that maternal mortality increased in the depressed areas and suggest that this was a direct result of economic depression and unemployment.[43] These assertions are based upon the findings of the Ministry of Health's investigation into maternal mortality in Wales published in 1937. It found that puerperal mortality in the Special Areas of south Wales increased from 5.16 deaths per 1,000 live births in the period 1924–8 to 6.50 deaths in 1929–33.[44] The report concluded that while puerperal mortality rates had decreased or remained stationary in the rest of Wales during the inter-war period, mortality rates in the Special Areas had increased 'considerably'.

The significance of these findings is contentious. Many of the more 'pessimistic' interpretations have utilized this material to suggest the dire consequences of the Depression. Alternatively, while not disputing the accuracy of the 1937 report, Winter has argued that south Wales was exceptional and that maternal mortality decreased in other parts of Britain during the period.[45] More importantly, Irvine Loudon has focused on the determinants of maternal mortality and has questioned the importance of socio-economic factors. Loudon attributes the high and increasing puerperal mortality rates in the depressed areas of south Wales as, in the words of the Ministry of Health report, 'the cumulative result of a variety of unfavourable factors working in association', rather than the effects of malnutrition alone.[46] In a more general consideration of the determinants of maternal mortality during the inter-war period, Loudon emphasizes the quality of obstetrical care, the virulence of streptococcal infection and increased levels of abortion.[47] Moreover, Loudon supports his contention that clinical factors were of greater importance than maternal nutritional status as a determinant of maternal mortality by arguing that had nutritional status been the crucial factor, then the decrease in maternal mortality that occurred after 1935 would have been more marked in relation to accidents of childbirth and not in relation to puerperal sepsis. That the decrease in maternal mortality was primarily due to a decrease in puerperal sepsis, Loudon contends, demonstrates that it was the quality of obstetrical care and, in particular, the introduction of sulphonamides from 1937 onwards that was the crucial factor.[48]

However, while Loudon focuses upon areas of high maternal mortality he does not satisfactorily explain the increase in puerperal mortality in the Special Areas of Wales. His assertion that the migration of the healthiest young women from the region served to increase mortality rates is tenuous and, at best, only a partial explanation.[49] While mortality from puerperal sepsis in Wales exceeded the rates for England and Wales, excess mortality from 'other puerperal causes', which Loudon associates with social and economic factors, was much greater. Moreover, whereas mortality from puerperal sepsis increased slightly for England and Wales as a whole in the period 1924 to 1935, mortality from 'other' puerperal causes decreased slightly. This suggests that the generally improving economic situation in England and Wales as a whole was reflected in a slight decrease in mortality from 'other' puerperal causes but that changes in the quality of obstetrical care led to a small increase in puerperal sepsis. In contrast, the Special Areas of south Wales experienced an increase in all forms of puerperal mortality suggesting that social and economic determinants played a greater role than in the rest of England and Wales.

In support of Loudon's contentions, it is important to note that, of the increases in the different forms of maternal mortality in south Wales, the greatest increase was in relation to maternal deaths from puerperal sepsis.[50] Nevertheless, while Wales experienced a fall in puerperal sepsis mortality from 1937 onwards as a result of the introduction of sulphonamides, mortality from other puerperal causes remained high.[51] Therefore, while the Special Areas of Wales, in common with the rest of England and Wales, experienced an increase in mortality from puerperal sepsis, which Loudon associates with clinical factors, they also experienced an increase in those forms of maternal mortality that Loudon associates with social and economic determinants. Loudon's emphasis on obstetrical factors can explain the fall in maternal mortality in England and Wales as a whole after 1935 but fails to account for the increase in 'other' puerperal causes of maternal death in the Special Areas before this date.

Infant mortality and stillbirths

While the use of maternal mortality as an indicator of maternal health is contentious and problematic, certain forms of infant mortality more clearly reflect standards of maternal health and female nutritional status. In particular, neonatal infant mortality (that is, mortality in the first thirty days of life) has been used by historical demographers to reveal prenatal causes of infant mortality or mortality due to the birth process. These 'endogenous' causes of infant mortality included developmental problems experienced in the womb, injury at birth, prematurity and other congenital causes of death, and were primarily determined by maternal nutritional and health status. Poor or deteriorating maternal nutritional status increases neonatal mortality through increased likelihood of developmental problems in the womb, greater prematurity, an increased likelihood of difficult labour and lower birth weights.[52]

It is evident that neonatal mortality was consistently higher in south Wales than the England and Wales average but also that, in common with the rest of England and Wales, during the inter-war years neonatal mortality rates in south Wales were more resistant to improvement than death rates for infants over the age of one month. Quinquennial neonatal mortality averages show that the decrease in England and Wales was only very small during the inter-war period from 33.6 deaths per 1,000 live births in 1921–4 to 29.4 in 1935–9.[53] The neonatal mortality rates for the two administrative counties and the county boroughs of Cardiff and Swansea similarly fell during the same period but the decreases were even smaller. However, the county boroughs of Merthyr and Newport, and the Rhondda Urban District, experienced increases in this form of infant mortality from the early 1920s to the early 1930s, while in smaller geographical units such as the urban districts of Abertillery and Mountain Ash, and the Penybont Rural District, neonatal mortality rates increased by even larger margins during the course of the inter-war period.[54] The neonatal mortality rate for the Abertillery Urban District increased from 38.2 deaths per 1,000 live births in 1920–4 to 42.3 in 1935–8, while the comparable rates for Mountain Ash were 28.4 and 40.5, and for Penybont 36.5 and 38.6. In the cases of Penybont and Mountain Ash these increases occurred despite the highly developed and energetic nature of the infant welfare services in these localities.[55]

The neonatal mortality rate is a particularly sensitive indicator of the nutritional status and health of expectant mothers and it is significant that neonatal mortality rates increased in districts that experienced high levels of unemployment and poverty in the inter-war period. It is evident that south Wales experienced a different trend in neonatal mortality to England and Wales as a whole. Figure 3.2

demonstrates that neonatal mortality rates in south Wales closely approximated, or marginally exceeded, the England and Wales rate during the early-to-mid 1920s. Towards the end of the decade, neonatal mortality in south Wales began to increase and began to exceed the England and Wales rate by a larger margin. The rise in neonatal mortality rates in south Wales, demonstrated by Figure 3.2, is most clearly demonstrated in the cases of the administrative counties of Glamorgan and Monmouthshire where sufficiently large numbers of deaths produced a smoother trend line. In these cases neonatal mortality rates rose during the late 1920s, peaked during the early 1930s and declined thereafter. The same general trend can be observed for Merthyr and Rhondda but the greater annual fluctuations disguise this to some extent. Therefore, levels of neonatal mortality in south Wales during the inter-war period closely reflected the economic fortunes of the region as levels of unemployment and poverty similarly increased during the late 1920s, peaked during the early 1930s and decreased during the mid-to-late 1930s.

Figure 3.2: Neonatal mortality rates for selected areas of south Wales and England and Wales as a whole, 1920–39[56]

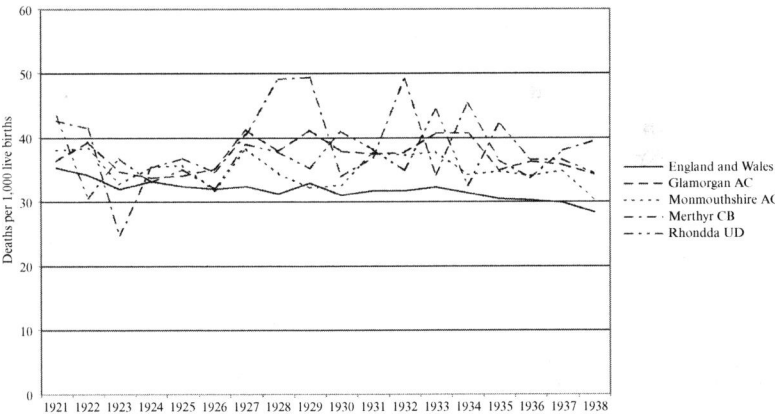

Patterns of stillbirth mortality in south Wales shared many of the same characteristics as those for neonatal mortality. As Nicky Hart has pointed out, stillbirths were a significant aspect of 'reproductive mortality' and yet have not received the same amount of attention from historical demographers as infant mortality.[57] While neonatal mortality is a useful indicator of the nutritional and health status of expectant and nursing mothers, the stillbirth rate reveals even more starkly the health status of child-bearing women in inter-war south Wales. As Hart comments:

> Stillbirth is ... a valuable health status indicator ... Where death occurs in utero the external environment is mediated by the mother's body, which is the foetal lifeline and a means of environmental insulation. The female body is the instrument of human procreation, and stillbirth is a good indicator of its capacity, its vitality. Since female physique reflects material conditions and the distribution of subsistence between the sexes, stillbirth is also an important potential indicator of inequality between them.[58]

Stillbirths and neonatal deaths share many of the same determinants. Both are primarily determined by the nature of the foetal environment in the period two to nine months after conception. The stillbirth mortality rate for England and Wales decreased from about 40 deaths per 1,000 total births in the late 1920s to about 37 per 1,000 by the end of the 1930s.[59] The rates for south Wales were consistently, and often considerably, higher than the England and Wales aggregate.[60] Merthyr, in particular, experienced one of the highest stillbirth mortality rates in the whole of England and Wales during the 1930s.[61] The greater levels of stillbirth mortality in south Wales are clearly demonstrated in figure 3.3. Stillbirths were made notifiable from 1 July 1927 and so reliable figures for the period before 1928 are not

Figure 3.3: Stillbirth rates in south Wales and for England and Wales, 1928–39[62]

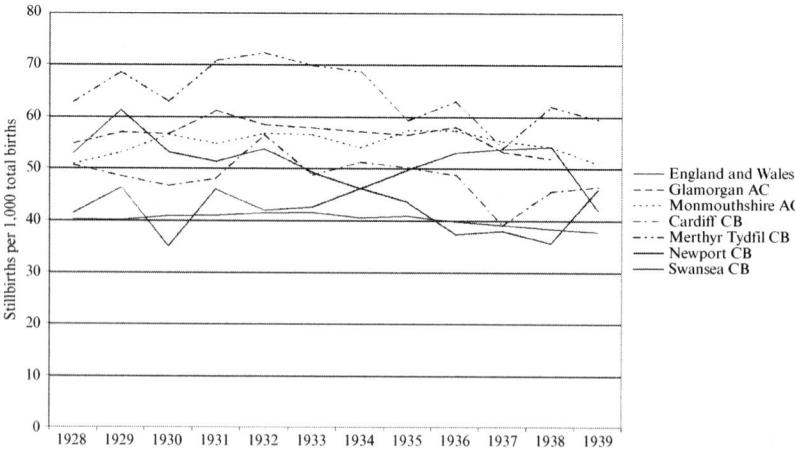

available for the areas illustrated by figure 3.3. Nevertheless, some local medical officers in south Wales recorded the numbers of stillbirths in their annual reports before this date. Figure 3.4 demonstrates that stillbirth rates in these depressed areas increased during the course of the inter-war period. This increase, however, might have been because of the more effective registration of these deaths. The stillbirth figures for the Rhondda in the 1920s, for example, were supplied to the medical officer by the sextons of the three local cemeteries and, since newspapers contained occasional reports of stillborn infants found in rivers, canals and other places, it seems likely that figures for the 1920s underestimate the true extent of stillbirth mortality in south Wales.[63] Countering this to some extent was the fact that, prior to 1927, in cases where infants died soon after birth, doctors or midwives often counted them as stillbirths so as to avoid the formalities of registration, thereby exaggerating the true extent of stillbirth mortality.[64] Similarly, it is possible that stillbirths continued to go unreported during the 1930s. Nevertheless, from 1928 onwards the statistics are more reliable and they clearly show an excess of stillbirths in south Wales over the England and Wales average and a rise in stillbirths in south Wales in the early 1930s over the late 1920s.

Figure 3.4: Stillbirths in certain districts of south Wales, 1920–39[65]

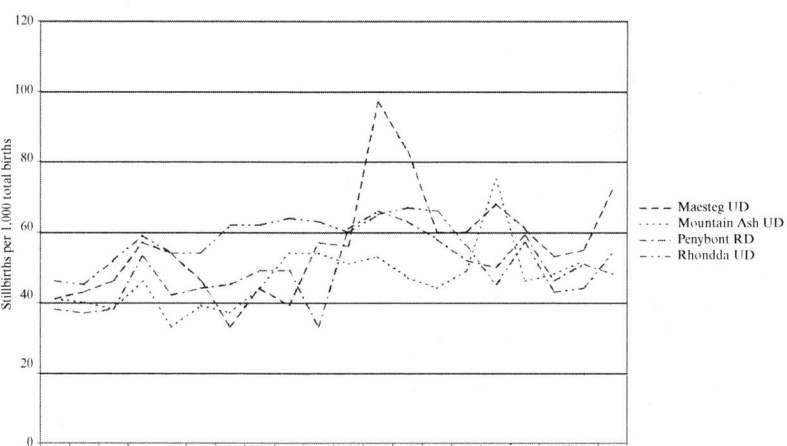

Developments in scientific medicine and improvements in the public physical environment failed to make a significant impact on neonatal mortality and, for the same reasons, made little difference to levels of stillbirth mortality. Expectant mothers – at the mercy of economic conditions that determined their nutritional status and a culture that ensured that a household's resources were devoted to the male 'breadwinner' – paid a heavy price during the inter-war depression as a large and increasing proportion of pregnancies resulted in stillbirths. Nicky Hart's assertion that neonatal and stillbirth mortality did not change appreciably during the economic depression of the 1930s, based as it is upon the aggregate England and Wales rates, reflects the improvements experienced in more affluent areas of Britain. It neglects the very different experience of south Wales and, possibly, other depressed areas where stillbirth mortality increased during the Depression.[66] The patterns of neonatal and stillbirth mortality emphasize once again that it was the women of south Wales who bore the brunt of the economic difficulties faced by families during the inter-war depression. Women's inability to meet the demands placed on their bodies by pregnancy, exacerbated by the consequences that economic conditions had for their nutritional intake, was reflected in the higher levels of stillbirth and neonatal mortality.

Conclusion

Therefore, the material and analysis presented above demonstrates that the nature of industrial communities in south Wales had a profound influence on the lives and health of working-class women. While mortality levels in industrial south Wales exceeded those for England and Wales as a whole, it is evident that female death rates exceeded corresponding female death rates for England and Wales to a greater extent than male death rates. This was as true of the late Victorian and Edwardian periods as it was of the inter-war years. However, such regional disparities in female mortality levels intensified during the Depression as improvements in female mortality in south Wales were retarded by economic depression and, indeed, as increases occurred in certain types of female mortality, including young adult female mortality and maternal mortality. Disaggregated death rates reveal that not only did women in south Wales experience higher levels of mortality than women elsewhere but also that certain forms of mortality, and in particular those forms of mortality closely associated with social and economic determinants, increased as a result of economic depression. Therefore, economic depression, unemployment and poverty did cause standards of health to deteriorate during the inter-war period and levels of mortality to increase. Moreover, if health and mortality in the inter-war period were 'rooted in economic disadvantage',[67] then it is also true to say that such economic disadvantage was also rooted in gender roles specific to industrial communities. Patterns of female mortality were determined by the social, economic and cultural factors that were, in turn, the product of specific ideas about gender. Women in south Wales were assigned a subordinate and, indeed, inferior status within their society by the nature of capitalist development, and in particular the coal-mining industry, that required large amounts of unpaid female labour within the home. The work was particularly onerous and the workplace decidedly unhealthy. This was exacerbated by gendered conceptions of duties, responsibilities and requirements that meant that women suffered the effects of unemployment and poverty to a greater extent than their male counterparts. Poverty and deprivation were gendered experiences and it was the women of south Wales that suffered disproportionately the effects of economic depression in the form of poor and deteriorating standards of health and increased mortality levels.

Notes

[1] For brief overviews of the historiography in relation to health see A. Crowther, *Social Policy in Britain 1914–1939* (London, 1988), pp. 66–72; A. Thorpe, *Britain in the 1930s* (Oxford, 1992), pp. 110–19; H. Jones, *Health and Society in Twentieth-Century Britain* (London, 1994), pp. 74–6.

[2] J. Stevenson and C. Cook, *The Slump* (London, 1977), pp. 19–21, 38–46, 78–81; J. Winter, 'Infant mortality, maternal mortality and public health in Britain in the 1930s', *Journal of European Economic History*, Vol. 8, no. 2 (1979), 453–60; Charles Webster, 'Healthy or hungry thirties?', *History Workshop Journal*, Vol. 13 (1982), 110–29; J. Winter, 'Unemployment, nutrition and infant mortality in Britain, 1920–50', in J. Winter (ed.), *The Working Class in Modern British History* (Cambridge, 1983), pp. 232–55; Margaret Mitchell, 'The effects of unemployment on the social condition of women and children in the 1930s', *History Workshop Journal*, Vol. 19 (1985), 105–27.

[3] Deirdre Beddoe, *Out of the Shadows: A History of Women in Twentieth-Century Wales* (Cardiff, 2000), p. 93; eadem, 'Munitionettes, maids and mams: women in Wales, 1914–1939', in Angela V. John (ed.), *Our Mothers' Land: Chapters in Welsh Women's History 1830–1939* (Cardiff, 1991), p. 206; Mari A. Williams, 'Yr ymgyrch i "achub y mamau" yng nghymoedd diwydi-

annol de Cymru, 1918–1939', Geraint H. Jenkins (ed.), *Cof Cenedl XI: Ysgrifau ar Hanes Cymru* (Llandysul, 1996), 117–46; Mari A. Williams, '"In the wars": Wales 1914–1945', in Gareth Elwyn Jones and Dai Smith (eds), *The People of Wales* (Llandysul, 1999), pp. 192–3; K. O. Morgan, *Rebirth of a Nation: Wales 1880–1980* (Oxford, 1981), pp. 233–4; Chris Williams, *Capitalism, Community and Conflict: The South Wales Coalfield 1898–1947* (Cardiff, 1998), p. 76; John Davies, *A History of Wales* (Harmondsworth, 1994), p. 580.

[4] Winter, 'Unemployment, nutrition and infant mortality', 252.

[5] J. Landers, *Death and the Metropolis: Studies in the Demographic History of London 1670–1830* (Cambridge, 1993), p. 3.

[6] Steven Thompson, 'A social history of health in inter-war south Wales' (unpublished Ph.D. thesis, University of Wales, 2001); see also idem, '"That beautiful summer of severe austerity": health, diet and the working-class domestic economy in south Wales in 1926', *Welsh History Review*, Vol. 21, no. 3 (2003), 552–74; Steven Thompson, *Unemployment, Poverty and Health in Interwar South Wales* (forthcoming, 2006).

[7] Crowther, *Social Policy in Britain*, p. 70.

[8] For the best account of women's lives in the south Wales coalfield see Dot Jones, 'Counting the cost of coal: women's lives in the Rhondda, 1881–1911', in John, *Our Mothers' Land*, pp. 109–33; see also Beddoe, *Out of the Shadows*, pp. 16–18; Carol White and Sian Rhiannon Williams (eds), *Struggle or Starve: Women's Lives in the South Wales Valleys between the Two World Wars* (Dinas Powys, 1998), pp. 14–17.

[9] Neil Evans and Dot Jones, '"A blessing for the miner's wife": the campaign for pithead baths in the south Wales coalfield, 1908–50', *Llafur*, Vol. 6, no. 3 (1994), 6; Beddoe, 'Munitionettes, maids and mams', pp. 203–4.

[10] Jones, 'Counting the cost of coal', pp. 124–6.

[11] See for example H. Jennings, *Brynmawr. A Study of a Distressed Area* (London, 1934), p. 156; A. Hutt, *The Condition of the Working Class in Britain* (London, 1933), pp. 29–30; *Men Without Work: A Report made to the Pilgrim Trust* (Cambridge, 1938), p. 135; A. Fenner Brockway, *Hungry England* (London, 1932), pp. 167–8.

[12] L. Fontaine and J. Schlumbohm, 'Household strategies for survival: an introduction', *International Review of Social History*, Vol. 45 (2000), Supplement 8, 5–6.

[13] White and Williams, *Struggle or Starve*, pp. 128, 133, 134.

[14] See for example J. Hanley, *Grey Children: A Study in Humbug and Misery* (London, 1937), p. 19.

[15] Jennings, *Brynmawr*, p. 157; E. Ginzberg, *A World Without Work* (London, 1942), p. 37; *Men Without Work*, pp. 112, 133; Gelligaer UDC, *Annual Report of the Medical Officer of Health* (1926), pp. 38–9; government investigators came to the same conclusions: Public Record Office (PRO), MH55/629, Ministry of Health, J. Pearse, T. W. Wade, O. Evans and J. E. Underwood, 'Report of an Inquiry into Conditions Affecting Health through Unemployment in South Wales and Monmouthshire', 23 October 1936, pp. 10–11, 49–50;

Ministry of Health, *Report on an Investigation in the Coalfield of South Wales and Monmouthshire*, PP 1928-9 (VIII, Cmd. 3272), p. 6.

16 Maggie Pryce Jones, *Kingfisher of Hope* (Llandysul, 1993), pp. 61, 32; see also *Men Without Work*, pp. 112, 126-8, 139-41.

17 Rhondda UDC, *Annual Report of the School Medical Officer*, 1935, pp. xlvi-xlvii; ibid., 1936, pp. xliv-xlv; ibid., 1937, pp. xlix-liii; ibid., 1938, p. xlix.

18 Stevenson and Cook, *The Slump*, pp. 79-80; Irvine Loudon, 'On maternal and infant mortality 1900-1960', *Social History of Medicine*, Vol. 4, no. 1 (1991), 49.

19 S. H. Preston, 'Population studies of mortality', *Population Studies*, Vol. 50 (1996), 525.

20 A. J. Taylor (ed.), *The Standard of Living in the Industrial Revolution* (London, 1975); J. G. Williamson, *Coping With City Growth During the British Industrial Revolution* (Cambridge, 1990); and the many articles in *Economic History Review*, *Explorations in Economic History* and *Journal of Economic History*.

21 J. Winter, *The Great War and the British People* (London, 1986); Linda Bryder, 'The First World War: healthy or hungry?', *History Workshop Journal*, Vol. 24 (1987), 141-57; J. Winter, 'Public health and the political economy of war: a reply to Linda Bryder', *History Workshop Journal*, Vol. 26 (1988), 163-73.

22 Webster, 'Healthy or hungry thirties?', 125.

23 See B. Benjamin, *Population Sources: A Review of UK Sources* (Aldershot, 1989), pp. 41-3; J. Winter, 'The decline of mortality in Britain 1870-1950', in T. Barker and M. Drake (eds), *Population and Society in Britain 1850-1950* (London, 1982), pp. 104-5.

24 The statistics in this paragraph are calculated from data obtained from *Registrar-General's Statistical Review* (1920-39) and the annual reports of medical officers of health for Glamorgan Administrative County (AC), Monmouthshire AC, Cardiff County Borough (CB), Merthyr Tydfil CB, Swansea CB and Newport CB (all 1920-39). The mortality rates quoted in this study have been collated in Thompson, 'A social history of health in inter-war south Wales', in which the methodologies employed in the calculation of these statistics, and the methodological problems inherent in their use, are explored in greater detail.

25 Figures calculated from Glamorgan County Council (CC), Annual Reports of the Medical Officer of Health (1920-39). It must be remembered that the standardized male and female death rates used in the table are not comparable in an area but only to the England and Wales sex-specific rates. Therefore, the male rates in the table are comparable to the England and Wales male death rate and the female rates are comparable to the England and Wales female death rates. Crude death rates or death rates standardized according to the direct method need to be used to compare male and female death rates.

26 Calculated from statistics obtained from *Registrar-General's Statistical Review*, medical officer of health reports for Glamorgan AC, Monmouthshire AC, Cardiff CB, Merthyr Tydfil CB, Swansea CB and Newport CB (all 1920-39), Census of England and Wales, 1921, and Census of England and Wales, 1931.

27 *New Statesman and Nation*, 23 November 1935, p. 759.

[28] A point also made by E. Lewis-Faning, *A Study of the Trend of Mortality Rates in Urban Communities of England and Wales, with Special Reference to 'Distressed Areas'* (London, 1938), p. 4.
[29] Jones, 'Counting the cost of coal', pp. 124–6.
[30] Calculated from statistics obtained from annual reports of medical officers of health for Rhondda UD and Merthyr Tydfil CB, *Registrar-General's Statistical Review* (all 1931–3), and Census of England and Wales, 1931.
[31] W. D. Johnston, 'Tuberculosis', in K. Kiple (ed.), *The Cambridge World History of Human Disease* (Cambridge, 1993), p. 1060.
[32] *The Registrar-General's Decennial Supplement, England and Wales 1931, Part II a Occupational Mortality* (London, 1938), pp. 329, 333, 337–8.
[33] L. Bryder, *Below the Magic Mountain: A Social History of Tuberculosis in Twentieth Century Britain* (Oxford, 1988), pp. 99–100; Johnston, 'Tuberculosis', p. 1060.
[34] Johnston, 'Tuberculosis', p. 1060.
[35] Rhondda UD, *Annual Report of the School Medical Officer*, 1936, pp. xliv–xlv; ibid., 1937, p. lii.
[36] G. Cronjé, 'Tuberculosis and mortality decline in England and Wales, 1851–1910', in R. Woods and J. Woodward (eds), *Urban Disease and Mortality in Nineteenth-Century England* (London, 1984), p. 89; Rhondda UD, *Annual Report of the Medical Officer of Health*, 1937, p. 155.
[37] For further evidence of increasing tuberculosis death rates see Bryder, *Below the Magic Mountain*, pp. 114–16, 124.
[38] Lewis-Faning, *A Study of the Trend of Mortality Rates*, pp. 23, 35, 57, 65; for a critique of the methodologies employed by Lewis-Faning and his conclusion that unemployment did not cause an increase in mortality in the depressed areas of south Wales see Thompson, 'A social history of health in interwar south Wales', pp. 293–4.
[39] PRO, MH79/336, J. Pearse, J. Alison Glover, A. P. Hughes Gibb and T. W. Wade, 'Inquiry into the Present Conditions as Regards the Effects of Continued Unemployment on Health in Certain Distressed Areas', 3 July 1934, pp. 2–4; see also Bryder, *Below the Magic Mountain*, p. 116.
[40] *Annual Report of the Chief Medical Officer of the Ministry of Health* (London, 1932), p. 17; Ministry of Health, *Report of an Investigation in the Coalfield of South Wales and Monmouth*, p. 5.
[41] Cardiff CB, *Annual Report of the Medical Officer of Health*, 1930, p. 7; Glyn Cox, *Report of an Investigation into the Incidence of Tuberculosis in the County of Anglesey and the Urban District of Barry* (Cardiff, 1937), pp. 32–3; Rhondda UD, *Annual Report of the Medical Officer of Health*, 1931, p. 57; Nantyglo and Blaina UD, *Annual Report of the Medical Officer of Health*, 1925, p. 4.
[42] W. Williams, 'Puerperal mortality', *Transactions of the Epidemiological Society of London* (1895–6), pp. 100–33; W. Williams, *Deaths in Childbed* (London, 1904); *Forty-fourth Annual Report of the Local Government Board, 1914–15, Supplement Containing a Report on Maternal Mortality*, PP 1914–16 (xxv, Cd. 8085), pp. 32–3, 36, 40.
[43] Webster, 'Healthy or hungry thirties?', p. 117; Mitchell, 'The effects of unem-

ployment on the social condition of women and children', pp. 111, 115–16; Morgan, *Rebirth of a Nation*, p. 233; Williams, 'Yr ymgyrch i "achub y mamau"', pp. 121–2; Beddoe, 'Munitionettes, Maids and Mams', p. 206. A notable aspect of many of the pessimistic interpretations of maternal mortality in inter-war Britain is reference to the feeding experiments of the National Birthday Trust Fund in the Rhondda valley but, as A. Susan Williams, *Women and Childbirth in the Twentieth Century: A History of the National Birthday Trust Fund 1928–93* (Stroud, 1997), pp. 81, 90–1, 98 demonstrates, these experiments were methodologically flawed and cannot be used as evidence of low maternal nutritional status with the confidence that has hitherto been placed upon them.

44 Ministry of Health, *Report on Maternal Mortality in Wales*, PP 1936–7 (XI, Cmd. 5423), p. 88.
45 Winter, 'Unemployment, nutrition and infant mortality', p. 243; Winter, 'Infant mortality, maternal mortality and public health', pp. 454–5.
46 Irvine Loudon, 'Maternal mortality: 1880–1950. Some regional and international comparisons', *Social History of Medicine*, Vol. 1, no. 2 (1988), 183–228 (197).
47 Irvine Loudon, *Death in Childbirth: An International Study of Maternal Care and Maternal Mortality 1800–1950* (Oxford, 1992), pp. 243–4, 251; see also Loudon, 'On maternal and infant mortality'.
48 Loudon, 'Maternal mortality: 1880–1950', pp. 197–8.
49 Ibid., p. 197.
50 Ibid., p. 190.
51 *Twentieth Annual Report of the Ministry of Health*, PP 1938 (XI, Cmd. 6089), p. 325.
52 R. Lee, 'Infant, child and maternal mortality in Western Europe: a critique' in A. Brändström and L.-G. Tedebrand (eds), *Society, Health and Population during the Demographic Transition* (Stockholm, 1988), pp. 15–16.
53 Calculated from statistics from annual reports of medical officers of health of Glamorgan AC, Monmouthshire AC, Cardiff CB, Merthyr Tydfil CB, Swansea CB, Newport CB, and *Registrar General's Statistical Review* (all 1920–39).
54 Annual Reports of Medical Officers of Health for Abertillery UD, Mountain Ash UD, Penybont RD (1920–39). It is only possible to obtain neonatal infant mortality rates for certain administrative districts. Penybont was largely a rural district but its population was largely concentrated in the northern part of the district and primarily engaged in industrial activities.
55 See Penybont RD, *Annual Report of the Medical Officer of Health*, 1920–39; Mountain Ash UD, *Annual Report of the Medical Officer of Health*, 1920–39.
56 Annual reports of medical officers of health for Glamorgan AC, Monmouthshire AC, Merthyr Tydfil CB, Rhondda UD, and *Registrar-General's Statistical Review* (all 1920–39).
57 N. Hart, 'Beyond infant mortality: gender and stillbirth in reproductive mortality before the twentieth century', *Population Studies*, Vol. 52 (1998), 215–29.

[58] Ibid., p. 227; a point also made by D. Graham, 'Female employment and infant mortality: some evidence from British towns, 1911, 1931, 1951', *Continuity and Change*, Vol. 9, no. 2 (1994), 315.
[59] *Registrar-General's Statistical Review* (1928–39).
[60] Ministry of Health, *Report on Maternal Mortality in Wales*, pp. 16–17; see also Winter, 'Unemployment, nutrition and infant mortality in Britain', p. 239.
[61] Graham, 'Female employment and infant mortality', 315.
[62] *Registrar-General's Statistical Review* (1928–39).
[63] See also E. Baker, *'Yan Boogie': The Autobiography of a Swansea Valley Girl* (Pretoria, 1992), pp. 49–50.
[64] Rhondda UD, *Annual Report of the Medical Officer of Health*, 1923, pp. 28–9.
[65] Annual reports of medical officers of health for Maesteg UD, Mountain Ash UD, Rhondda UD and Penybont RD (1920–39).
[66] Hart, 'Beyond infant mortality', 227.
[67] Webster, 'Healthy or hungry thirties?', p. 125.

4

'The Growing Toll of Motherhood':[1] Maternal Mortality in Wales, 1918–1939

MARI A. WILLIAMS

As many of the papers included in this volume illustrate, discussions relating to the history of Wales during the period between the two World Wars seem inevitably to include references to terms such as unemployment, poverty and ill health. Our collective memory of life during the period is loaded with images of a desperate people living on the breadline and facing a constant struggle against all odds. Some historians, however, have argued that this is a misleading and one-sided representation of life during the inter-war period, which fails to acknowledge that great improvements were achieved in the living conditions of the majority of the population. It is claimed that the 1930s in particular was not such a miserable decade after all, as significant advancements in the fields of housing, health and employment improved the lives of many people.[2] The fact remains, however, that such general trends were of little comfort to a significant proportion of the Welsh population.

Despite many important developments in the fields of medicine and health care, Wales continued to be blighted by serious health problems, not least of which was that of maternal mortality. Although general death rates in England and Wales fell during the inter-war years, deaths in childbirth remained high and actually increased in some instances. Indeed, as Irvine Loudon, the author of several authoritative studies on the problem of maternal mortality, has noted: 'the risk of a woman dying of puerperal fever in Britain in the first half of the 1930s was as high as it had been in the 1860s, and actually higher than in 1910.'[3] As will become evident, the problem was particularly acute in Wales where the maternal mortality rate exceeded the rate in England by 35 per cent between 1924 and 1933.[4] The situation was particularly grave in industrial south Wales where an increase of 14.2 per cent was recorded in Glamorgan and a staggering 42 per cent in Monmouthshire.[5] During this period (1924–33), between 2,500 and 3,000 women lost their lives as a result of childbirth, while many more suffered serious illnesses, diseases or disabilities. When compared with the number of females who died as a result of infectious diseases such as tuberculosis, maternal mortality was perhaps not regarded as a major problem; however, the great tragedy was that the death rate was allowed to increase at all, for the reality was that the deaths of a significant proportion of those women who died in childbirth could quite easily have been prevented.

The beginning of the inter-war period heralded a new era in the administration and provision of health care in England and Wales. Following the devastation of the First World War, immediate action was taken to alleviate some of the pressing problems of health and housing. These new post-war measures were accompanied by important administrative changes which saw the formation of the Ministry of Health and the Welsh Board of Health in 1919, and the granting of considerable powers to local authorities to administer and deliver health services. The loss of so many young lives on the battlefields of Flanders and elsewhere, as well as growing concern for the falling birth rate, placed renewed emphasis on ensuring the well-being of the nation's mothers and children. The maternity and child-welfare movement was thus given a new impetus which resulted in the passing of two important Acts in 1918, namely the Maternity and Child Welfare Act and the Midwives Act.

One of the most important features of the new Maternity and Child Welfare Act was that it authorized local authorities to establish maternity and child-welfare centres, while the Midwives Act ensured greater control of the midwifery service and required local authorities to pay 'medical aid' fees to doctors called in by a midwife. Hopes were high that a new era was dawning but in Wales, as elsewhere, the sense of optimism which accompanied these new developments was soon to be dashed by a combination of economic and social forces. The post-war mood of prosperity proved to be short-lived and from the early 1920s both the industrial and rural communities of Wales were struck by a series of economic crises, bringing any talk of progress to a sudden halt.[6] In addition to these financial obstacles, health campaigners also found themselves waging a constant battle against the apparent indifference and prejudice of local authority officials, councillors and members of the medical profession, the vast majority of whom were male.[7] Despite the many important advancements which were made in the field of maternal welfare during the inter-war period, the scale and speed with which assistance was provided to expectant mothers in Wales was thus to prove extremely disappointing. Indeed, writing in 1935, G. F. McCleary, formerly a Deputy Senior Medical Officer in the Ministry of Health, maintained that the continued high maternal mortality rate should be regarded as the outstanding failure of the maternity and child-welfare movement during the inter-war period.[8]

Before moving on to examine in greater detail the factors which contributed to this situation, it is appropriate to consider how the maternal mortality rate was calculated. From 1915 onwards, when an Act was passed making it compulsory to notify every birth officially, the maternal mortality rate was based on the number of mothers who died for every 1,000 births.[9] After 1927, following legislation which made the registration of stillbirths compulsory, this basis was changed to every 1,000 total births (that is whether the births were live or stillbirths). Maternal deaths were generally recorded as falling into two categories: puerperal deaths, that is deaths which were directly due to childbearing and usually caused by infection or sepsis (bloodpoisoning); and secondly, non-puerperal deaths caused by accidents of pregnancy or where childbirth was a contributory factor. When it is considered that the Ministry of Health regarded areas where the maternal mortality rate exceeded 5 deaths per 1,000 live births as 'problem areas', it is immediately evident that the situation in many parts of Wales gave cause for great concern (see table 4.1). Between 1924 and 1933, the puerperal mortality rate for Wales was 35 per cent in excess of the rate for England.[10] During this period, there were only two counties and two county boroughs in Wales where the maternal mortality rate fell below the average for England and Wales, while four Welsh counties recorded the exceptionally high puerperal mortality rate of 6 or more deaths per 1,000 births. On a more local level, the statistics revealed that the situation was particularly serious in some parts of the country. For example, between 1929 and 1933, when a significant increase was recorded in the number of puerperal deaths in England and Wales as a whole, the death rate in the economically depressed regions of south Wales was 54.8 per cent higher than in England. In some communities, the rate was double that recorded in

Table 4.1: Number of deaths and puerperal mortality rate per 1,000 live births, 1924–33

Area	Puerperal deaths	
	No. of deaths	Rate per 1,000 births
Counties		
Anglesey	54	6.79
Brecknockshire	45	4.48
Caernarfonshire	89	5.05
Cardiganshire	48	6.39
Carmarthenshire	193	6.34
Denbighshire	171	6.56
Flintshire	107	5.63
Glamorgan	873	5.85
Merioneth	40	5.84
Monmouthshire	350	5.18
Montgomeryshire	40	4.76
Pembrokeshire	84	5.70
Radnorshire	19	5.27
County Boroughs		
Cardiff	193	4.75
Merthyr Tydfil	76	5.84
Newport	70	4.04
Swansea	164	5.52
Wales	2616	5.57
England and Wales	27664	4.21
England	25043	4.11

Source: Ministry of Health, *Report on Maternal Mortality in Wales* (1937).

England and Wales as a whole: in 1934, a rate of 10.7 was returned in the Ogmore and Garw Urban District and 11.99 in the Rhondda Urban District.

Given the gravity of the problem, it was not surprising that a great deal of public attention was focused on the issue of maternal mortality both in England and Wales. Many health workers, charitable organizations and political groups voiced their concerns publicly, and openly criticized the authorities for failing to address the severe health problems faced by women in many parts of Great Britain.[11] Such was the pressure to find a solution to the matter that the Ministry of Health was compelled to commission a series of official reports and inquiries from the mid-1920s onwards. In addition to examining the situation prevailing in parts of England, the special problems faced in Wales were given particular attention. In an investigation conducted in 1924, Dr Janet M. Campbell, Senior Medical Officer in the Department of Maternity and Child Welfare at the Ministry of Health, provided a detailed examination of the situation in five rural counties, namely Cumberland and Westmorland in England, and Brecknockshire, Montgomeryshire and Pembrokeshire in Wales. Following on from this report, a departmental committee was set up by the Ministry of Health in 1928 which produced an interim report in 1930 and a final report in 1932. Again, Wales received special attention and Dr Dilys M. Jones of the Welsh Board of Health was given the task of reporting on the Welsh situation. Finally, in 1934, two special reports were commissioned by the Ministry: the first examined the problem of maternal mortality in certain parts of England, while the other considered the situation in Wales. The *Report on Maternal Mortality in Wales* was conducted by officials of the Welsh Board of Health and was published in 1937.[12]

Although the government was to be congratulated for undertaking such detailed research, one of the most depressing features of these investigations was the fact that they highlighted the same problems time and time again and repeated many of the previous recommendations. It would appear, therefore, that the official reports were either consistently failing to address the real causes of maternal mortality or that very little attention was paid to their findings by local authorities and health practitioners. One of the preventative measures continually stressed by health officials was the importance of antenatal care. Although provision had been made for the establishment of antenatal clinics in the Maternity and Child Welfare Act of 1918, their crucial role in ensuring the well-being of the expectant mother and unborn child was not fully appreciated in all parts of the country. In 1935, seventeen years after the passing of the Act, only a third of expectant mothers attended antenatal clinics in Wales.[13] Although the situation compared favourably with that which existed prior to 1918, the services provided were extremely patchy and were unevenly distributed. Only five of the thirteen administrative counties of Wales had established antenatal clinics by 1934, namely Glamorgan (43), Monmouthshire (16), Flintshire (6), Denbighshire (2) and Carmarthenshire (1). No antenatal clinics existed in the predominantly rural counties of Anglesey, Brecknockshire, Caernarfonshire, Cardiganshire, Merioneth, Montgomeryshire, Pembrokeshire and Radnor.

The lack of facilities in the rural areas was certainly not a reflection of a lack of demand. In their annual reports, the Medical Officers of Health who served these rural communities continually called for services such as antenatal clinics and maternity hospitals to be provided, but their requests appear to have fallen on deaf ears. For example, in 1927, D. Arthur Hughes, the Carmarthenshire Medical Officer of Health, unveiled schemes to establish antenatal clinics at six of the county's larger infant-welfare clinics. Four years later the plans had not been carried out, a situation which he described as 'deplorable'.[14] His successor, William M. Lloyd, also had little success in persuading local councillors and officials to press ahead with the plans; the decision to adopt a scheme providing antenatal and postnatal care was again deferred by the authority in 1937.[15] Even in the counties of Glamorgan and Monmouthshire, where the greater number of clinics had been established by the early 1930s, the situation was far from satisfactory. Local women such as Elizabeth Andrews, Rose Davies and Eliza Williams, who campaigned tirelessly for improved maternity services in their communities in the Rhondda and Aberdare, found that there was much prejudice and ignorance to be overcome, both on the part of local councillors, general practitioners and expectant mothers. In 1924, the local health official at Aberdare claimed that he had not come across one general medical practitioner who showed any sympathy towards antenatal clinics: 'the attitude of the majority is apathetic, whilst some are frankly antipathetic'.[16] Meanwhile, according to the Glamorgan Medical Officer of Health, expectant women showed little enthusiasm for the clinics: 'The women themselves do not yet know what antenatal care may be able to do for their comfort and health and safety at the time of pregnancy and confinement, and it is natural that they should be shy of consultation or examination that they do not think necessary.'[17]

In those areas where clinics had not been established, the responsibility for providing antenatal care fell to the midwives, nurses and health visitors who paid home visits to expectant mothers. Standards of midwifery had certainly improved greatly by the inter-war years as a result of the Midwives Acts of 1902 and 1918.[18] Following the passing of the Midwives Act of 1918, only women certified by the Central Midwives Board could lawfully call themselves midwives. Furthermore, it became the duty of a midwife in the case of an emergency to call in a doctor herself, rather than asking the patient's relatives to do so.[19] Nevertheless, many problems remained, particularly in the isolated rural districts where there was a severe shortage of trained midwives. The distances which the midwives were called upon to travel in such areas, sometimes in the worst possible weather, was a great deterrent in attracting suitably trained recruits.[20] Women working in rural communities could also not hope to make a living as professional midwives unless subsidized by the local authority or nursing associations. Not all Welsh local authorities provided financial support (the county of Merioneth being one example), and large areas of rural Wales thus went without the services of trained midwives.[21] Moreover, none of the Welsh local authorities provided financial assistance to allow midwives to attend post-certificate courses in training institutions. It was not surprising, therefore, as was the case in some parts of the Rural District of Newtown and Llanidloes, that expectant mothers had no choice but to 'resort to the old-fashioned and unqualified midwife'.[22] In Caernarfonshire in 1920, it was reported that sixteen untrained midwives were in practice, five of whom had no knowledge of antiseptics.[23] Clearly, there were considerable risks involved in the practice of employing untrained midwives or 'handy-women', as became apparent in Carmarthenshire in the mid-1920s. Following the deaths of seven mothers from puerperal fever, the source of infection was traced to an untrained woman who had attended at their confinements.[24]

Although clearly justified in some instances, the growing number of puerperal deaths could not solely be attributed to 'meddlesome' and 'ignorant' midwives, as some members of the medical profession claimed.[25] The general lack of investment in the provision of maternity services, coupled with the decline in the birth rate, meant that practical experience and knowledge of obstetric practice among general practitioners was not as high as it should be. Moreover, specialist obstetric advice was often not readily available, particularly in smaller towns and rural areas.[26] For example, in Brecknockshire, a county served by three small cottage hospitals, the medical staff were general practitioners who were said to have no more than 'an ordinary knowledge of obstetrics'.[27] Both Brecknockshire and Radnor relied on hospitals in Cardiff and Swansea for their consultant services, and it could therefore take hours to obtain the assistance of a specialist. As one local health official from the area noted in 1938: 'To put the matter in a nutshell, Wales is short of obstetric specialists who can serve the interior of the country at a moment's notice.'[28]

The lack of designated maternity hospitals was a serious deficiency in the provision of health care in Wales. The 1937 *Report on Maternal Mortality in Wales* noted that only six maternity homes were provided by local authorities in Wales; no accommodation for maternity cases, apart from that provided in poor law institutions, existed in the following counties – Anglesey, Brecknockshire, Carmarthenshire, Denbighshire, Merioneth, Pembrokeshire and Radnor. Furthermore, only four local authorities paid a subsidy to voluntary institutions for the use of maternity beds.[29] The overwhelming majority of Welsh mothers thus gave birth in their own homes, often in circumstances which made it extremely difficult to maintain a high standard of hygiene and of clinical care. The situation was far from satisfactory in the thickly populated industrial communities, where the incidence of puerperal sepsis was most prevalent. Speaking in 1935, Councillor Eliza Williams from the Rhondda urged the local authority to press ahead with the establishment of a maternity hospital. In her opinion, far too many babies were being born in overcrowded houses in the district and she cited the case of a family of four living in one room where the mother was shortly expected to be confined.[30] Under such circumstances, the risk of infection was particularly acute. As a local medical officer from Monmouthshire noted in 1921: 'It is impossible for even the most careful mother to bring up children in a hygienic manner, and to observe the common decencies of life, when five or six of a family have only one living room and one sleeping room at their disposal.'[31] Conditions in the rural areas were equally unsatisfactory, if not worse. During the 1930s, the Ministry of Health's report on tuberculosis in Wales collected damning evidence of the appalling living and sanitary standards prevailing in many parts of rural Wales.[32] Commenting on the primitive condition of a house in Llannor, Caernarfonshire, the authors noted that 'there was nothing to equal it in the industrial areas of South Wales'.[33]

The nature of the daily chores undertaken by Welsh working-class women around the home was also the cause of great concern. In the coal-mining communities of south and north-east Wales, miners' wives waged a constant battle against the coal dust which penetrated every corner of their homes. In the opinion of a correspondent who wrote to the *Aberdare Leader* in 1937, the women in many homes in the area were nothing more than 'household slaves' who washed 'over and over again the same dirty clothes, dirty dishes', and undertook 'an endless round of drudgery'.[34] Before the establishment of pithead baths, they were also responsible for the heavy work of fetching and carrying water in preparation for the miner's return from the pit.[35] As Dot Jones has argued, there is little doubt that the health problems of miners' wives were exacerbated by their poor living conditions and their continued heavy domestic workload.[36] Women in the agricultural districts fared equally badly in this respect. As a local health official from Cardiganshire noted in 1923, females were responsible for carrying out a number of heavy duties around the farm, and many women continued with such work during their pregnancy: 'She is the household, or farm drudge, and, instead of reasonably resting, works harder than ever.'[37]

Bearing large families and caring for their growing children placed an additional strain on expectant mothers. Although the Welsh birth-rate had fallen dramatically since the beginning of the twentieth century, from 30.1 in 1901–10 to 15.6 in 1934, large families remained common, notably in the industrial communities. For those working-class women who were already struggling to make ends meet, frequent pregnancies proved both physically and emotionally demanding. The evidence presented by Margery Spring Rice in the publication *Working-Class Wives: Their Health and Conditions* (1939), featured the experiences of many mothers from south Wales and revealed a grim picture of the impact which excessive child-bearing had on their general health.[38] The unfavourable economic and social conditions of the inter-war years merely served to exacerbate the difficulties facing many expectant and nursing mothers. In her study of the experiences of Welsh miners' wives during the 1926 General Strike and subsequent nine-month lock-out, Marion Phillips cited the distressing cases of several large unemployed families who were finding it hard to survive: in one example from the Rhondda, a family with nine children under the age of sixteen was living on the seventeen shillings a week received from the Board of Guardians; elsewhere, a family with four children under the age of five and another on the way was said to be 'sinking for want of a good meal'.[39] Given the circumstances, it was not surprising that some women viewed their pregnancies with considerable fear and dread. Indeed, the daunting prospect of having another child to feed and clothe, coupled with anxieties relating to their own well-being, drove some mothers to take the drastic action of procuring their own abortions.

One of the striking features of the problem of maternal mortality in south Wales during the inter-war years was the dramatic increase in the number of deaths from puerperal sepsis. Although this increase could be related to a number of causes, it was widely acknowledged that deaths due to abortion were of considerable importance in the increased incidence of puerperal sepsis. The 1937 *Report on Maternal Mortality in Wales* estimated that the ratio of abortions to childbirths ranged from 14 to 25 per cent, and that abortions were most common in the industrial counties of Glamorgan and Monmouthshire.[40] However, as doctors or midwives were not always called in to assist in cases of abortion (both natural and criminal), it proved extremely difficult to assess exactly how many women had abortions and it is likely that their numbers were greatly under-recorded. As the Medical Officer of Health for Glamorgan noted in 1929, the only cases which usually came to light were those which had resulted in the serious injury or death of the female: 'It is to be feared that the practice of criminal abortion is much more general than is commonly known ... Apart from partially known results in death, we have no real knowledge of its prevalence or the ill-health caused by it.'[41] It was also apparent that a large number of the stillbirths in the region were the direct result of some form of 'interference'. Such was the opinion expressed by many local health officials, including the Rhondda Medical Officer of Health who noted in 1932: 'As experienced in recent years the still-births are relatively more numerous and it is suspected that, in many instances, are due to artificial means applied for the purpose of inducing abortion.'[42] Autobiographical evidence also suggests that the incidence of procured abortions was on the increase, with women resorting to the use of instruments such as knitting needles or crochet hooks, the administration of syringes to inject irritant fluids, such as soap and water, or the swallowing of drugs and other preparations.[43] There is no doubt that the straitened social and economic circumstances of working-class families had a bearing upon the decision to interfere with pregnancies. As Dr R. Llewellyn Williams of Mountain Ash maintained in his annual report for 1935, many expectant mothers procured abortions for the simple reason that they could not afford to have children.[44] Lady Juliet Rhys Williams, an active campaigner in the field of maternal and child welfare in south Wales, who also served on the Ministry of Health's Inter-Departmental Committee on Abortion which was established in 1937, thought it not at all surprising that so many local women resorted to such extremes:

While thousands of married women had less than 4s. a week for food, could it be wondered at if a few of them preferred to face the horrors of illegal abortion rather than continue the unequal struggle to survive, burdened by another child to maintain.[45]

The numerous reports of court cases which appeared in local newspapers as a result of such actions, provide further evidence of the desperate circumstances and hard choices facing expectant mothers during this period. The case of a 37-year-old miner's wife from Abercynon, who died in 1921 following an attempt to procure an abortion, was typical of many others. Her husband of eighteen years knew that she was worried about her pregnancy and having already borne eight children she had told him that she did not want to have another baby.[46]

The lack of official information available to Welsh women regarding family planning meant that many continued to regard abortion as an efficient method of birth control. Although some local health officials supported the establishment of birth control clinics and advice centres, their demands often met with considerable opposition when presented before councillors, local authority officials and senior Medical Officers of Health.[47] In the Rhondda, members of the Urban District Council voted against the recommendation of their local Medical Officer of Health to establish birth control clinics on numerous occasions during the 1920s. At a meeting of the authority which was held in 1926, councillors expressed the opinion that such institutions were both 'immoral and irreligious'.[48] One of the main opponents of the service, Dr W. E. Thomas, repeated his objections some months later at a meeting of the Glamorgan Public Health and Housing Committee, when he claimed that 'contraceptive practices were detrimental to the health of the woman'. Councillor Rose Davies of Aberdare disagreed and argued that the health of local mothers was being put at risk precisely because of the lack of birth control clinics. The women of Aberdare had themselves already made it clear, at a meeting held in the town earlier that year, that there was a real need for such facilities in the area. Dr W. E. Thomas remained unconvinced, however, and the women of Aberdare eventually had to wait another five years before their wish was granted and a birth control clinic was established in the town in 1931.[49]

This conflict between the needs of local mothers and the prejudices of their elected male representatives was a recurring feature during the inter-war period. More often than not, important decisions relating to housing and health were made by men who were not always best qualified to judge on such matters. Gradually, however, an increasing number of women were elected to local housing and health committees. Women such as Elizabeth Andrews in the Rhondda and Rose Davies in Aberdare had played an active role in the work of their respective local authorities since the early 1920s. A decade later, several more women had joined their ranks and assisted in the important work being carried out in the fields of health and housing. In 1932, Councillor Eliza Williams was elected the first female chairman of the Rhondda Urban District Council and was followed in 1932 by Councillor Annie Price. Yet, despite these important gains, female representatives continued to wage a constant battle for greater recognition within their local authorities and were often sidelined. For example, when a special conference was held in February 1935 to discuss the need to establish a maternity hospital in the Pontypridd area, only male delegates were sent to the meeting from Pontypridd, Rhondda, Mountain Ash, Aberdare, Llantrisant and Llantwit Vardre councils. In the opinion of Eliza Williams, this was 'an insult to the women of the Rhondda'.[50]

By the early 1930s, however, in the face of increasing pressure to find a solution to the problem of maternal mortality, the government granted local health authorities permission to provide birth control advice to married women in 'cases where further pregnancy would be detrimental to health'. However, as there was no obligation on local authorities to act, very few actually pressed ahead to establish such centres. The first birth control advice centre which was established in Pontypridd in 1930 was in fact initially set up by a voluntary organization from London.[51] It was not until 1935, however, following a protest by local women, that a centre 'for married women who had been specially recommended' was finally opened under the auspices of the local authority in the neighbouring district of the Rhondda.[52] The negative attitude expressed towards birth control clinics contrasted sharply with the considerable support given to antenatal clinics and maternity centres in the area by that period. By 1934, seventy-eight such centres had been opened in the counties of Glamorgan and Monmouthshire and their crucial role in ensuring the well-being of pregnant mothers had been recognized. Writing in 1939, D. Rocyn Jones, the Monmouthshire Medical Officer of Health, commented that:

> We definitely declare that many an expectant mother would have been in her grave to-day but for the attention and advice given her at these ante-

natal centres. These centres have been a godsend to the motherhood of this country, and particularly in areas where obstetric practice is slip-shod, and sometimes incompetent.[53]

In assessing the success of such centres, medical commentators frequently referred to the invaluable contribution which they made, not only to the health of the mothers but also to their children. At a time when considerable anxiety was voiced regarding the dramatic fall in the birth rate, many believed that one of the best means to halt the trend was to make pregnancy and motherhood a more attractive experience. Indeed, some commentators went as far as to suggest that the negative attention given to the maternal mortality 'problem' had contributed in some way to the fall in the birth rate by 'tending to terrify child-bearing women'.[54] The secretary of a nursing association in the Swansea valley accused some political groups of 'scare-mongering' and feared that many young Welsh women would be deterred from having children in the future:

> What with birth-control propaganda, the dissemination of 'informative' literature, our falling birth-rate, and what I have heard some medical men describe as 'this bogey of maternal mortality', we shall soon be forced to emulate our neighbours across the Channel and give a bonus for every baby born.[55]

As the body of medical and social evidence collated during the 1920s and 1930s testifies, however, there can be no doubting the reality of the situation and the fact that a large proportion of women in both industrial and rural Wales had suffered greatly as a result of their difficult experiences during pregnancy and childbirth. Indeed, the authors of a report conducted by the Pilgrim Trust in 1937 suggested that as many as 3,200 Welsh mothers had died as a direct result of the economic depression of the inter-war years.[56] As D. Rocyn Jones of Monmouthshire noted in 1935, the straitened economic experiences of the previous decade had a deletrious effect on the physical condition of many women:

> There were many predisposing causes at work, especially in South Wales, where they had long continued poverty in those counties which had resulted from unemployment. That poverty must lower the standard of the mother's health and make her less able to resist infection.[57]

Although not appreciated by all medical experts, there can be little doubt that social and economic factors had a direct bearing on the high maternal mortality rates of inter-war Wales. After all, working-class women in both the industrial and rural areas endured great hardships as a result of the crises in the coal and agricultural industries. The lifestyle of many working-class women was simply not conducive to good health and vitality, and their resistance to disease and infection was low. Tuberculosis was a major problem in Wales during the inter-war period, and the female death rate was particularly high: during the period 1931–5, the death rate among females aged 15–35 was 70 per cent higher in south Wales than in England and Wales as a whole; in Merthyr Tydfil, the figure was nearly $2\frac{1}{2}$ times that average.[58] Anaemia and 'general listlessness' were regarded as common female ailments, while malnutrition in expectant mothers was frequently remarked upon by local health officials and cited as one of the causes of premature and stillbirths.[59] The health of new-born babies also suffered, as many nursing mothers were unable to breastfeed their children because they were malnourished.[60] Writing in 1938, O. Vaughan Jones, part-time County Obstetrician for Caernarfonshire, noted that the 'type of mother' found among the 'local working-class' was:

> of a poor constitution, probably because of under-nourishment. I am of the opinion that this pitiful state of affairs is due mainly to poverty, ignorance and their mode of living. The Liverpool slums and working class (amongst whom I worked for years) are of infinitely better physique.[61]

Working-class families rarely ate meat, fruit, green vegetables or fresh milk, and survived on a staple diet of white bread, butter or margarine, potatoes, sugar and jam.[62] In agricultural districts, where perhaps one might have expected greater variation in the diet, eating habits were no better. Speaking at Welshpool in 1932, A. W. Ashby, Professor of Agricultural Economics at Aberystwyth University, declared that 'the limitation and lack of variety in the dietary in many farms was a disgrace'.[63] Families in rural Cardiganshire were said to survive largely on stewed tea, bread and butter and *cawl* (broth) – a concoction which one health official described as having the nutritional value of 'boiled bricks'.[64] Local medical officers of health also frequently chastized the farming population for selling their fresh produce in return for tinned groceries, such as condensed milk, which had become part of the staple diet in many rural households.[65]

Despite the body of evidence which lends support to the argument that poverty, resulting in poor housing and poor diet, was the root cause of the poor physical condition of so many Welsh women, the

'THE GROWING TOLL OF MOTHERHOOD' 137

authorities seemed loath to admit that economic factors had played a crucial role in the high incidence of maternal mortality. Whilst acknowledging that there had been 'an increase in sickness and ill-health among the mothers in the industrial areas of South Wales', the 1937 *Report on Maternal Mortality in Wales* maintained that 'the influence exerted by poor nutrition in producing maternal mortality' could not be 'accurately estimated'. The authors of the report acknowledged, however, that 'an excess of ill-health among expectant mothers increases the risks at childbirth'.[66] On reading their findings, columnists writing in the journal *Medical Officer*, were left dumbstruck and retorted: 'We are left convinced that [the reduction of maternal mortality] is more likely to be achieved by a herd of cows than by a herd of specialists.'[67] In their opinion, the achievements of a feeding scheme for necessitous and expectant mothers, run by the National Birthday Trust Fund in parts of the south Wales valleys, which had resulted in a dramatic decrease in the local maternal mortality rate, pointed towards a very different conclusion.[68] The authors of a report on health services in Britain, published in 1937, agreed: 'The evidence from these experiments is most striking: moreover, their conclusion that insufficient food leads to lowered vitality and consequent inability to bear the strain of child-birth seems logical and reasonable.'[69]

The debate has raged on among historians, some of whom have cast doubt on the relevance of poverty and prevailing standards of nutrition, and stress the importance of clinical aspects as opposed to social, economic and environmental factors.[70] In trying to address the reasons why maternal mortality rates remained so high in inter-war Wales, it seems one must accept that a combination of factors was at work. Wales certainly had its fair share of both clinical and administrative problems: in the large, densely populated industrial areas the risk of infection was great, while the quality and availability of obstetric and maternity services were extremely poor in the isolated and sparsely populated rural districts. Moreover, across the whole of the country, working-class women faced considerable economic hardship and grave social problems throughout the inter-war period. The high incidence of maternal mortality in both rural and industrial Wales was testimony to the fact that large parts of the country were home to seriously disadvantaged communities, where expectant mothers were deprived of many basic public health and welfare services and of a satisfactory standard of living. Thankfully, by the late

1930s, the situation showed some signs of improvement, both as a result of new legislation (notably the 1936 Midwives Act which required local authorities to establish a salaried midwifery service), the introduction of powerful new drugs (sulphonamides) to tackle infection, and belated measures on the part of local and central government to provide more services and greater financial and material assistance to necessitous mothers. Such changes, however, would not have been achieved without the tireless campaigning and behind-the-scenes work of many unsung Welsh heroines. It was largely thanks to the unstinting work and efforts of female councillors, charity workers and campaigners that during the 1940s, pregnancy and childbirth became occasions to be celebrated rather than feared.

Notes

[1] *Western Mail*, 29 March 1935.
[2] See, for example, C. L. Mowatt, *Britain Between the Wars 1918–1940* (2nd edn, London, 1968).
[3] Irvine Loudon, *The Tragedy of Childbed Fever* (Oxford, 2000), p. 192.
[4] *Hansard*, HC (Series 5), vol. 325, col. 755 (18 June 1937).
[5] Ministry of Health, *Report on Maternal Mortality in Wales*, PP 1936–7 (XI, Cmd. 5423), p. 18.
[6] See, Mari A. Williams, '"In the wars": Wales 1914–1945', in Gareth Elwyn Jones and Dai Smith (eds), *The People of Wales* (Llandysul, 1999), pp. 179–206.
[7] See the evidence of Elizabeth Andrews, the Labour Party's women's organizer in Wales from 1919, who campaigned tirelessly to establish maternity and child welfare clinics in the Rhondda and elsewhere, in Elizabeth Andrews, *A Woman's Work is Never Done* (Ystrad Rhondda, 1956), pp. 30–1.
[8] G. F. McCleary, *The Maternity and Child Welfare Movement* (London, 1935), p. 168.
[9] Alison Macfarlane and Miranda Mugford, *Birth Counts: Statistics of Pregnancy and Childbirth* (London, 1984).
[10] Deirdre Beddoe, *Out of the Shadows: A History of Women in Twentieth-Century Wales* (Cardiff, 2000), p. 93.
[11] See, for example, Labour Committee of Inquiry, *The Distress in South Wales: Health of Mothers and Babies Imperilled* (London, 1928); D. Llywelyn-Williams, *Cyflwr Iechyd yng Nghymru* (Wrexham, 1930); The Pilgrim Trust, *Interim Reports of Unemployment Inquiry*, no. IV, H. W. Singer, 'Unemployment and Health' (London, 1937); idem, *Men Without Work* (Cambridge, 1938); also Jacqueline Jenkinson, *Scotland's Health 1919–1948* (Bern/Oxford, 2002), pp. 188–208 for a discussion of the Scottish maternal mortality problem during the inter-war years.

'THE GROWING TOLL OF MOTHERHOOD' 139

12 Janet M. Campbell, *Maternal Mortality* (London, 1924); Ministry of Health, *Interim Report of the Departmental Committee on Maternal Mortality* (London, 1930); idem, *Final Report of the Departmental Committee on Maternal Mortality and Morbidity* (London, 1932); Ministry of Health, *Report on Maternal Mortality in Wales*.
13 Political and Economic Planning (PEP), *Report on the British Health Services: A Survey of the Existing Health Services in Great Britain with Proposals for Future Development* (London, 1937), p. 96.
14 *Annual Report of the Carmarthenshire Medical Officer of Health, 1932* (Llanelly, 1933), p. 71.
15 *Annual Report of the Carmarthenshire Medical Officer of Health, 1937* (Carmarthen, 1938), p. 6.
16 National Library of Wales (NLW), Welsh Board of Health Collection, *Annual Report of the Aberdare UDC Medical Officer of Health and School Medical Officer of Health, 1924*, p. 75.
17 *Annual Report of the Glamorgan Medical Officer of Health, 1925* (Cardiff, 1926), p. 20. Similar points were also made by several local health officials in the Welsh rural areas; for example, writing in 1923, the Medical Officer of Health for the Llandysul Rural District Council noted that antenatal services were ignored by local women 'mainly owing to ignorance and indifference, and occasionally from a false sense of modesty'. NLW, Welsh Board of Health Collection, *Annual Report of the Llandysul RDC Medical Officer of Health, 1923*.
18 See Nicky Leap and Billie Hunter, *The Midwife's Tale: An Oral History from Handywoman to Professional Midwife* (London, 1993).
19 McCleary, *The Maternity and Child Welfare Movement*, p. 155.
20 For example, in the parish of St Asaph, Denbighshire, which was described as a 'very mountainous and scattered' area where 'roads were almost impassable in winter', district nurses undertook a great deal of midwifery work and were called upon to travel long distances, usually on bicycles. *Denbighshire Free Press*, 6 August 1932.
21 Such was the case in many parts of Carmarthenshire and Radnor throughout the 1920s.
22 NLW, Welsh Board of Health Collection, *Annual Report of the Newtown and Llanidloes RDC Medical Officer of Health, 1927*.
23 *Annual Report of the Carnarvonshire Medical Officer of Health, 1920* (Carnarvon, 1921), p. 39.
24 *Quarterly Report of the Carmarthenshire Medical Officer of Health, July 1929* (Llanelly, 1929), p. 6.
25 For example, in the opinion of Gilbert I. Strachan (professor of Obstetrics and Gynaecology, Welsh National School of Medicine, Cardiff), 'meddlesome midwifery' was the 'most important single cause of puerperal sepsis'. *The Lancet*, 30 November 1935, 1255.
26 *Y Genedl Gymreig*, 7 November 1932.
27 *Annual Report of the Medical Officer of Health for the year 1938* (Brecon, 1939), p. 19.

28 Ibid.
29 *Report on Maternal Mortality in Wales*, p. 37.
30 *Rhondda Gazette*, 16 February 1935.
31 *Monmouthshire County Council, Report upon Maternity and Child Welfare for the year 1921* (Newport, 1922), p. 17.
32 Ministry of Health, *Report of the Committee of Inquiry into the Anti-Tuberculosis Service in Wales and Monmouthshire* (London, 1939).
33 Ibid., p. 153.
34 *Aberdare Leader*, 20 February 1937. For a similar viewpoint, see the autobiographical account of Walter Haydn Davies, *The Right Place, The Right Time* (Swansea, 1975).
35 See Neil Evans and Dot Jones, '"A blessing for the miner's wife": the campaign for pithead baths in the south Wales coalfield, 1908–1950', *Llafur*, Vol. 6, no. 3 (1994), 5–28.
36 Dot Jones, 'Counting the cost of coal: women's lives in the Rhondda, 1881–1911', in Angela V. John (ed.), *Our Mothers' Land: Chapters in Welsh Women's History 1830–1939* (Cardiff, 1991), pp. 109–33.
37 *Annual Report of the Llandysul RDC Medical Officer of Health for the year 1923* (Llandysul, 1924).
38 Margery Spring Rice, *Working-Class Wives: Their Health and Conditions* (Harmondsworth, 1939).
39 Marion Phillips, *Women and the Miners' Lock-out: The Story of the Women's Committee for the Relief of Miners' Wives and Children* (London, 1927), p. 73.
40 *Report on Maternal Mortality in Wales*, p. 68.
41 *Annual Report of the Glamorgan Medical Officer of Health, 1929* (Cardiff, 1930), p. 16.
42 NLW, Welsh Board of Health Collection, *Annual Report of the Rhondda Medical Officer of Health for the year 1932*, p. 24. See also the comments of the following: Monmouthshire Medical Officer of Health, *Maternity and Child Welfare* (May 1917), p. 229; *Annual Report of the Rhondda Medical Officer of Health for the year 1920*, p. 22; the comments of the Glamorgan Medical Officer of Health, *Western Mail*, 11 December 1926; and *Annual Report of the Rhondda Medical Officer of Health for the year 1930*, p. 25; *Annual Report of the Carmarthenshire Medical Officer of Health, 1933* (Llanelly, 1934), p. 7.
43 See Beatrice Wood, *Wednesday's Child: An Autobiography* (Port Talbot, 1989), p. 50; Eileen Baker, '*Yan Boogie': The Autobiography of a Swansea Valley Girl* (Johannesburg, 1992), p. 49; Carol White and Sian Rhiannon Williams (eds), *Struggle or Starve: Women's Lives in the South Wales Valleys between the Two World Wars* (Dinas Powys, 1998).
44 *Aberdare Leader*, 1 August 1936.
45 *Western Mail*, 13 June 1936.
46 *Glamorgan Free Press*, 26 August 1921.
47 For example, D. Arthur Hughes, the Medical Officer of Health for Carmarthenshire, and D. Rocyn Jones, the Medical Officer of Health for Monmouthshire, were both vehemently opposed to the establishment of birth control clinics. For a more detailed examination of this issue, see Kate Fisher,

'"Clearing up misconceptions": the campaign to set up birth control clinics in south Wales between the wars', *Welsh History Review*, vol. 19, no. 1 (1998), 103–29; Margaret Douglas, 'Women, God and birth control: the first hospital birth control clinic, Abertillery 1925', *Llafur*, Vol. 6, no. 4 (1995), 110–22.

48 *Rhondda Gazette*, 20 March 1926.
49 *Aberdare Leader*, 3 April 1926; *Western Mail*, 11 December 1926.
50 *Rhondda Gazette*, 16 February 1935.
51 *Glamorgan Free Press and Rhondda Leader*, 7 June 1930. The clinic was taken over by the Pontypridd Urban District Council in 1933.
52 *Rhondda Gazette*, 27 October and 15 December 1934; *Annual Report of the Rhondda Medical Officer of Health, 1935*, p. 44.
53 D. Rocyn Jones, 'Public health in Wales: a survey', *Welsh Review*, Vol. 1, no. 1 (1939), 23.
54 *British Medical Journal*, 26 January 1935, p. 175; *Western Mail*, 2 February, 22 and 23 July 1935.
55 *Western Mail*, 8 February 1935.
56 The Pilgrim Trust, *Interim Reports of Unemployment Inquiry*, no. IV; H. W. Singer, 'Unemployment and Health', p. 12.
57 *Western Mail*, 29 March 1935.
58 Ministry of Health, *Report of the Committee of Inquiry into the Anti-Tuberculosis Service in Wales and Monmouthshire*, pp. 24–5; Carnarvonshire County Council, *Annual Report of the County Medical Officer of Health for the year 1938* (Carnarvon, 1939), p. 49.
59 See, for example, the comments of the following Medical Officers of Health: County of Anglesey, *Annual Report of the Medical Officer of Health for the year 1930* (Llangefni, 1931), p. 7; report of the Maesteg Medical Officer of Health, *Glamorgan Gazette*, 4 October 1935; report of the Caerphilly Medical Officer of Health, *Rhondda Gazette*, 8 October 1938; Carnarvonshire County Council, *Annual Report of the County Medical Officer of Health for the year 1938* (Carnarvon, 1939), p. 11; report of the Vaynor and Penderyn Medical Officer of Health, *Merthyr Express*, 2 September 1939.
60 Such was the opinion expressed by local Medical Officers of Health at Maesteg, Mountain Ash, Caerphilly, Vaynor and Penderyn between 1935 and 1938.
61 Carnarvonshire County Council, *Annual Report of the County Medical Officer of Health for the year 1938*, p. 49.
62 Ministry of Health, *Annual Report of the Chief Medical Officer of Health for the year 1928* (London, 1928), p. 246; Maesteg UDC, *Annual Report of the Medical Officer of Health for the year 1926* (Maesteg, 1926).
63 *Caernarvon and Denbigh Herald*, 29 January 1932.
64 Llandysul RDC, *Annual Report of the Medical Officer of Health for the year 1928* (Llandysul, 1929).
65 Llandysul RDC, *Annual Report of the Medical Officer of Health for the year 1924* (Llandysul, 1925); NLW, Welsh Board of Health Collection, 'Report on the health and sanitary condition of the Cardigan rural district' by Dr T. W. Wade, July 1925 in *Annual Report of the Cardigan Medical Officer of Health*,

1925; *Y Genedl Gymreig*, 7 November 1932; *Annual Report of the Medical Officer of Health of the Merioneth County Council for the year 1933* (Dolgelley, 1934), p. 89.

66 *Report on Maternal Mortality in Wales*, pp. 92, 94.

67 Cited in Charles Webster, 'Healthy or hungry thirties?', *History Workshop Journal*, Vol. 13 (Spring 1982), 118.

68 For further details regarding the National Birthday Trust campaign in the Rhondda, see Lady Williams, 'Malnutrition as a cause of maternal mortality', *Public Health* (October 1936), 11–19; Mari A. Williams, 'Yr ymgyrch i "achub y mamau" yng nghymoedd diwydiannol de Cymru, 1918–1939' in Geraint H. Jenkins (ed.), *Cof Cenedl XI: Ysgrifau ar Hanes Cymru* (Llandysul, 1996), pp. 117–46; A. Susan Williams, *Women and Childbirth in the Twentieth Century: A History of the National Birthday Trust Fund 1928–93* (Stroud, 1997).

69 PEP, *Report on the British Health Services*, p. 99.

70 For a detailed discussion of these issues, see Loudon, *The Tragedy of Childbed Fever*; idem, 'Some international features of maternal mortality, 1880–1950', in Valerie Fildes, Lara Marks and Hilary Marland (eds), *Women and Children First: International Maternal and Infant Welfare, 1870–1945* (Oxford, 1992), pp. 5–28.

5

'Teach the Miners Birth Control':[1] The Delivery of Contraceptive Advice in South Wales, 1918–1950

KATE FISHER

The first municipally run birth control clinic in Britain was opened in Abertillery, south Wales, in 1926. Local authorities were barred from providing birth control information until 1930, but in 1925, the Abertillery and District Hospital capitalized on a little known clause in the 1912 Maternity Act which allowed birth control advice to be given in hospitals. It was the only hospital in the country to take advantage of this loophole.

However, the clinic was short-lived. At first it was very popular. Nurse Naomi Jones wrote:

> You will be delighted to hear we had a glorious success on the 15th at the opening of our new department at the Hospital quite a crowd came ... we did not close until 1.50 p.m. and then the maid had to fetch me for lunch. Too funny really about 20 mothers asked if they might come on Monday morning to be fitted up. I had to explain I could not possibly see to so many in one morning.[2]

Nine months later, however, the birth control clinic was much less popular: 'very few attend to my disgust. I cannot think what steps to take to try and induce women to attend.' A further seven months later Nurse Jones wrote once more having 'decided to leave Abertillery and take up nursing again. I am sorry really. It seems useless remaining here after the huge effort I have made in trying to educate the working mothers to no avail.'[3] It is unclear why the clinic was so short-lived, closing within a year of opening. Writing in 1937, Marie Stopes claimed it was 'killed by gossip, the women who went there were gossiped about' and Nurse Jones blamed the 'Welsh religious element'. Direct evidence of this opposition is more difficult to find. The Welsh wing of the Anglican Church made no comment on birth control during this period. However, Welsh bishops were present at the 1930 Lambeth Conference which cautiously, and with many reservations, sanctioned birth control.[4] The free churches' official line was that birth control was a matter of individual conscience. In practice, the Abertillery Free Church Council in 1925 passed a resolution opposing the opening of the clinic and local preachers may well have used the pulpit to oppose the clinic. Most strikingly, upon its opening, Revd Ivor Evans, the local Nonconformist preacher, wrote 10,000 words of protest to the local paper, the *South Wales Gazette.* Yet the strength of his protest should not blind us to the fact that his was a lone voice in the documentary archives. His exchange of correspondence in the press with Ivor Griffiths, secretary of the clinic, did not spark any contributions from any other readers.

Moreover, there is also reason to suspect that birth control activists retrospectively exaggerated the degree of opposition that they had faced. Joyce Daniel, who helped set up fourteen clinics in south Wales between 1930 and 1939, stressed the extraordinary resistance she encountered, both from the general public and the councils she lobbied.[5] In a later interview with the *Western Mail* she explained: 'There was no ground gained without a fight ... The attitudes were quite incredible. I'll never forget one woman who wrote and said, "How can you mention such a subject in a world where daffodils blow?"'[6] 'A storm of opposition' she claimed greeted the opening of a clinic in Pontypridd, with letters written to the local papers 'calling us "a band of misguided females"'.[7] However, only one Catholic woman, Hilda Porcher, wrote to the local newspaper, calling the campaigners 'absolutely wrong, psychologically, religiously and morally'.[8]

A striking example of the exaggeration of the opposition to birth control is the case of the burning of the Marie Stopes caravan clinic, which toured Wales between May 1929 and June 1930.[9] Joyce Daniel reported that 'the Welsh people set fire' to the caravan in a retrospective of her work in Wales in *Family Planning* in July 1964.[10] The story is repeated in a 'History of Family Planning in Wales' published in the Glamorgan GPs' newsletter, though the source was probably Joyce

Daniel.[11] Perhaps more independently, however, Dr Evelyn Fisher, a doctor who moved from south Wales in 1928 and worked for many years at the Marie Stopes clinic in Holloway, also reported that it was burnt down.[12] However, no newspapers mentioned the caravan being 'set alight by an angry crowd'.[13] Neither did Marie Stopes, and this is particularly significant as she was never shy of publicizing the misfortunes and injustices she suffered, and her journal, *Birth Control News*, reported every minor happening at the caravan clinics. Clearer evidence comes from the correspondence between Marie Stopes and the nurses in charge of the caravan. These letters provide a complete itinerary and weekly report of the caravan and, from these, it seems quite clear that the caravan did not in fact burn down in Wales, though it was vandalized and ransacked in Tredegar in 1930. Very little was taken and it was thought to have been the action of one of the 'gangs of unemployed youths'.[14] The caravan was burnt down in Bradford.[15] It seems that we have evidence of the creation of a modern myth. It is possible that Joyce Daniel remembered that something happened to the caravan in Wales and also that it was burnt down and, in retrospect, conflated the two incidents.

It is important not to discount such stories as false or as highlighting the problems with retrospective analysis and memory. Rather, the false account of the burning of the caravan in south Wales perhaps reveals an underlying historical reality obscured by the facts of the matter. The telling of certain stories including (or especially) fictionalized ones is plausibly indicative of palpable social antagonism, of opposition that was subtle and indirect, that resulted, for example, in minor skirmishes which do not find record in remaining documents. While there may not have been direct sabotage of clinics or large-scale organized objections in south Wales, hostility was nonetheless persistent and powerful. In seeking to illustrate the problems experienced in establishing birth control clinics, campaigners retrospectively adapted and manipulated their narratives. However, such stories reveal the extent to which evidence of attitudes towards birth control and the problems faced by some birth control clinics have not made it into the historical record. The true extent of opposition to birth control clinics is not tangibly revealed through documentary sources because discussion of the rights and wrongs of birth control would largely have occurred in oral and not written contexts.

The documentary source material on the impact and success of birth control clinics is limited.[16] Little actual clinic data or case records remain and reports on the running of clinics frequently feature colourful incidents rather than typical cases. There are very few follow-up studies of clinics, thus it is even more difficult to ascertain what happened to patients in the years following a clinic visit.[17] Finally, such data tell us little about the attitudes of those unaware of birth control clinics, or those who were unwilling to attend. The great advantage of oral history is that it allows these silent voices and wider contexts to be revealed. Much of the evidence in this paper will be drawn from interviews conducted between 1993 and 1995 with fifty-nine people in south Wales about various aspects of family, contraceptive use, knowledge and attitudes. Forty-one were women, and eighteen were men.[18]

It will be argued that reluctance to take advantage of the reproductive technology available at birth control clinics was significant, but took a form which clinic campaigners rarely acknowledged or documented. Evidence suggests that while clinics were appreciated by a number of the working-class women targeted, the failure rate was significant as was general antagonism to clinics and the methods they promoted. It will be argued that a number of key principles held by clinic campaigners were at odds with the attitudes towards family planning common in working-class communities. These were not primarily the religious or moral objections to interfering with procreation, as frequently claimed by campaigners. Rather, alternative methods of birth control were chosen by working-class respondents in Wales as more suited to their own contraceptive aims, desires and preferences. This testimony draws attention to the continued preferences for 'traditional' methods of birth control, notably withdrawal, contrary to the family planning, sex and marriage guidance advice of the period.

'Wales presents ... very special need for our movement'[19]

South Wales had a high profile in the literature of inter-war birth control campaigners. There were a number of groups and organizations agitating for birth control information to be more freely available, from a number of different ideological standpoints. Birth control information, particularly for the working classes, was variously advocated as a solution to poverty, overpopulation, racial degeneration or maternal and infant morbidity and mortality. For all birth control campaigners, south Wales, seen as paradigmatic of deprivation in Britain, epitomized the need for municipal birth control clinics. Yet, most of the discussion of south Wales used the situation in the mining valleys simply as propaganda to impress upon the government the need for municipal clinics run as part of local authorities' maternity and child-welfare services. During the 1920s, there were only a few concerted efforts to provide practical birth control assistance for Welsh women.[20]

The strategy of birth control campaigners and the distribution of clinics in south Wales changed, however, after 1930, when the government issued Memo 153/MCW which stipulated that local authorities were permitted (but not mandated) to provide birth control advice in 'cases where further pregnancy would be detrimental to health'.[21] The main focus of the birth control movement shifted from the national to the local; the main aim became to persuade local authorities to implement the new government directive, and south Wales was one of the areas particularly targeted by the newly formed National Birth Control Council (later the National Birth Control Association) which was an amalgamation of various birth control organizations. The NBCA appointed Joyce Daniel, who had been instrumental in setting up the Pontypridd clinic, as Area Organizer for south Wales. She proved to be exceptionally active and dedicated. The executive committee minutes of the NBCA frequently noted the amount of unpaid overtime she put in. She tirelessly approached councils and lobbied Medical Officers of Health, health committees and maternity committees in the attempt to persuade local authorities to set up birth control clinics alongside their maternity and child-welfare clinics, frequently revisiting areas where she did not meet with immediate success. It was easy for local authorities to ignore birth control especially given that the government did not initially publish the new Memorandum, supplying copies only to authorities that asked for it.[22] Joyce Daniel thus forced those authorities who were either unaware of their new powers or reluctant to implement them to discuss the establishment of birth control clinics. Her achievements were impressive.[23] In September 1932, after only two years' activity, Joyce Daniel reported that she had succeeded in getting eight clinics established. By 1939 fourteen local authorities had set up clinics (Aberdare, Barry, Caerphilly, Gelligaer, Llanelli, Llantrisant and Llantwit Fadre,

Mountain Ash, Ogmore and Garw, Pontardawe, Pontypridd, Port Talbot and Rhondda); Maesteg was in the process of setting up a clinic, Glycorrwg Urban District Council had made arrangements to send women to the clinic at Pontypridd while financially desperate Merthyr had opened a clinic in cooperation with the NBCA. A private clinic was set up by the NBCA in Pontypool as the Monmouthshire County Medical Officer refused to set up any birth control clinics in the county. Marie Stopes, having left the NBCA, set up her own private clinic, in a run-down area of Cardiff – Splott – in 1937.

'"The men" should be talked to'[24]

All early birth control clinics and most family planning initiatives reflected the dominant assumption that successful family limitation was generally initiated and maintained by women. Marie Stopes's Committee for Constructive Birth Control reported in *Birth Control News* its conviction that 'where possible the wife should be properly fitted at a Clinic with the contraceptive best for her own use'.[25] This determination to provide family limitation advice to women rather than men has had a crucial influence on the promotion in fertility literature of female methods of birth control, especially caps, pessaries, diaphragms (and later the pill), all of which might be used without the knowledge of the husband. Indeed, clinics presented themselves as battling against men, and their propaganda portrayed them almost as refuges where women who had been mistreated by either male doctors or husbands could go. Such stories of suffering were prominent in clinic literature. The Cardiff clinic reported cases such as:

> Mrs ——, who between 1934 & 1937 had 5 pregnancies: 1 miscarriage, 2 premature, 2 full term. 'Husband suffering from V.D. refused treatment. Contracted by wife who is a wreck! One child lost an eye & another saved only by hospital treatment. Husband refuses to limit this pitiful family. Wife came here feeling desperate.'[26]

Although many women benefited from this approach, such as Mrs James, who said on leaving the Splott clinic, 'Thank God, I can keep myself safe now and not have to trust to him',[27] there is reason to believe that this anti-male stance may have deterred other women from attending, and done nothing to encourage husbands to send their wives. The evidence of unfortunate women who did not have cooperative husbands should be interpreted not simply as evidence of women's desire and need for methods of contraception that did not require male cooperation, but also as evidence of the widespread assumption that a husband's expected role was to take the initiative with regard to contraceptive use. The horror expressed at these cases can also be read as implying that most men were generally expected to take a more proactive role. It was perhaps only the minority of women who, unable to rely on their husbands to take responsibility for contraception, turned to birth control clinics as a last resort.

Evidence suggests that men frequently played a significant role in finding out about clinics and encouraging wives to attend or even coming to the clinic with them. Eva's husband heard about the Stopes Cardiff clinic at work: 'when they were having meal breaks ... they would talk about the babies ... And he came home one day, full of excitement, he said, "well I understand that there's a family planning clinic out in Splott."'[28] Nurse Gordon was surprised by the interest expressed by men when she attended a public meeting to advertise the Cardiff clinic in 1938: 'The men seemed equally anxious to take our slips, many asked for them after we had got inside the Hall.' One man turned up at the Cardiff clinic with his wife: 'A man brought his wife here for advice, he had been using sheaths but she did not like them.'[29] Indeed, some men appear to have been far more interested in the issue of birth control than their wives. Mrs Cosker, for example, who attended the caravan clinic when it was stationed in Treorchy had been 'too nervous' to use the sponge provided but resolved to try again because 'her husband wished her to do so'.[30]

Clinic staff did not always welcome enquiries from husbands, and men who tried to get advice were frequently turned away and invited to send their wives instead. While the caravan clinic was stationed in Swansea in April and May 1929, Nurse Williams reported having been 'besieged ... by husbands' wanting information for their wives who 'didn't want to be seen coming to the caravan', and certainly not during daylight hours. She 'of course...told them I would be very pleased to help their wives if they would visit the caravan and gave them the hours'.[31] Similarly, when in 1943 a man went to the Cardiff clinic seeking advice, the nurse commented that there was little she could do unless his wife attended, which he doubted she would: 'I asked him to get his wife to come in and have a talk with me, but he does not think she will. I let him have some sheaths & solubles and gave him some literature for her to read, which was about all I could do.'[32]

Oral testimony suggests that husbands played a very significant role in all aspects of contraceptive use: in initiating discussions about birth control, in determining which methods to use, in finding out about methods, obtaining any appliances used, in making sexual advances and in deciding how frequently contraception would be employed.[33] The vast majority (both women and men) of those interviewed asserted that men were expected to take responsibility for birth control. Women played down their involvement in birth control decisions and frequently presented such action as having been 'up to their husbands'. Ernest, for example, was adamant that it was 'the man's duty':

> Oh well, we used, we used to use the err french letters we used to call 'em, I don't know, what's the official thing call? What was the expression? Sheaths. The sheath, that's right. It was the man's option ... It was the man, it was the man's job.[34]

Doris was also typical in emphasizing her husband's role:

> *So what did you use, in order not to get pregnant, during those 12 years?*
> Oh, he used something. Not me.
> *What did he use?*
> Well, the usual, whatever you call 'em, french letters we used to call them.
> *And where did you first find out about those?*
> Oh, that was up to him ... oh, men knew all about those things long before they got married, don't worry.

She later revealed that she had, in fact, used a female method, but she preferred leaving it to her husband:

> Yeah, I did use some sort of pessary in the beginning. I forget what they were, so long ago. Gosh. But um, he started using something then, see, didn't bother.
> *So which did you prefer, you preferred french letters to pessaries?*
> Oh, yeah.
> *And why was that?*
> I thought it was safer. He had all the stuff then, I didn't [laughs].

Such a woman would not have been easily wooed by birth control clinics which wanted women to take control of their own fertility. Indeed, she attested that she had not been interested in attending her local clinic, because she and her husband 'just used our own methods'.[35] Clinic methods demanded that women challenge male responsibility for the regulation of sexual behaviour. Moreover, such a challenge also required her to subvert traditional sexual roles and anticipate or prepare for sexual activity instead of responding to male initiative. Clinics' requirement that women upset traditional gender roles was one of the clearest reasons why many women rejected birth control clinics and the methods they promoted. Clinic records frequently reveal women's dislike of female methods and their preference for male ones, such as Mrs Burgess who abandoned her sponge because she 'felt quite safe using "coitus int" as husband is very careful'; or Mrs Jones whose 'husband objects' to the sponge and 'prefers coit.int'.[36]

'Feels nervous for fear of failure'[37]

Clinic campaigners felt that one great advantage of clinic methods was their technological superiority. Clinics sought to provide 'medical' methods of birth control in a clinical environment. Ostensibly, the interior of the clinic was also carefully constructed to put patients at their ease.[38] Marie Stopes instructed her nurses to 'rub in the homely atmosphere' when informing others of the clinics and all clinics were decorated to her specifications; even the caravan clinic was painted in her favoured shade – 'botticelli blue' – and had printed curtains.[39] Yet, far more crucial was the medicalization of the environment. Clinics sought to be associated with professional health-care services and to be distinguished from what they saw as disreputable, quack, commercial outlets, rubber shops, hygienic stores and the like, and promoted scientific methods that were supposed to be far removed from traditional practices such as withdrawal and abortion. Most local authorities held their birth control clinic in Maternity and Child Welfare Centres thereby connecting birth control with municipal health services.[40] Private clinics were often hampered by their venues and generally had to find other ways of associating their clinics with professional medicine. Marie Stopes established a clinic in a house in a run-down residential area of Cardiff and her travelling caravan was set up wherever possible. Notice was given, for example, in May 1930 that its whereabouts were 'near the dirt track, Park Road, Tredegar'.[41] In such circumstances, clinics had to proclaim their clinical respectability. Inside the clinics was an array of medical equipment and uniformed staff whose qualifications were displayed.[42] Nurse Naomi Jones, of Abertillery, was clearly impressed with the apparatus in her clinic:

> I am very proud of my clinic everything so compact waiting room fitting room and sterilyzing [sic] room lavatory and w.c. all next door to each other, sinks, *two* in the fitting room hot and cold water, heated by electricity, polished floors as you know. The sweet picture Dr so kindly gave me I have framed and hung, also my two certificates.[43]

Most patients were provided with cervical caps: devices which were not easily available and required medical intervention to determine the size needed.[44] The importance of medical supervision of contraception was further promoted by the requirement that patients return for regular check-ups.

Caps were presented as safe, modern, medically tested and reliable. Nurse Daniels advertised the clinic she set up in 1924 in Cardiff as providing instruction 'which is absolutely reliable and is judged by the highest medical authorities to be the best known'.[45] Other methods, especially withdrawal, were denigrated as having severe physical and psychological side effects as well as being likely also to result in unwanted pregnancies.

Yet the medical environment did not necessarily convince clients of the dangers of traditional methods nor of the reliability of clinic appliances. Rather, health and safety fears dominated responses to clinics and framed many contraceptive choices. A number of people were suspicious about the efficacy of the devices provided by clinics and would not 'trust' them. Other common worries included fears that a cap or sponge would be impossible to remove or that it might be harmful. Evelyn Fisher, who worked at a Marie Stopes clinic in London, failed to get a clinic set up in south Wales in the late 1920s because she found 'the women were afraid to use' caps because the 'idea was totally new'.[46] Nurse Gordon found 'the prejudice against the use of Caps seems great', when trying to set up a clinic under the auspices of Marie Stopes in Swansea in the early 1940s: 'at every meeting the same questions are asked and repeated, the chief one is, don't caps cause cancer!'[47] Clinic workers found a number of patients like one woman who 'couldn't fancy the idea' or another who was 'too nervous to use sponge. I discussed things with her but failed to assure her.'[48] Similarly, Mrs Heard simply 'couldn't fancy the idea'.[49] As Lella Secor Florence also found, 'even after instruction at the Clinic, a patient will write in great anxiety to know whether it is possible for the pessary to get lost inside, or whether this or that story she has been told about the ill-effect of contraceptives is true'.[50] Similar dislikes and suspicions of unfamiliar new appliances were also revealed by interviewees. Leslie, for example, explained that his wife would not go to the clinic in Pontypridd that his sisters went to:

> Ooh, my wife never went any like that. Oh no, no, no. But she didn't believe in anything like that.
> *Why was that?*
> Oh well, she don't know, she didn't believe in it. Perhaps, I was so much of a dead nut against it, causing cancer, things like that.[51]

Such fears were, in fact, not alleviated by some clinic campaigners. Marie Stopes also declared that caps caused cancer, excepting her own 'pro-race' version, and frequently denigrated the appliance methods chosen at rival clinics as less efficacious or as positively harmful.[52] Doubts about the reliability and safety of methods were not confined to the suspicions of clinic clients, for whom information about such methods was relatively new. Dr Mizzen who worked at the Maternity and Welfare Clinic in Swansea resisted the establishment of a birth control clinic on the grounds that she did not 'believe caps are safe or reliable' or that 'women should be taught to fit caps themselves'.[53]

When assessing the impact of family planning services on users it is important to recognize that barrier methods of contraception are not self-evidently safe. Barrier methods, particularly pessaries, caps and diaphragms, were novel, tricky to learn how to use and worked according to a rather sophisticated principle. It was not obvious that a cap covered the necessary area, that it might not easily slip out of place or invite infection, or that the spermicidal cream that was used as an accompaniment would effectively kill sperm. The use of appliance methods required acceptance and understanding of their physiological effects. By contrast, withdrawal was an intuitively understandable and harmless 'natural' method. For many, withdrawal worked according to a simple, observable principle and seemed more reliable than an internal, unseen and unfelt barrier. Elizabeth is a good example:

> *Which do you prefer of those? [methods tried]*
> Withdraw, oh yes, you knew you were safe then, you know.[54] 'Cos it was a worrying time though they got protection.
> *So would you trust withdrawal more than caps?*
> Definitely, oh yes. Yeah.

Why was that?
I don't know, you felt safer, you know, not so messy, no.[55]

Moreover, the failure of an appliance method of birth control was understood quite differently from the failure of withdrawal. When pregnancy occurred despite the use of withdrawal such instances were predictable, expected 'slip ups'. They were not seen as a sign that the method itself had failed but rather that the user had made a mistake. Pregnancies were not therefore wholly unexpected. Nora used withdrawal so as 'not to have babies' but recalled that they 'missed many times'. She praised rather than condemned her husband's failure to use the method successfully, 'he was cooperative, only many times we slipped up. Never mind, he was good and we were happy'.[56] By contrast births accompanying the use of other methods of contraception were more likely to be seen as the fault of the appliance and not the user. That the risk of the pregnancy had not necessarily been apprised at the time (since the user would not automatically be aware of any problem with the method of contraception used) would make a resultant conception all the more surprising and unexpected. When respondents talked about the unreliability of withdrawal it was always in terms of user failure. The method itself was not perceived as risking pregnancy; rather it was the likelihood that one might fail to practise the method properly which was recognized.

For such couples withdrawal was a convenient and suitable method of reducing the frequency of conception while not preventing it altogether. It is a mistake to assume that those who use birth control are inevitably or primarily looking for a thoroughly reliable method of contraception. Henry explained that withdrawal was a suitable method of birth control for him and his wife (they also used condoms) as they were not aiming to prevent pregnancy but to limit their eventual family size to a reasonable number. Rather than planning births, or avoiding births, they were aiming to keep the total number of pregnancies 'in perspective'.

You were telling me about the size of your family and ...
No we just took things as we went, both of us, I think, never really planned anything, whatever was to come, we accepted it ... make your life around whatever your family turns out to be, that's the way Dee and I have taken it ...
But you were using contraceptives to try not to have too many?
Oh, well, I suppose, yes, yes, you were trying like not to, you know, just to have it and have as many as you can in that sense of it, you were trying to keep it in perspective like ...[57]

Many early providers of birth control advice were surprised by the trust placed in withdrawal. Lella Secor Florence thought that 'the amazing thing about *coitus interruptus* is the reliance which couples continue to place on it even after they have had a number of failures'.[58] Such comments indicate the enduring misconception about the role of withdrawal in the fertility-reduction strategies of working-class communities. Far from being unreliable or unsafe, its principle was obvious and occasional failures were expected and not necessarily unwanted.

'She was difficult to teach'[59]

Many women found cervical caps and sponges rather difficult to insert, and teaching patients to use them correctly proved a major difficulty.[60] Enid Charles's survey of contraceptive practice among primarily middle-class women found that the 'most frequent source of dissatisfaction' with the cap 'is fitting and adjusting'.[61] Marie Stopes rather uncharitably noted that 'there is always a percentage of extremely stupid and unreliable women whom it is difficult to instruct'.[62] In fact, her preferred method of birth control was the most complex available, required the most elaborate fitting procedure and, moreover, was, by the clinics' own reckoning, unsuitable for many. Sylvia Dawkins, a family planning doctor interviewed by Television History Workshop, explained the complex procedures of examination and the difficulties experienced in determining which method was suitable and finding the right size:

> If you gave a barrier method you had to instruct the people how to use it. You fitted them with, say a diaphragm, instructed them, asked them to go home and practise putting it in and out, come with it in, so that we could be sure they got it right, you see, and knew what they were doing. Then we gave them the cap, and we didn't on the first occasion because you couldn't fit them properly the first occasion, they were tense. When they'd come back with the cap in they were relaxed and you found the size wasn't anywhere near right.[63]

Those who had been physically affected by frequent pregnancy and/or poor gynaecological care found the cap most difficult to use. Clinic records are dotted with similar examples. One woman, for example, 'is very stout and found it awkward to place and remove sponge', while another 'was too tender to use a sponge' as she had been 'badly lacerated after severe labour and delivery'.[64] Gertrude, who attended a birth control clinic in Aberdare, was tried first with a cervical cap, which appears to have been entirely unsuitable despite the clinic's apparent determination to try and fit one:

> couldn't wear what the woman did, I couldn't hold it. I went, I don't know how many times they tried to fit me, and you had to go on the table and be examined and all that, see, before they would er. But I couldn't, I wasn't, I should have been stitched and I wasn't, so I couldn't hold it.[65]

Sometimes those who had problems inserting caps and sponges were given other methods, such as the sheath. Nurse Williams wrote to Marie Stopes while the caravan was stationed in Swansea in May 1929 that 'the uterine conditions of the mothers on the whole is not good. The sponge and the sheath being practically the only suitable methods.'[66] However, patients who found it difficult to insert female methods were expected to keep trying. Many were sent away, sometimes with written instructions, told to practise and come back for further instruction. Many lost patience, as Nurse Gordon found to her frustration: 'some of these women expect to be safe without the slightest effort on their own part'.[67]

Patients were also required to return for regular check-ups. It proved difficult to persuade many women that they needed continued medical supervision of their contraceptive practices (some women had to travel considerable distances to get to their nearest clinic). In north Kensington it was found that 'hundreds of them were never heard from after their first or second visits'.[68] Gertrude clearly illustrated the difficulties of keeping up regular attendance. To travel to the clinic involved a considerable journey, on foot, with children in tow. In addition, if she met anyone she knew in the waiting room she would leave.

> Oh, and we used to have to take the babies up to Aberdare to the clinic see, didn't have a place near 'ere, had to go, had to take the pram and walk up and back ...
> *Were there many people in the clinic?*
> Oh, there was a lot, well yes there'd be a lot there, but you'd be in a little room and they'd take all your notes, privately, you wouldn't be among those people and then you'd go in [the waiting room], and you wouldn't go back in there! You'd go home! ... I had the shock of my life when I seen this one woman [an acquaintance], and I went out and I tried to hide until she'd gone, 'cos I know she was there before me and of course you'd go in the waiting room, see.[69]

Even conscientious and content users found it difficult to keep attending. At first, Eva, who started going to Marie Stopes's clinic soon after it opened in 1937, would revisit regularly: 'every now and again – I would say, "well I've had this x amount of time do you think it's time I had a new one?"' However, she did not maintain this level of devotion to the regime and eventually stopped using the method in favour of another: 'after a while we stopped going [to the clinic] so often. I stopped using it after the war.'[70]

'It was too much trouble'[71]

Clinics also presented female methods as easy and convenient to use. For them, caps interfered least with the spontaneity of the sex act and had the least effect on the physical pleasures of sexual intercourse. Historians have continued to endorse this view.[72] The assumption here is that withdrawal was so intrinsically unsatisfactory that it should inevitably have fallen into disuse once more efficient and pleasurable methods became available. Evidence suggests, however, that a considerable number of those exposed to modern methods rejected them in favour of traditional ones, people like Mrs Jones who 'has not used sponge, threw it away. She and her husband are satisfied with coitus interruptus.'[73]

However, in assessing the relationship between birth control methods and sexual pleasures, we need to recognize that constructions of what is pleasurable and important about sex vary considerably and that there are no 'natural' or obvious responses to birth control methods.[74] Instead we have to examine the interaction between the changing constructions of sexual preferences and the connotations of various birth control methods in order to understand the dominance of withdrawal among those surveyed.

Caps were sometimes viewed as having had distinct disadvantages in terms of sexual enjoyment. The claim that they were easy and practical to use was frequently rejected. Mrs Jones of Maesteg, for example, reported that she would not 'bother with it' as it was 'too much trouble'. Birth control campaigners were exasperated to find women in 'a state of apathy ... many were too indifferent to make the effort'.[75] Enid Charles also found distaste for contraceptive devices among her respondents and a preference for coitus interruptus because it involved no trouble, preparation or expense.[76] Lella Secor

Florence also found that husbands 'do not seem to mind withdrawal – they prefer this method, with its freedom from preparation'.[77] The practicalities of using a female method of birth control meant that women had to anticipate or prepare for sex. Lella Secor Florence, for example, found in her clinic that many women were resistant to using caps because they were 'an unwomanly invitation to pleasures which are supposed to have been designed for her husband alone'.[78] Such an open embracing of sexual activity was clearly behind a number of respondents' dislike of birth control clinics and the methods they provided. Gwen was clearly very unhappy with the cap because she had to play a proactive role in sex. She had to prepare for intercourse and deal with the cap afterwards. Withdrawal was much more spontaneous and meant she could leave all consideration for birth control to her husband.

What was it like to use?
Well, it wasn't very, you know [pause] I don't like talking about it really, but you had to put it in so long, you know, you didn't have intercourse until you put it in – so long – and then take it out and all that business. It was horrible, really.
So what didn't you like about it? Was it,
I didn't like it at all. I don't [pause] I mean, we had been married two and a half years and didn't have any children, so, er, I thought it was quite safe anyway. Fortunately we never had any more anyway.
So what had you done during those two and a half years to try and not get pregnant?
No, I didn't try. I trusted him really. [laughs]
And what did you trust him to do? What did he do that?
Oh! [faintly, as if sharp intake of breath]
You see I don't really know.
Withdrawal they call it, don't they? [pause][79]

Integral to oral history respondents' construction of sexual pleasure was the idea that the experience should be uncontrived. The key positive words used to describe sex were 'spontaneous', 'normal' and 'natural'. Sex was to be engaged in when the mood emerged in the right circumstances and was framed as the result of ordinary desires. It was not to be routine, planned or predictable. Caps directly conflicted with such a construction of sexual pleasure. Gladys thought that Marie Stopes was unpopular because she advocated an 'unnatural' approach to the planning of families, reliant on artificial as opposed to natural methods of birth control.

'TEACH THE MINERS BIRTH CONTROL'   159

Had you ever heard of a woman called Marie Stopes?
Oh I heard about her, she was this c— birth control woman, wasn't she? She was very unpopular. Ah, I remember her, but er it was terrible thing what she was doing then. We were narrow minded ... people didn't believe in it then, no they believed in natural families ... she was very unpopular.[80]

Thus, for respondents who valued spontaneous and uncontrived sexual experiences, withdrawal had a clear advantage over methods advocated by birth control clinics. Not only was no technology involved, but equally significantly it was felt to be a method which required no prior knowledge, experience or education. Many respondents described withdrawal as a natural act, rather than a deliberate attempt to interfere with the natural process of conception.[81]

And how did you stop yourself getting pregnant when you didn't want any more children?
Didn't do anything. Just natural.[82]

Conclusion

This paper has highlighted the disjunction between the attitudes of those promoting female methods of birth control in clinics and of those in Wales they sought to help. Those setting up and running clinics were frequently surprised and disappointed by the low attendance and the failure of some who did attend to learn and use the clinics' preferred methods of birth control successfully. Three main factors dominated clinics' public assessment of the difficulties they faced: the perception that too few people knew about clinics; the expectation that appliances were expensive; and finally moral or religious disapproval of birth control in principle. A closer look at clinic records and at oral history testimony suggests that other factors were at least relevant if not more important in framing contraceptive choices and in fuelling dislike of the clinics and the methods they predominately advocated. Clinics rarely openly acknowledged such reactions, but across the UK several contemporary birth control advocates were surprised to find that even after exposure to scientific alternatives, patients preferred using withdrawal.[83] In Wales in 1930, of the 133 women who found a clinic nurse on their doorstep six months after having attended the Marie Stopes caravan clinic, 25 per cent admitted to having been unable or unwilling to use the method advised and to have abandoned it, usually in favour of withdrawal. Oral history similarly attests to the popularity of withdrawal, even among those who had access to other appliance methods, such as caps. Of those interviewed, almost all respondents used some form of birth control. Withdrawal was by far the most commonly used method, with 78 per cent practising it. There was significant evidence of use of other methods: 29 per cent used condoms, 16 per cent used pessaries. Only 11 per cent used caps obtained from birth control clinics. Moreover, most disliked their cap and either abandoned it, or only used it occasionally, continuing to rely primarily on other methods, predominantly withdrawal.

This paper has investigated the criteria by which birth control methods were judged. Many sought methods which were easy to use and understand; they found caps complex to fix, difficult to insert correctly, and worryingly novel. Others sought methods which required no preparation, either in obtaining the appliance or in the procedure required before or after sexual intercourse. For these people caps were extremely demanding in terms of time, effort and money. Finally and crucially, many appear to have favoured methods which left the responsibility, if not also the control, in the hands of the husband. The opinion held by clinic campaigners that female methods were bound to be more popular was based on the assumption that women, who tended to bear the brunt of the burdens of pregnancy, childbirth and childcare, cared more about contraception than men (this commonsense has also influenced leading histories of birth control during the twentieth century).[84] Yet, oral history testimony suggests not only that we need to revise this image of female-centred birth control choices and pay attention to the vital part played by the husband in contraceptive strategies, but also to recognize that attitudes towards methods were also affected by the gendered culture of contraception. One factor behind the reluctance of many to embrace female methods and the continuing popularity of withdrawal was the perception that withdrawal was a male method of contraception and a dislike by many, both women and men, of methods which actively involved women.[85] For men and women in south Wales, clinics' promotion of female methods of birth control and active exclusion of husbands from clinics was a further factor hampering their success. Far from being opposed to birth control in principle, as many clinic campaigners feared, many people in south Wales were content to continue with the contraceptive practices they already knew and understood.

Notes

1. *The New Generation*, Vol. 8, no. 1 (January 1929), p. 1.
2. Naomi Jones to Sister Roberts, 16 June 1925, from the Marie Stopes papers in the Contemporary Medical Archives Centre (CMAC is now known as Archives of Manuscripts (A&M) at the Wellcome Library for the History and Understanding of Medicine (hereafter A&M, PP/MCS/C.16) (All quotations are as found, no punctutation added, or spelling changed).
3. Naomi Jones to Marie Stopes, 23 February 1926, A&M, PP/MCS/C.16; Naomi Jones to Marie Stopes, 14 September 1926, A&M, PP/MCS/C.16.
4. I am grateful to Dr Gwynfor Jones for his assistance in researching the Church in Wales's attitude towards birth control.
5. Her letters reveal a self-conscious delight at being involved in such a 'rebel activity' (as she called it).
6. 'A Daniel who fought for a family plan', *Western Mail*, 12 October 1976, p. 4.
7. Joyce Daniel, 'The wind of change', *Family Planning*, July 1964, cutting in the Family Planning Archive in the Archives of Manuscripts at the Wellcome Library for the History and Understanding of Medicine (hereafter A&M, SA/FPA/A14/19).
8. *Pontypridd Observer*, 26 September 1931, p. 5. I have not, however, undertaken a comprehensive survey of Welsh newspapers for this period and may have missed significant evidence of the opposition to birth-control clinics.
9. 'Behind the scenes', *Birth Control News*, Vol. XVI, no. 5, December 1937, p. 54.
10. Daniel, 'The wind of change'.
11. Glamorgan County Council newsletter to GPs, 1974, A&M, SA/FPA/A11/61E.
12. Alan S. Parkes and Dee King, 'The mothers' clinic', *Journal of Biosocial Science*, Vol. 6 (1974), 177.
13. 'A Daniel who fought for a family plan', p. 4.
14. Ellen Williams to Marie Stopes, 20 May 1930, BL, Add MS 58622.
15. 'Arson replaces argument', *Birth Control News*, Vol. 8, no. 5 (January 1929), 1.
16. For an important study of such data see Deborah A. Cohen, 'Private lives in public spaces: Marie Stopes, the mothers' clinics and the practice of contraception', *History Workshop Journal*, Vol. 35 (March 1993), 95–116.
17. See for example Lella Secor Florence, *Birth Control on Trial* (London, 1930); Marie Stopes, *The First Five Thousand* (London, 1925); Norman E. Himes and Vera C. Himes, 'Birth control for the British working-classes. A study of the first thousand cases to visit an English birth control clinic', *Hospital Social Services*, Vol. 19 (1929), 578.
18. Three of these also took part in a group interview which included twelve other women who were not interviewed individually. Most were widows or widowers, but there were thirteen interviews with couples. Dates of birth ranged from 1899 to 1925 and dates of marriage from 1918 to 1941. A self-selected sample was avoided and people were largely found in informal settings such as day centres. There, reminiscence would be encouraged, friendships made with potential respondents and those who were interested – the vast majority – were

then visited at a later date in their own homes. Interviews lasted up to four hours.
[19] Stella Browne, 'How the fight goes', *The New Generation*, Vol. 9, no. 1 (January 1930), p. 5.
[20] A number of prominent birth control campaigners such as Stella Browne, Richard Pennifold, Marie Stopes and Frida Laski lectured on the theory and practice of birth control to large and receptive audiences. A few clinics were also established in the 1920s: a clinic opened in Abertillery and District Hospital in 1925, although it closed, probably in 1926; Marie Stopes's caravan clinic spent a year touring south Wales between May 1929 and June 1930, and in 1930 a clinic was opened in Pontypridd.
[21] Ministry of Health, *'Birth Control', Memo 153/MCW* (London, July 1930).
[22] See for example R. A. Soloway, *Birth Control and the Population Question in England, 1877–1937* (Chapel Hill, NC, 1982), p. 311.
[23] On the establishment of birth-control clinics in south Wales and the activities of Joyce Daniel see Kate Fisher, "Clearing up misconceptions': the campaign to set up birth control clinics in south Wales between the wars', *Welsh History Review*, Vol. 18, no. 1 (June 1998), 103–29.
[24] Nurse Fowles to Marie Stopes, October 1930, BL, Add MS 58622.
[25] *Birth Control News*, vol. 17, no. 3 (February, 1939), 35.
[26] Nurse Gordon to Marie Stopes, July 1939, BL, Add MS 58625.
[27] Ibid., 29 April 1938.
[28] Oral history interview with Eva, code: bc1#1. Interview tapes and transcripts are currently in the possession of the author.
[29] Nurse Gordon to Marie Stopes, 8 February 1938, BL, Add MS 58625.
[30] Nurse Fowles to Marie Stopes, 22 March, 1930, BL, Add MS 58622.
[31] Nurse Williams to Marie Stopes, 6 May 1929, BL, Add MS 58621.
[32] Nurse Angeleri to Marie Stopes, 29 October 1943, BL, Add MS 58626.
[33] See Kate Fisher, "She was quite satisfied with the arrangements I made': gender and birth control in Britain, 1925–50', *Past and Present*, Vol. 169 (2000), 161–93.
[34] Ernest, code: bc3sw#2.
[35] Doris, code: bc3sw#6.
[36] Nurse Fowles to Marie Stopes, March 1930, BL, Add MS 58622.
[37] Ibid.
[38] Cohen, 'Private lives in public spaces', 98–9.
[39] Ibid., p. 113, n. 8.
[40] One exception was Llanelli where, due to the Medical Officer of Health's objection to using the Maternity and Child Welfare Centre, a clinic was held on one floor of Llanelly House, the home of Lady Stepney, A&M, SA/FPA/A11/76.
[41] *Birth Control News*, Vol. 9, no. 1, May 1930, 10–11.
[42] Angus McLaren, *A History of Contraception from Antiquity to the Present Day* (Oxford, 1990), p. 231.
[43] Naomi Jones to Sister Roberts, 16 June 1935, A&M, PP/MCS/C.16.
[44] Cohen, 'Private lives in public spaces,' 105. For Marie Stopes's views and disputes with birth-control campaigners about caps, see June Rose, *Marie*

Stopes and the Sexual Revolution' (London, 1992), p. 145; Audrey Leathard, *The Fight for Family Planning* (London, 1980), p. 14.
45 *Daily Herald*, 1924, cutting in A&M, PP/MCs/C.15.
46 Parkes and King, 'The mothers' clinic', 168.
47 Nurse Gordon to Marie Stopes, 1943 (?), BL, Add MS 58632.
48 Nurse Fowles to Marie Stopes, follow-up visits, 22 March 1930, BL, Add MS 58622; Nurse Fowles to Marie Stopes, follow-up visits, 8 July 1930, BL, Add MS 58622.
49 Ibid., 22 March 1930, BL, Add MS 58622.
50 Florence, *Birth Control on Trial*, p. 144.
51 Leslie, code: bc3sw#1.
52 See Ruth Hall, *Marie Stopes. A Biography* (London, 1977), p. 260; Marie Stopes, *Contraception: Its Theory History and Practice* (London, first published 1923, reprinted 1932), pp. 168–206.
53 Joyce Daniel report to Margaret Pyke, 1934, A&M, SA/FPA/A11/76.
54 Gigi Santow has also argued that the safety of withdrawal is generally underestimated. Gigi Santow, '*Coitus interruptus* in the twentieth century', *Population and Development Review*, 19 (1993), 770–2.
55 Elizabeth, code: bc3sw#12.
56 Nora, code: bc2#1.
57 Henry and Dee, code: bc2#27.
58 Florence, *Birth Control on Trial*, p. 100.
59 Angeleri to Marie Stopes, 4 October, 1940, BL, Add MS 58626.
60 Cohen, 'Private lives in public spaces', 105.
61 Enid Charles, *The Practice of Birth Control. An Analysis of the Birth-Control Experiences of Nine Hundred Women* (London, 1932), p. 53.
62 Marie Stopes to Victor Roberts, 12 December 1924, A&M, PP/MCS/C.15.
63 Derek Jones and Sharon Goulds (eds), *In the Club? Birth Control This Century* (Television History Workshop in association with Channel Four, 1988). The original interview transcripts are available at the Wellcome Library for the History and Understanding of Medicine, A&M, GC/105/26.
64 Nurse Fowles to Marie Stopes, 10 January 1930, BL Add MS 58622; Nurse Fowles to Marie Stopes, follow-up visits, 22 March 1930, BL Add MS 58622.
65 Gertrude, code: bc3sw#27.
66 Nurse Williams to Marie Stopes, 6 May 1929, BL Add MS 58621.
67 Nurse Gordon to Marie Stopes, 21 December 1945, BL, Add MS 58633.
68 Himes and Himes, 'Birth control for the British working-classes', p. 610.
69 Gertrude, code: bc3sw#27
70 Eva, code: bc1#1.
71 Nurse Fowles to Marie Stopes, 10 January, 1930, BL Add MS 58622.
72 See for example Michael Mason, *The Making of Victorian Sexuality* (Oxford, 1994), pp. 59–60; Wally Seccombe, *Weathering the Storm. Working-Class Families from the Industrial Revolution to the Fertility Decline* (London, New York, 1993), p. 181.
73 Nurse Fowles to Marie Stopes, 10 January 1930, BL Add MS 58622.
74 See Barbara J. Risman and Pepper Schwartz (eds), *Gender in Intimate*

Relationships. A Micro Structural Approach, (Belmont, CA, 1989); Joshua Gamson, 'Rubber wars: struggles over the condom in the United States', *Journal of the History of Sexuality*, Vol. 1 (1990), 263.

[75] Daniel, 'The wind of change'.

[76] Charles, *The Practice of Birth Control*, p. 52.

[77] Florence, *Birth Control on Trial*, p. 102.

[78] Ibid., p. 68.

[79] Gwen, code: bc3sw#18

[80] Gladys, code bc3sw#28.

[81] This argument is developed fully in Kate Fisher and Simon Szreter, "They prefer withdrawal': the choice of birth control in Britain 1918–1950', *Journal of Interdisciplinary History*, Vol. 34, no. 2 (2003).

[82] Harriet, code: bc3sw#19.

[83] See Himes and Himes, 'Birth control for the British working-classes', 612 and Florence, *Birth Control on Trial,* for example pp. 97, 143, 157.

[84] Angus McLaren, for example, is convinced that 'women were more anxious than men to limit family size'; McLaren, *A History of Contraception*, p. 203, and Susan Cotts Watkins acknowledges the assumption: "My friends and I believed that women had more reason than men to be concerned with the consequences of childbearing, and we took it for granted that their husbands simply would not co-operate' in 'If all we knew about women was what we read in *Demography*, what would we know?', *Demography*, Vol. 30 (1993), 557. Similarly Gigi Santow has asked whether we 'are correct ... in believing that men are always less concerned than women with the limitation of their families'. Santow, '*Coitus Interruptus* in the twentieth century', 769.

[85] For an opposing analysis see Clare Davey, 'Birth control in Britain during the inter-war years: evidence from the Stopes correspondence', *Journal of Family History*, Vol. 13 (1988), 332–4, 338.

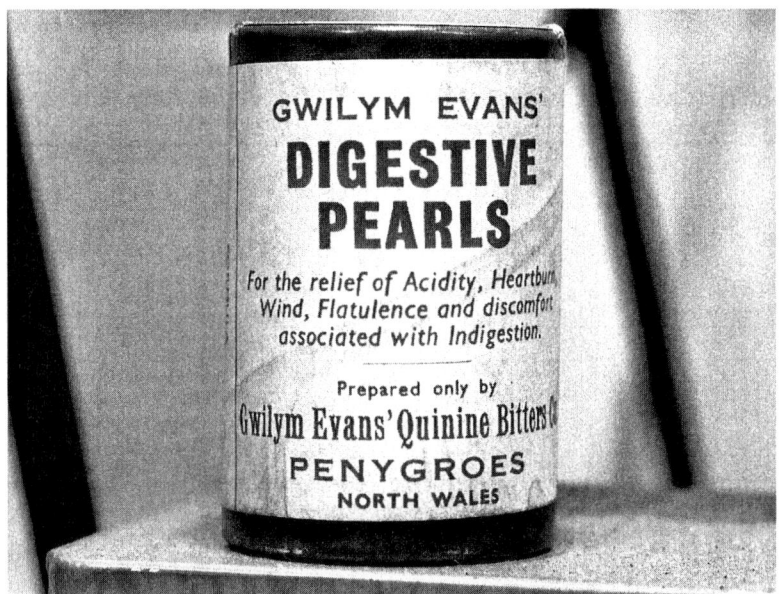

'The Penygroes Remedy' (photograph by Geoff Charles, permission NLW). Many proprietary remedies such as these 'Digestive Pearls' were produced locally in Wales between the wars and could be bought in village shops.

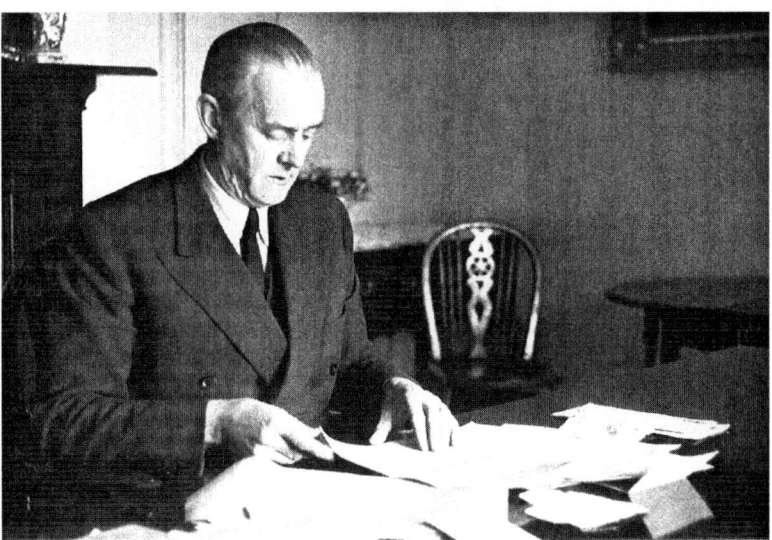

Mr Clement Davies at his desk at Plas Dyffryn (photograph by Geoff Charles, permission NLW).

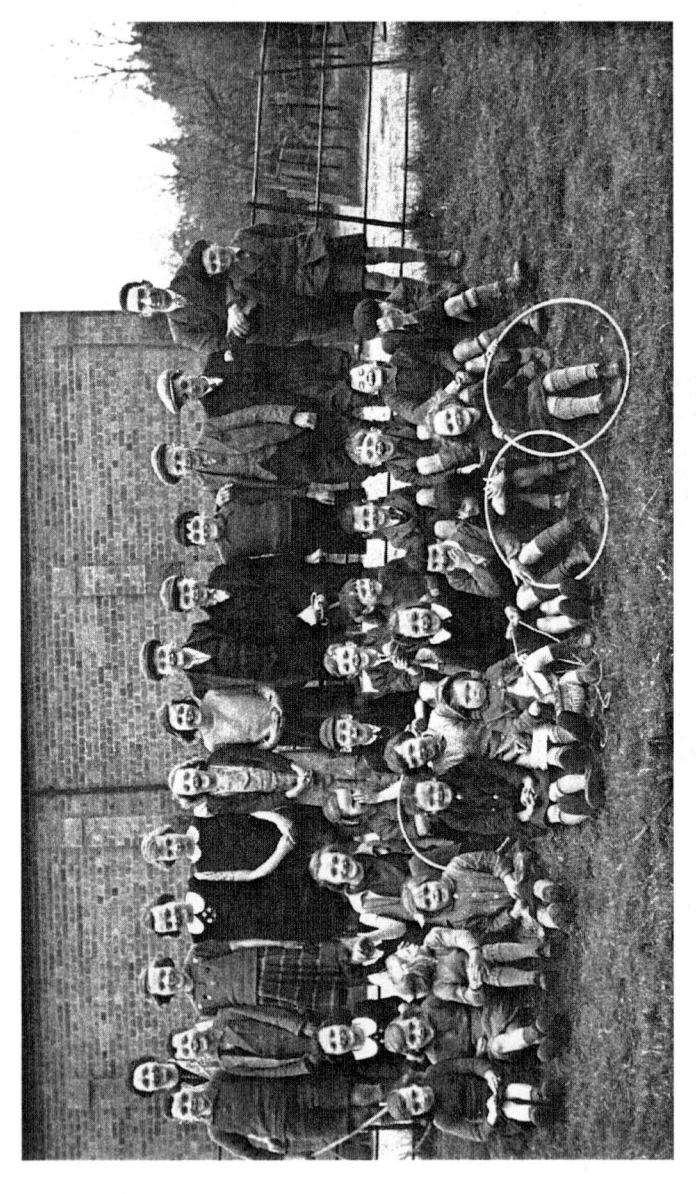

Children from Bettws Church of England school who had just been immunised against diptheria in May 1941 (photograph by Geoff Charles, permission NLW). The response rate from the scheme in Merionethshire was excellent, with 99.9% of children being immunised.

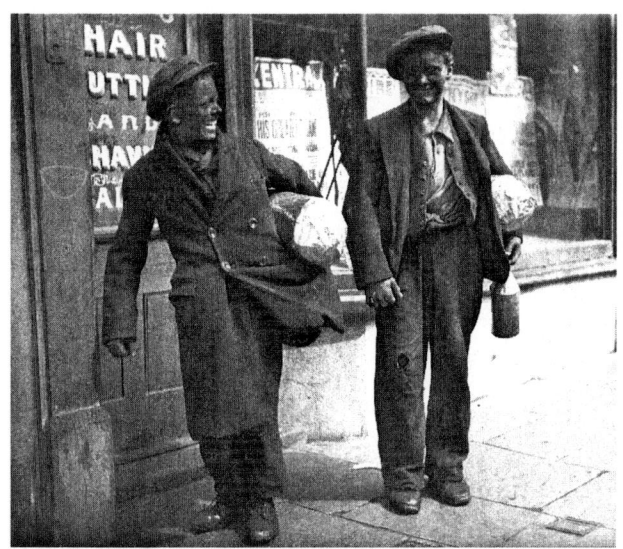

Young boys in south Wales started working in the coal mines as soon as they were old enough to leave school (photograph by Edith Tudor Hart c.1935, by kind permission of Wolf Suschitzky).

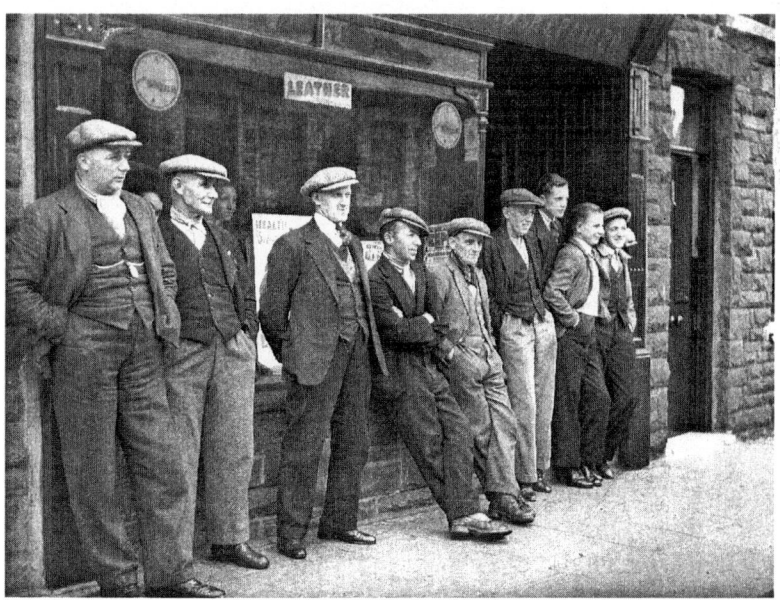

'Unemployed men in south Wales' (photograph by Edith Tudor Hart c.1935, by kind permission of Wolf Suschitzky).

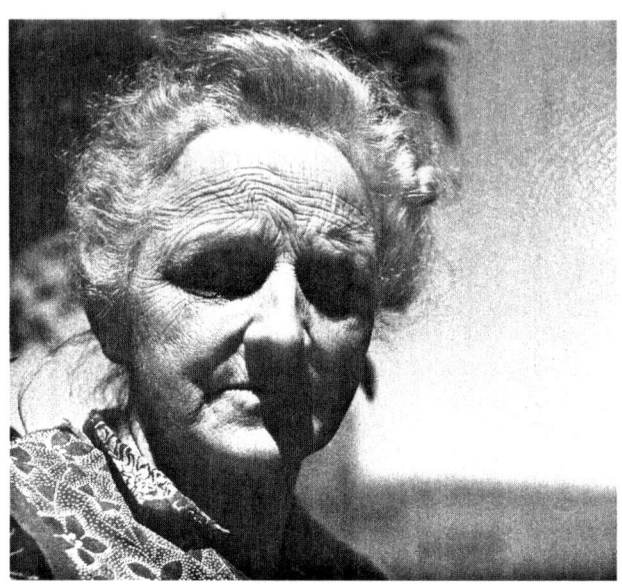

'A miner's wife in south Wales' (photograph by Edith Tudor Hart, c.1935, by kind permission of Wolf Suschitzky).

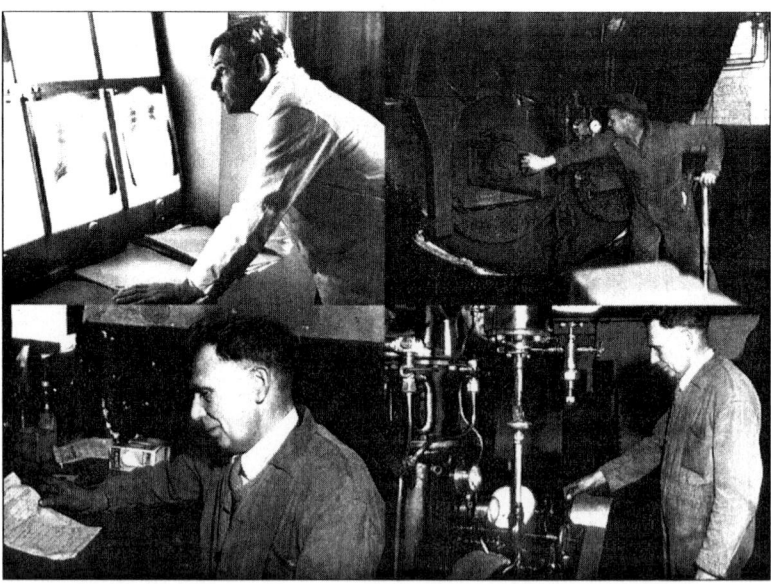

'The battle for health at Llangwyfan Hospital, Dyffryn Clwyd, 1955' (photographs by Geoff Charles, permission NLW). The hospital was established for the treatment of tuberculosis.

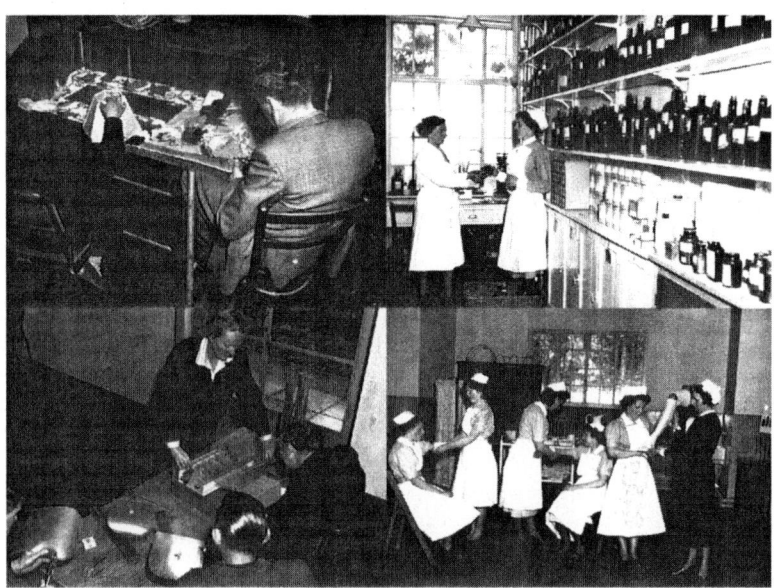

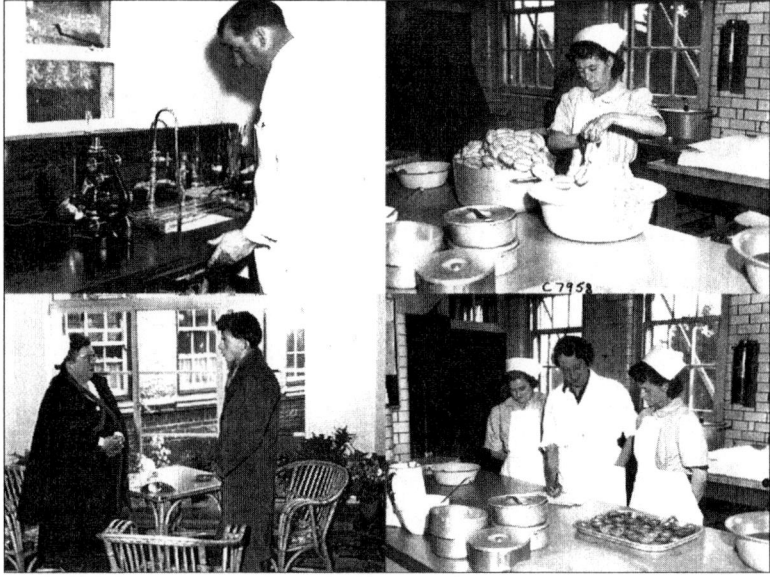

'Llangwyfan Hospital, 1955' (photographs by Geoff Charles, permission NLW). Occupational therapy and nurses' instruction were an important part of the daily activity at Llangwyfan Hospital.

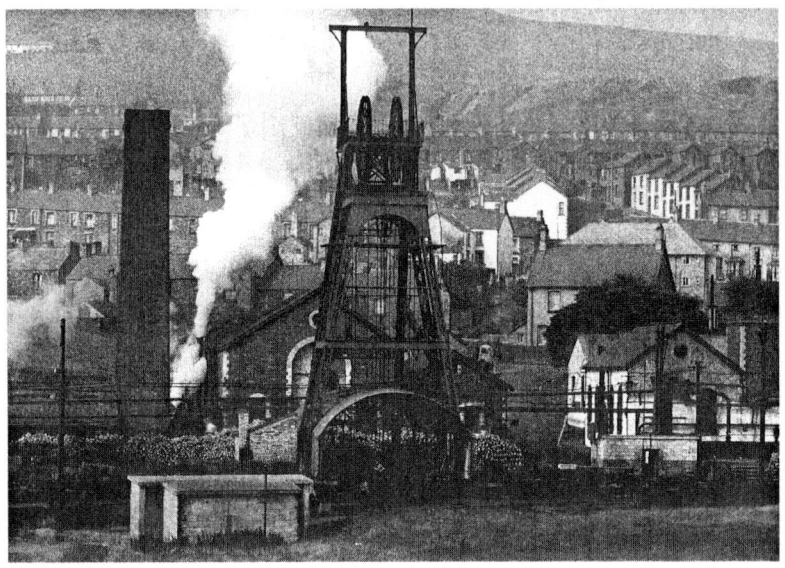

A south Wales village in the 1950s, indicating the close proximity of housing and industry (photograph by Wolf Suschitzky, by kind permission of Wolf Suschitzky).

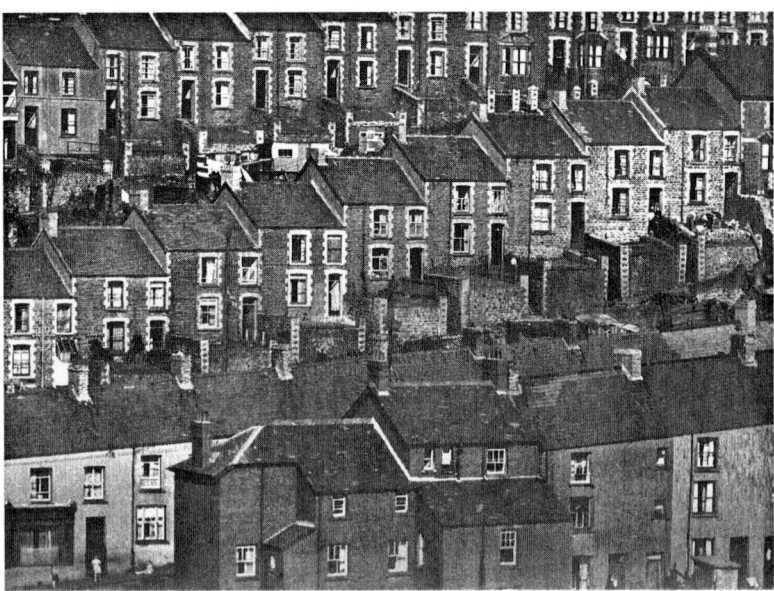

South Wales, Rhondda, 1955, where terraced houses lined the sides of the valleys (photograph by Wolf Suschitzky, by kind permission of Wolf Suschitzky).

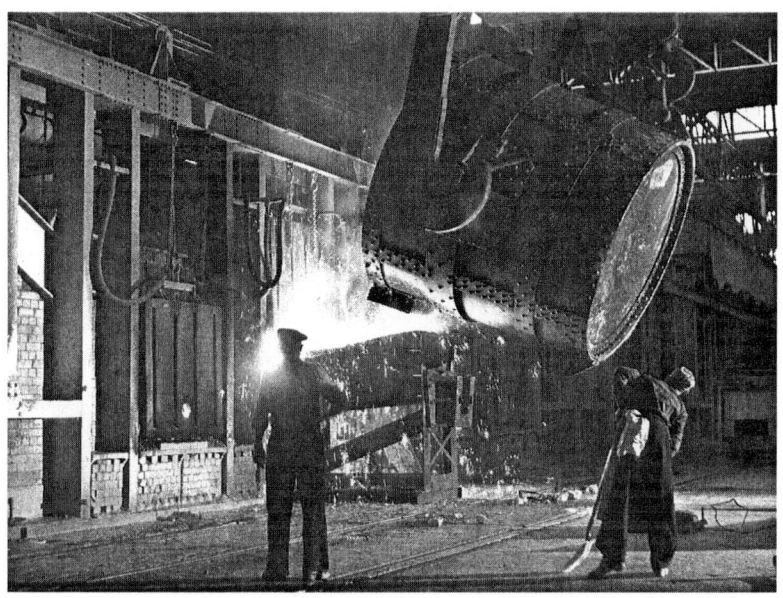

Abbey Works, 1953; the open hearth furnaces of the melting shop at the steel works (photograph by Wolf Suschitzky, by kind permission of Wolf Suschitzky).

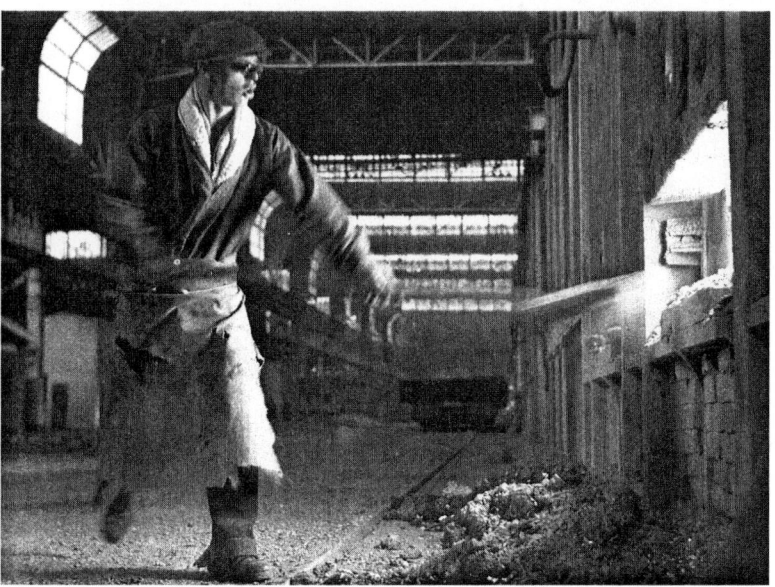

Abbey Works, 1953; a steel-worker wearing protective clothing (photograph by Wolf Suschitzky, by kind permission of Wolf Suschitzky).

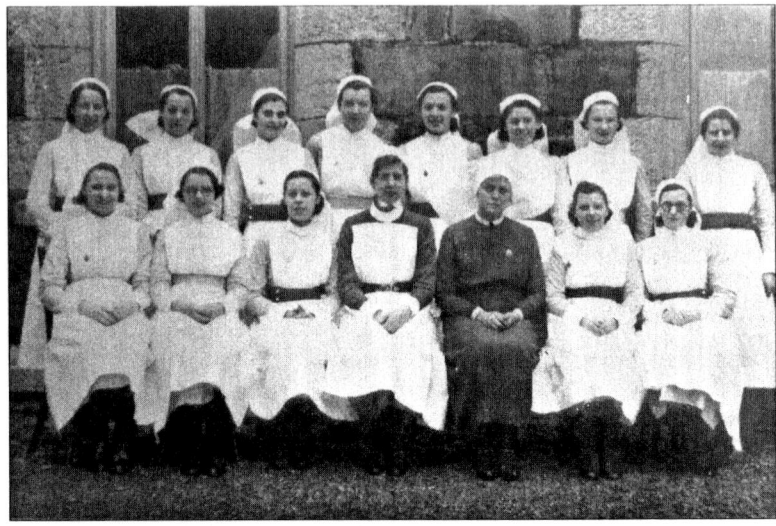

The first group of trainee State Registered Nurses to train at the Caernarvon and Anglesey Hospital, photographed in 1938 (O. V. Jones Collection, Archives Department, University of Wales, Bangor).

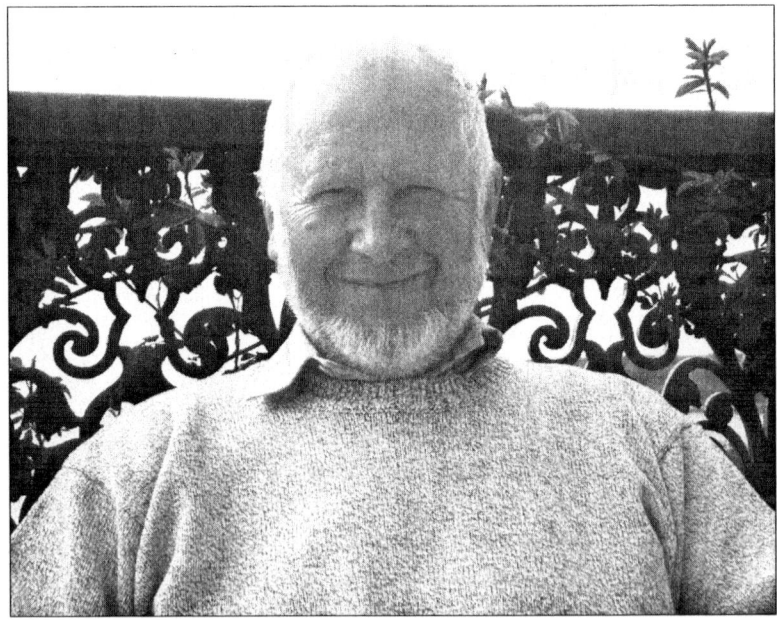

Julian Tudor Hart, general practitioner, researcher, citizen and scholar, at home in south Wales.

6

Nurse Training in the Caernarvon and Anglesey Hospital, 1935–1949

KATHERINE WILLIAMS

Nursing histories have frequently concentrated on the nursing elite. The lives of women of exceptional talent and influence, such as Florence Nightingale and Ethel Bedford Fenwick, interesting as they may be, provide only a distorted and uncharacteristic view of earlier nursing.[1] These celebrity nurses were often middle-class women fortunate enough to have access to a public world that was inaccessible for the majority. Representing nurses in this way has failed to give recognition to the 'rank-and-file' nurses in the UK. Moreover, stories of the nursing elite shed little light on the everyday world of nursing in Wales.

This chapter examines the patterns and practices of nurse training in a voluntary hospital in north Wales immediately prior to and during the Second World War. The hospital originated from a dispensary (the Carnarvon and Anglesey Loyal Dispensary) opened in 1810, the product of a subscription appeal launched in celebration of King George III's jubilee in 1809. The offspring infirmary was opened in 1845 and, from the beginning, employed a full-time physician and matron, as well as honorary physicians and surgeons. By 1851 the institution had already treated 3,255 patients. An elementary form of nurse training was introduced during the following decades and, by 1896, probationers were required to pay fees of £28 per annum for their training. As it became more difficult to find candidates willing and able to pay such a fee, a small salary was offered to probationers, in return for which they were required to remain as nurses at the infirmary for at least two years. In 1935 the Caernarvon and Anglesey

Infirmary (henceforth simply the C&A) was recognized by the General Nursing Council as a provider of nurse training and students were immediately recruited to this officially approved course. A record was kept on the progress of each candidate throughout her period of training. The hospital ledger maintained by the matron and containing the records of each probationer has formed the primary source for this study. This is the earliest source in relation to nurse training to be found in the School of Nursing in Bangor.[2] On a preliminary examination of the ledger, matron's subjective comments at the end of each personal record stood out as conveying a strong sense of either approval or disapproval and a picture emerged of the way matron viewed the probationers. However, some of the comments were ambiguous and vague in nature, so it proved necessary to explore other avenues of analysis to illuminate their meaning and place them in context.

It is from two exceptional studies in the field of nursing history that inspiration can be drawn for a detailed study of nurse records.[3] Accordingly, it was decided to create a coherent databank of all 315 cases utilizing each characteristic recorded in the ledger. These provided information on recruitment patterns, educational ability and examinations, discipline and resignation, duration of sickness and health, age and religion of probationers. The second step, following the analysis of the nurses' ledger, was to carry out interviews with retired nurses, who had trained in the hospital under the matron during the period covered by the ledger. An advertisement was placed in a local newspaper, and a small number of former nurses fulfilling this criterion responded. Two belonged to the original cohort who commenced training in 1935 and the other joined as a probationer in 1942. Three in-depth, semi-structured interviews were conducted through the medium of the respondents' first language, Welsh. Detailed notes were kept of the interviews and transcribed into English.

When the information from the ledgers was collated within a comprehensive databank a clearer picture began to emerge, offering a profile of the 'archetypal' nurse in Bangor. Matron's expectations of probationers indicate that there was an ideal model nurse that she was trying to mould. In the details that were recorded about probationers entering nursing, and thereafter updated throughout their training, a profile emerged that supported some of the impressions gained from an initial reading of matron's subjective comments. It was quite clear that matron would not have supported a probationer who appeared to question the system, and would see that she either resigned or was dismissed. This research outcome supports the assumption that matron did support the patriarchal forces in the hospital, by defining these young women in terms of expectations of subservience and adherence to narrowly defined gender roles. The interviewees' recollections confirmed that, as probationers, they were secured in roles of domesticity and subordination by matron's expectations of them.

The majority of recruits were very young on admission to training, with an average age of between seventeen and twenty. Some entered nursing straight from secondary school. This was the case with two of the three nurses interviewed. In the main, the trainees were local Welsh women, the daughters of small farmers, shopkeepers, quarry workers, railway employees and the like. Although not from well-to-do middle-class families, they were educated to secondary school level. Before the Second World War the nurses recruited came from Carnarfonshire and the neighbouring counties of Anglesey, Denbighshire and Merioneth, but during the war years, some came from further afield, for example Montgomeryshire, Flintshire, Cardiganshire, Chester and Wrexham. With regard to religion, most of the nurses belonged to local chapels, and were either recorded as 'Methodist' or 'Nonconformist', with a few recorded as 'C of E' (Church of England). Recruitment appears to have closely reflected the social, religious and linguistic characteristics of the region.

The records do not indicate whether the probationers' first language was Welsh or English, but from their place of origin and their surnames, it is probably fair to adduce from the records that the majority of them were Welsh-speaking. The former nurses who were interviewed recalled that matron spoke English and that the probationers on formal ward rounds and in ward reports spoke and wrote in English, only talking amongst themselves and with individual patients, through the medium of Welsh. 'Our work was mainly done in English,' said one informant, whilst another recalled: 'Welsh was not encouraged.'

Matron was responsible for nursing and nurse training. Her power and functions have been likened to those of an upper middle-class woman running a home with supreme authority over her servants. Matron used her power and influence to socialize nurses to endure hardships, to be obedient and above all to be subservient.[4] The apprenticeship system relied heavily on providing instruction through precept and example and great emphasis was placed on manual skills, obedience and discipline.[5] The emphasis in matron's comments in the nurse-training ledgers studied corresponds with all these characteristics. There does seem to be a noticeable lack of referral to the academic side of the course, favouring instead the practical side in matron's comments. One of matron's favourite comments could be noted as 'gave no trouble'. That comment could indicate a number of things, remembering the authoritative nature of matron's position within the hospital, and the junior nature of the probationer. It probably means that such candidates were quiet, submissive and followed instructions. The nurses studied only a limited amount of theory. One of the interviewees recalled that they had their lectures 'in a little room with little desks and a skeleton. The only textbook we had was Evelyn Pierce, we had "Aid to Hygiene" and an "Aid to Practical Nursing"'. If lectures fell on their day off they were still expected to attend.

All probationers would have to do a three-month trial and were expected to work under extremely difficult conditions by today's standards. It has been suggested that 'nurse training programmes were essentially low cost, low profile enterprises that produced skills and obedience'.[6] The recollections of the probationer nurses who trained at Bangor support this assertion. On commencement of training, probationers at the C&A were expected to give all their time to the hospital, enduring extremely long shifts. Every morning they were called at 6.00 a.m. to start at 7.00 a.m. and then they worked until 9.30 a.m. when they went for breakfast. They were given two hours a day of free time, either between 10.00 a.m. and 12.00 noon or between 2.00 p.m. and 4.00 p.m. As Nurse 'A' recalled 'you were expected to put 10 hours a day in of hard grind'. When the probationers were on day shifts they had one day off a month, but when on nights they had two days' leave a month. They spent six months on night duty, with shifts from 8.00 p.m. until 8.00 a.m. The nurses went in at 7.30 p.m. for a meal and then went on the ward, without a break during the night. There would be just one nurse on each ward, 'and what was called a runner between wards to help you'. This meant that nurses were regularly working in excess of seventy hours a week. In 1919 the College of Nursing had recommended 'an average week of 48 ... as a maximum for all nurses', but in 1939 the Lancet Commission report estimated that, as an average of all hospitals, nurses were working about 57 hours per week.[7] They noted, however, that at St Bartholomew's Hospital in London, nurses worked an 84-hour week. The hours worked by nurses at the C&A were therefore considerably longer than the average in the UK.[8] Sometimes, in cases of emergency or staff shortage, probationers at the C&A would be called upon to do additional hours. 'You often didn't go off on time – that was normal,' said one interviewee. Nurse B recalled that she always knew when matron was going to ask her to do an extra shift or work overtime, because matron would always begin by saying: 'You are one of my pillars . . .'[9] Unsurprisingly, probationers were invariably tired and often suffered from some form of illness during their training.

The nurse probationers were required to live in the nurses' home. When on nights, the nurses were allowed to go shopping, 'but not for long as the night sister would check you were all in your beds'.[10] Matron would also go around to check. Strict discipline was enforced in the home. 'Smoking in the bedrooms was a dreadful offence, you were removed from training it was such a dreadful thing. One warning and then you were dismissed if caught again.'[11]

As noted at the beginning of this chapter, fewer than 40 per cent of the recruits survived the course to qualify over the fifteen-year period analysed for this study. Thirty-one probationers were not kept on after their initial trial period of three months. Five of these were recorded as not returning after their days off. A heavy loss came at the end of the first twelve months with many failing their State Preliminary examination. Out of 202 candidates who sat the preliminary examinations over the fifteen-year period, around 20 per cent (forty-one) failed. This matches evidence nationally that a high number of recruits actually left their course at the end of the first year.[12] This probably reflected the quality of women's education during the period. However, the pass rates did improve over the period of this study, going from eleven out of eighteen in 1940, to twenty out of twenty-one passing in 1948. This is attributed to two factors, the educational calibre of the probationer and the matron's selection process. A number of candidates are made to resign because they are 'poor in theory' according to the entry written by matron in the ledger.

Examinations certainly presented a major challenge for nurse probationers. Many of these young student nurses were tired and worn out because of the long hours they put in. This, together with the fact that they had to sit the examination through the medium of English, when many of them were first-language Welsh speakers, resulted in their being at a double disadvantage. As one nurse recalled 'we just couldn't express ourselves, you came down because of it'.[13] It was not possible to take the practical examinations in Bangor at that time and so probationers had to go to Liverpool or Chester, where the language was English and the environment and ward layout unfamiliar. Students had to sit the written examinations at Bangor in English. For those probationers who stayed the course the pass rate at the finals of the State Registration examinations was almost 100 per cent, and 112 nurses succeeded at this final hurdle. This was very impressive, because the Lancet Commission Report of 1932 had found that on average about 40 per cent of candidates failed the final examinations.[14] Passing finals still meant spending a further fourth year as a probationer in the hospital that trained them – and on a third-year student's pay! This was in order to achieve the hospital badge, as without it a nurse could not obtain work elsewhere, despite having passed the State Registration examination.

Although practically all of the C&A nurses who sat their qualifying examinations passed, there was considerable wastage between the preliminary and final examinations. After getting through the hurdle of their State Preliminary examinations the things that would prevent them from finishing the course were the probationer's health, marriage or a disciplinary reason.

Beginning with a cohort of twelve in the first intake in 1935, the size of the probationer entry ranged from just four in 1937, to a peak of thirty-three entrants in 1941. The majority of the smaller groups were in the early days. Early recruitment patterns can be linked to two influencing factors, the growth of the training school and the influence of the war on the hospital. Initially, students were accepted sporadically after applying directly to the matron. In 1940 the pattern of intake changed to small groups of two and three being accepted together. In January 1944 there were three groups, two of six and then a group of ten. This then remained the consistent pattern until 1947, when eleven probationers were taken on in the September. Following this, the last three years show intakes of ten and eleven probationers, three times a year.

Most areas were increasing their number of recruits in preparation for war in 1939, and Bangor would seem to have followed this national picture. During the war though the hospital suffered a drop in recruits in 1943 (down to nineteen), possibly due to the relocation to the area of industries involved in the war effort and the advent of female conscription. Recruitment wasn't helped by pre-war reports that in some hospitals, nurses were working up to anything between 100 and

140 hours or more. Some hospitals were not giving nurses the leave to which they were entitled.[15] The experiences of nurse probationers at the C&A confirmed how exhausting these long hours of work could be. One of the nurses interviewed described being 'too tired to actually get changed when I went off duty'. Another one spoke about sleeping in her uniform, falling asleep on the bed after coming off duty and sleeping right through to the next morning. They all spoke of how on their day of leave they slept the 'whole day off, you were so tired'. The probationers were taught to pay particular attention to hygiene and cleanliness. 'Every Monday morning we used to do extra cleaning, all the beds were done everyday anyway. It was clean, clean all the time. Kitty the ward maid was always cleaning the kitchen, brushing and polishing.'[16] On enrolment they were each given seven white aprons and four caps, to be made up like a butterfly, and two blue and white striped dresses.[17] Everything would be carefully washed, starched and ironed. Items were washed which would simply be disposed of today. Cotton bandages were boiled during the day, and the night-staff would iron them.[18] Matron was very particular about cleanliness and presentation. 'Matron had a thing about fluff,' recalled one nurse. 'All the pillow openings had to be away from the door ...' Another remarked on how 'hygiene was of the utmost'.[19] It was all organized with regimental precision. In a published account of her early years at the C&A, Sister Laura Chesterton recalled that 'Matron did a round every morning, and everybody had to stand to attention. The patients were like dead bodies in their beds, the corners of the beds were just so, and the wheels had all to be straight.'[20]

The length of stay for operations at the turn of the twentieth century was often very long. It demanded skilled nursing to prevent infection, as staff had no resources other than scrupulous hygiene and the use of physical care. This made the day a very laborious and demanding one for the nurses. In 1905–15 the average stay in the C&A hospital was thirty days, by the mid-1920s it was reduced to twenty-one days, decreasing even further to eighteen days by 1940–6.[21] A total of 197 operations were carried out in the C&A Hospital in 1913, and with risks associated with both anaesthetics and surgery it meant that the demand on nurses was a far greater one than we can appreciate in relation to today's surgery. The number of in-patients nursed each year rose considerably to 1,047 in 1928 and to 3,205 in 1947.[22] In his history of the hospital, O. V. Jones recognized that it was not until 1930 that a significant reduction in mortality rates occurred in the hospital.[23] No antibiotics were available in the 1930s, and infectious diseases (scarlet fever, diphtheria, tuberculosis) were still prevalent in the local communities of Anglesey, Caernarfon and Bangor. Therefore it would seem that doctors and nurses were becoming better equipped to deal with the health problems of the day. The probationers were not given training in fever nursing, which was a separate qualification. Cases of infectious diseases were sent to the nearby Minffordd Isolation Hospital, opened in 1895. However, patients in the C&A would occasionally run high temperatures and Nurse B recalled the use of leeches on the forehead to reduce a patient's temperature.

Nursing with its practical base, was seen to prepare women for domesticity, and this was often advanced as a reason for parents to allow their daughters to enter training. Matron was promoted as a surrogate mother, and the nursing skills that she would teach the young probationers were considered a good preparation for motherhood and marriage.[24] This was one of the consequences of living in a patriarchal society, and the fact that, in the 1930s, all general nurses were women. One of the interviewees revealed that her father was so pleased that all of his three daughters had gone into nursing, as they would be able to look after him in old age![25]

Nurse training required a great deal of stamina. The retired nurses who were interviewed explained that it was not the practice to give applicants a full medical. Matron's only concern was to check if they were flat-footed and unable to stand for long periods. Screening consisted of being asked to take their shoes off in matron's office and stand on a bath mat. During training, the nurses could seek advice from one of the hospital doctors, who was given responsibility for their welfare.[26] Dr Davies, the person nominated, worked in casualty and also ran the venereal disease unit, but the nurses did not find him approachable. One interviewee summed up how she and other probationers felt in relation to this Doctor – 'you just wouldn't go to him however ill you felt'.

The wastage rates were high in some cohorts of trainees and the work could also prove hazardous to their long-term health. The main illnesses suffered by the apprentice nurses were appendectomy, scarlet fever, diphtheria, septic fingers and toes, jaundice and tuberculosis. In addition the probationers appear to have picked up all the childhood illnesses, like mumps and measles. The time spent recovering from illness, and particularly operations, was considerable. Whilst people today still have appendectomies, one can be out of hospital in a very short span, some cases only being in two to three days at the most. In 1937, however, one probationer had sick leave for forty-five days following an appendectomy. Another in 1938 was warded with appendicitis on the second of April and was still off in the middle of June. When suffering from any less serious ailment, probationers were simply expected to carry on, however ill they felt. If they did have time off for more serious illnesses, then they were automatically given their holiday time in which to recover. One of the interviewees recalled matron as saying: 'holidays were not for our benefit but for the benefit of the hospital'.[27]

Of course, patients may have been put at risk if probationers were working when they were unwell. One nurse is noted in the records as being a diphtheria carrier! A number of students were not only warded whilst on duty but were also recorded as transferred to the local sanatorium for infectious diseases. These particular probationers never came back to nursing. On the other side of the coin, the nurses were also prepared to put their own lives at risk by coming into nursing, as these were pre-immunization days. So they actually faced patients daily with very little protection themselves. One of the respondents quite painfully described how one fellow student died whilst on the ward in horrendous circumstances, from a massive gastric bleed following tuberculosis.[28] There was no counselling or support on offer for the probationers. In all, during the fifteen-year period covered by the records, fifty-three probationers left because of illness.

Some probationers' records clearly show that they were dismissed. The rationale is usually made explicit in these cases, mainly being associated with misconduct, as defined by matron. Some examples of dismissal include: 'cautioned for misbehaviour on the Penrhyn ward and for smoking in her bedroom. Temperamental. Dismissed after repeated complaints from the nursing staff – aprons etc. found in her possession and did not belong to her.' 'Suspended for not sleeping in the Nurses Home.'

In analysing this category of data a difficulty arose in defining the distinction between what actually occurred when the termination of employment was recorded as 'dismissal' and what happened when the word 'resign' was appended. It appeared, on initial readings of this latter category, that the interpretation was straightforward; but on further examination it began to appear that this might not have been the case. The comments often read 'asked to resign'. Who asked? Were they persuaded or coerced? There was suggestive evidence that it was not the probationer who was asking to resign, but possibly that it was matron doing the asking! In this ambiguous area of 'resigned' or 'requested to resign' fifty-seven probationers can be accounted for during the fifteen-year period. In relation to their records, the evidence is too ambiguous really to decide whether they went of their own accord.

Interestingly, Olson and Maggs had the same problem in their studies.[29] Olson develops the idea that, rather than dismissal, a compromise was reached whereby the student was allowed to resign. This alters the scenario, from the student choosing to leave to the student being made to leave, or possibly choosing to leave voluntarily after pressure was brought to bear, but it is a fine line between the two. Olson goes on to make the point that strong-willed women were more likely to resign, leaving less-forceful women behind. In his study, the main reasons he gave for women leaving, in relation to dismissal and resignation, arose from 'breaking the rules'.[30] To be dismissed would also have implications for future employment and references, which is possibly why they were made to resign, since it would be in their interest. Matron would then write 'request to leave' on the record, followed by 'resigns'.

In many cases, negative comments were written by matron, placing the blame directly on the student, for example 'Did not wish to continue training', 'bad influence' or 'resigned, resented correction'. These women were often young, lacking support and possibly were powerless to put their case, in the sense that they had had little previous employment experience. It was evident that matron was not going to have her power threatened by any who questioned her, or anyone who was to have associations with the trade unions. Everyone in the hospital knew how matron was against the unions, as one interviewee recalled. Probationers were labelled if they spoke out of turn. The documented comments by matron reflect this. Their characters were noted as 'difficult little person', 'surly out for women's rights' and despite some like this qualifying they were not kept on; another was recorded as 'temperamental – capabilities above the average – instigator of the trade unions'. Matron stamped her authority, by not employing her when she qualified; a clear message to the rest of the workforce!

There are indications that, over time, matron found it an increasing battle, as women began to question her authority, especially as they became more emancipated during the war years. The nurses interviewed made references to the army personnel, who were based in the grounds during the war, influencing the women's attitude to work and to trade unions. Matron was possibly finding it difficult to keep control. Comments begin to filter through the records, showing matron to be ill at ease with the situation. In August 1943 matron excels herself in 'power' writing, 'weak willed – easily led . . . made her resign, hospital certificate was then forfeited'. This harsh response is difficult to judge, as there is no previous evidence on this trainee, only to say that she had no recorded prior problems and had completed three years and seven months at this point. It has to be remembered that this probationer could not work elsewhere without her hospital certificate. This was not an isolated incident. Such cases of instant dismissal served to remind women of their insecure positions and how they were cheap pairs of hands, easily replaced.

The ruthless dismissal of young recruits was only possible as long as there was a stream of fresh replacements. During the 1930s there were, as one of the interviewees pointed out, only three choices for women in north Wales – domestic service, teaching or nursing. During the post-war years the options for women slowly began to expand and fewer women were waiting in the sidelines to obtain a post. Fewer women were willing to remain a spinster simply in order to have a career. Therefore, not only was it more difficult to recruit probationers, it was more difficult to recruit matrons and senior staff to a life in the former mould. In the words of one nurse: 'When I think back it must have been a very lonely life for matron – she lived in the hospital. Her sitting room was upstairs off ENT ward, with her bedroom nearby . . . Her life was fully devoted to the hospital, it was her life, she can't have had any private life outside of the hospital.'[31] Matron had a demanding role to fulfil. 'Everyone did respect her, even the medical staff,' recalled one former nurse.[32] 'Matron used to gather us like lambs – she was firm but fair – not cruel,' said another.[33] The probationers under her tutelage respected as well as feared her.

All three interviewees referred to the power of matron by saying you could be called to the office at any time to be reprimanded and sacked on the spot. This had obviously stayed in their minds well over fifty years later. There was no greater fear than having this held over you during training. They all knew what it was like to be told off for misdemeanours, such as running in the hospital during emergencies. 'Nurse, you only run in the case of fire and haemorrhage!'[34] Matron 'ran a very tight ship', and would do spot checks to keep everyone on their toes. At times she would appear to take almost an *in locus parentis* role, not allowing them out late, or sleeping out, and checking with the home sister that they were in bed during the day when they were on night duty.[35] She was renowned for punishing the probationers as if they were naughty children; those deemed to have done wrong were made to stand outside matron's office. 'You would shake in your shoes, she would start with "Words fail me . . ." for something like being caught out after 10.00 p.m.'[36] Her disapproval of any transgression is exemplified when she writes about one probationer who had qualified, but applied to work elsewhere: 'Good practical nurse, but poor in theory. Rumours of friendship with night porter – proved to be true.' Conduct is a key issue that comes to the surface throughout the records. Matron had failed in her role of segregating the sexes in the hospital in this instance!

Probationers had to request formal permission to get married. Nurses were well aware of the fact that a 'marriage bar' applied and that, conventionally, being married prevented women from carrying on nursing. Interviewee B, who married in 1948, recalled that 'once you married you gave up, you had to – you had your husband and children to look after'.[37] Amongst the fifteen-year cohort, twenty probationers left to get married, thirteen of whom had passed their State Preliminary examinations. This practice of excluding married women persisted for long after the Second World War in north Wales. Interviewee C recalled that these assumptions still applied in the early 1960s:

> In 1961, I went to say to Matron that I was getting married, and to apply to carry on working. But this wasn't allowed by Matron. It just wasn't the done thing, you were expected to stay at home and look after your family and home, husband, etc.[38]

It was recognized that, occasionally, personal caring obligations would take precedence over a nurse's career, even when she was unmarried. A dozen of the nurses left for personal reasons. In one case matron recorded that the probationer was 'called home' and in another that she 'left to nurse her mother'.

The C&A was a voluntary hospital and like many similar institutions was faced with increasing costs in the 1930s.[39] Many hospitals during this period were moving into a deepening financial crisis.[40] Originally, admission as a patient to the C&A Hospital was restricted and depended on obtaining nomination from one of the trustees. By the time these probationers joined, the hospital was running a health scheme, one nurse recalling that 'You had to put a penny in every pound to be in the health scheme.'[41] The charges were complicated, and Mr Williams, the hospital secretary, kept the books. Patients not covered by a scheme had to pay directly for their treatment. 'You had to pay at the end of your stay, it was very hard on some. Mrs Dan Jones came to you with her book, to the actual patients to see how you were going to pay.' The probationers were also expected to pay £5 for a ticket to attend the fund-raising hospital ball. The interviewees all referred to the local women's committees that appeared to have played a major role in raising funds for the hospital. Local working men contributed to hospital funds, one former nurse recalling that: 'The quarrymen's pennies were collected; without them the committee couldn't have run the hospital.'[42] Another interviewee recalled being sent in her afternoon break to stand with her collecting box on the Menai Suspension Bridge, to try and boost subscriptions. Students at the local Bala-Bangor theological college also helped to raise money.[43]

The extent and nature of local patronage is illustrated by the way in which some of the local ladies of influence showed a special concern for the probationers, arranging for food to be sent from local gardens. One recalled that 'Lady Vivian used to be really good to us taking us on boat trips and strawberry teas.'[44] Such days out were particularly memorable and could be vividly recalled over fifty years later: 'a Mrs Johnson ... would bus us to Plas Newydd – we went on the river and Nellie fell in.'[45]

During the Second World War many industries, services and personnel were relocated to north Wales, and the hospital became very much busier.[46] To relieve pressure on beds, patients would be transferred to convalesce in the Heath House and Parciau at Marianglas.[47] As one nurse recalled: 'it was pretty grim during the war – we never had enough beds.'[48] When the Liverpool Royal was 'bombed out', patients and staff were transferred to the C&A Hospital. Nurses from Liverpool 'had to come to us to finish their training in Bangor', recalled another informant – 'we were that busy!'.[49]

Many changes occurred during the war, but the patronage of local families remained a significant factor, as another interviewee recalled: 'We had hampers of rabbits from Miss Vivian. There was also Miss Johnson in Llandegfan who sent eggs for the soldiers. Plas Newydd also sent things for the soldiers.'[50] Food shortages and rationing meant that extra rations were highly valued: 'There was an egg collection in Anglesey and Caernarfon ... and we used to have to have egg cleaning sessions.'[51] Helen Davies, who joined the X-ray department of the C&A as a radiographer in 1943, recalled that the local aristocratic families supplied all of the linen required by the wards during the war.[52] In recognition of their goodwill there was an element of reciprocity. Lady Vivian kept Pekinese dogs, and Helen Davies remembered 'on more than one occasion giving a barium meal to one of the dogs to locate swallowed bones' in return for fund-raising activities.[53]

The inauguration of the National Health Service in 1948 changed this relationship, as it altered the funding structure and the dependence of the hospital on local charity. Towards the end of the voluntary system the C&A was dealing with almost 20,000 patients a year, as inpatients and outpatients.[54] Large-scale provision of this sort was unsustainable on the basis of rattling tins on the Menai Bridge. The hospital was henceforth financed by central government funding and administered under the jurisdiction of the Welsh Hospitals Board. The climate in which nurse training was conducted also began to change, albeit more slowly. Megan Lloyd Williams, the last matron to hold this position at the C&A, who was appointed to the post in 1963, commented on the great change which took place in the aftermath of war: 'Up to this point, single women living in residential accommodation had dominated the profession.'[55] By the 1960s women's expectations were changing and the patriarchal system that had so dominated the hospital was beginning to weaken.

This case study has illustrated the high level of commitment and dedication required of those probationers who survived the three-year training course and the fourth year of internment. In the evidence derived from the ledgers it became apparent that matron did have a 'prescriptive model' informing her outlook and her expectations of probationers. Matron's treatment of the probationers under her tutelage confirms that the approach highlighted by the Lancet and Athlone investigations, whereby training was represented as 'a mortifying experience during which girls were purified for their training',[56] was employed in north Wales during the period of this study.

As this chapter has illustrated, trainee nurses were key contributors to the health care offered in hospitals during the 1930s and 1940s. Yet the nursing profession has often failed to appreciate what was achieved during this period. Nurses have consistently deprecated their own worth, often allowing volumes of documentary evidence to be destroyed. Possibly this is because what is recognized as routine care is regarded as being mundane and therefore less worthy of being recorded as history.[57] In a history of the C&A which gives full attention to improvements in 'medicine' and the role of the medical men involved, nursing gets only a modest note of recognition, when it is commented that: 'The Training school undoubtedly added to the efficiency of the nursing service at the "C&A"'.[58]

The move within nursing to higher education and away from 'traditional and ritualistic' care to a more evidence-based care system has only exaggerated the lack of value placed on the past. It has made it difficult for nurses to review their past, as there is little research or teaching in this area within current nurse education.[59] This chapter has aimed to give a place in history to the many women who toiled away under often very difficult circumstances in Welsh hospitals. These women formed the backbone of the developing health-care system, during a period that was opening new avenues in women's working lives.

Notes

[1] Accounts of the life and work of Florence Nightingale for long dominated the field; see for example E. T. Cook, *The Life of Florence Nightingale*, 2 vols (London, 1913); Cecil Woodham Smith, *Florence Nightingale* (New York, 1951); L. Seymer, *A General History of Nursing* (London, 1932); idem, *Florence Nightingale's Nurses: The Nightingale Training School 1860–1960* (London, 1960); M. Baly, *Florence Nightingale and the Nursing Legacy* (London, 1986). Winifred Hector, *The Work of Mrs Bedford Fenwick and the Rise of Professional Nursing* (London, 1973).

[2] As Lesley Hall has noted, 'Nursing tends to be less well-documented than medicine'; Lesley Hall, 'Nurses in the archives: archival sources for nursing history', in Anne Marie Rafferty, Jane Robinson and Ruth Elkan (eds.), *Nursing History and the Politics of Welfare* (London, 1997), pp. 259–73 (259). However, as Hall noted, some hospitals have retained nursing records, and the C&A was one such example. The records must have been transferred to St David's Hospital, Bangor, either when nurse training was moved there in 1969, or when the C&A closed in 1984. The records then moved with the nursing library to the Institute of Nursing, University of Wales, Bangor. They are now located in the nursing library at Fron Heulog.

[3] T. Olson, 'History case study of apprenticeship nurses in Minnesota' (unpublished Ph.D. thesis, Minnesota University, 1991); idem, 'Numbers, narratives and nursing history methodology', *Journal of Nursing Scholarship*, Vol. 30, no.

1   (1998); C. Maggs, 'Nurse recruitment to four provincial hospitals, 1881–1921', in Celia Davies (ed.), *Rewriting Nursing History* (London, 1980).
4   C. M. Chapman, *Sociology for Nurses* (London, 1977); J. Salvage *The Politics of Nursing* (London, 1985); P. Smith, *Nursing Research: Setting New Agendas* (London, 1988).
5   M. Baly, *Nursing and Social Change* (London, 1995, 3rd edn.), p. 299.
6   R. McMahon and A. Pearson, *Nursing as a Therapy* (Cheltenham, 1998), p. 238.
7   Brian Abel-Smith, *A History of the Nursing Profession* (London, 1960) p. 137.
8   They were similar to those in Australia, where nurses worked an average of 72 hours per week, see Judith Godden, 'For the benefit of mankind: Nightingale's legacy and hours of work in Australian nursing, 1868–1939' in Anne-Marie Rafferty, Jane Robinson and Ruth Elkan, *Nursing History and the Politics of Welfare* (London, 1997), pp. 177–91 (177).
9   Nurse A, 2nd interview.
10 Ibid.
11 Ibid.
12 In 1937 the government recognised the need for action. The shortage of nurses had been highlighted by the Athlone Report and the Lancet Commission of 1933. See S. M. Ferguson and H. Fitzgerald, *The History of the Second World War: Studies in the Social Services* (London, 1954), pp. 284–341.
13 Nurse A, 2nd interview.
14 Abel-Smith, *A History of the Nursing Profession,* p. 124.
15 Athlone Report on the hours nurses were working and not getting time off. The Athone Committee, Inter-departmental Committee on Nursing Services, *Interim Report* (1939).
16 Nurse B, 2nd interview.
17 Nurse C, 2nd interview.
18 Nurse B, 2nd interview.
19 Nurse C, 2nd interview.
20 W. Beer, *Portrait of the Carnarvon and Anglesey Hospital Bangor: The People and the Place (1948–1984)* (Mold, 2000), p. 72.
21 O. V. Jones, *The Progress of Medicine: A History of the Caernarfon and Anglesey Infirmary, 1809–1948* (Llandysul, 1984), p. 239.
22 Ibid., p. 230.
23 Ibid., pp. 239–42.
24 J. Muff (ed.), *Socialisation, Sexism and Stereotyping: Women's Issues in Nursing* (Illinois, 1988); M. Jolley and G. Brykczynska, *Nursing Beyond Tradition and Conflict* (London, 1995).
25 Nurse B, 1st interview.
26 Nurse B, 2nd interview.
27 Nurse C, 1st interview.
28 Nurse B, 2nd interview.
29 T. Olson, 'History case study of apprenticeship nurses in Minnesota'; C. Maggs, 'Nurse recruitment to four provincial hospitals'.
30 Nurse C, 2nd interview.

31 Nurse C, 1st interview.
32 Nurse A, 1st interview.
33 Nurse B, 3rd interview.
34 This was a role commonly assumed by matrons at the time. See 'Matrons at Work', *Nursing Times,* Vol. 62, no. 24 (17 June 1966), 811–12; R. M. Jones, 'Changing roles and communications: matrons or mums?', *Nursing Times,* Vol. 65, no. 23 (5 June 1969), 734.
35 Nurse C, 1st interview.
36 Nurse B, 2nd interview.
37 Nurse C, 2nd interview.
38 Jones, *The Progress of Medicine,* p. 00
39 C.Webster (ed.), *Caring for Health: History and Diversity* (Buckingham, 3rd edn., 2001), p. 138.
40 Jones, *The Progress of Medicine,* pp. 131–2. A number of the local quarries and industrial establishments ran schemes, whereby the workmen 'agreed to pay one penny for each pound of wages and the management contributed one penny for every three pence contributed by the men.' In 1932 a voluntary scheme was introduced for those whose income was under four pounds per week.
41 Nurse A, 2nd interview.
42 Nurse B, 2nd interview. The Coleg Bala-Bangor was a Baptist training college.
43 Nurse B, 2nd interview.
44 Ibid. She may be referring to the Menai Straits, which run alongside the Plas Newydd estate.
45 The infirmary was classified as the principal casualty hospital for the area, requiring at least thirty beds to be made available for war casualties. This greatly increased pressure on the hospital, but also brought with it a new source of revenue. Between 1939 and 1946 the Central War Committee paid the C&A a total of £31,261. See Jones, *The Progress of Medicine,* pp. 138–9.
46 Nurse A, 1st interview.
47 Nurse A, 2nd interview.
48 Ibid.
49 Nurse B, 1st interview.
50 Nurse A, 2nd interview.
51 A 'Linen League', founded in 1920, made arrangements for groups of ladies throughout Caernarfonshire and Anglesey to produce towels, pillowcases, sheets and so on for use by the hospital. Jones, *The Progress of Medicine,* pp. 134–5.
52 Beer, *Portrait of the Carnarvon and Anglesey Hospital,* p. 233.
53 Jones, *The Progress of Medicine,* p. 00.
54 Beer, *Portrait of the Carnarvon and Anglesey Hospital,* p. 50.
55 Robert Dingwall, Anne Marie Rafferty and Charles Webster, *An Introduction to the Social History of Nursing* (London, 1998), p. 118.
56 S. McGann, 'Archival sources for research into the history of nursing', *Nurse Researcher,* Vol. 5, no. 2 (Winter, 1997/8), 19–57.
57 Jones *The Progress of Medicine,* p. 229.

58 This void still exists, despite the fact that it is a quarter of a century since Marion Ferguson raised this as a serious issue to be addressed by the nursing profession. See Marion Ferguson, 'Reflections on teaching a history of nursing – 1', Occasional Papers, *Nursing Times,* 15 November 1979, and Marion Ferguson, 'Reflections on teaching a history of nursing – 2', Occasional Papers, *Nursing Times*, 22 November 1979.

7

The Jewish Medical Refugee Crisis and Wales, 1933–1945*

PAUL WEINDLING

Dr Paul Rothschild was perhaps the first of the medical refugees from Nazi Germany to practise in Wales. In 1934 Rothschild, newly requalified in Scotland, moved to a Welsh mining village.[1] In 1965 A. V. Hill, the Nobel-prizewinning physiologist, former Secretary of the Royal Society, and campaigner for refugees, published an eloge of Rothschild under the title, 'The good physician'. Hill explained that this paragon of virtue was expert on the pathology of muscle, having worked previously with the leading cardiologist Thomas Lewis.[2] Rothschild was also a dedicated physician, believing that general practitioners were needed in the Welsh mining valleys: 'One of his most treasured possessions was a miner's lamp, the one he had used in the pit in his Welsh village when emergency called him.' When he returned to London (becoming honorary physician of the Royal Society), he maintained Welsh links; some miners' daughters would at first stay with the Rothschilds, when they came to London for domestic service.[3] Rothschild's career was emblematic for Hill, demonstrating that a scientifically highly qualified physician was deeply humane, and could raise standards of health care. Rothschild fitted perfectly with the idea that there was a niche in Britain for medical refugees in areas which were undersupplied by doctors.[4] As independent MP for Cambridge University, Hill was an energetic campaigner for admitting medical refugees. He relished the fight with the restrictive British Medical Association (BMA), which lobbied the government to admit minimal numbers of refugee doctors, and to ensure that these practised outside metropolitan centres.[5] Hill saw that there was a skills shortage in British medicine, and that refugees had an important role to play in modernizing medical practice. More generally, historians have differed over British refugee policies. Alan Sherman has portrayed Britain as an 'Island Refuge', admitting per head of population larger numbers of Jewish refugees than the USA, and generously permitting the refugee *Kindertransport*.[6] In contrast, Louise London has argued that the Home Office was restrictive and often anti-Semitic, doing everything to ensure that Britain was at best a temporary refuge.[7] The refugees were a test of tolerance to outsiders more generally, and more particularly to Jewish incomers. These issues extended to Wales, which had received Jewish immigrants particularly since the 1880s. Anti-Semitism had flared in the Tredegar riots of 1911. In 1933 the *Western Mail* carried a heated controversy between a former Lord Mayor of Cardiff, Mr Forsdike, who praised Hitler, and rebuttals by a local rabbi, Revd Jerevich, who condemned Germany as 'a plague spot'.[8]

The admission of medical refugees was a litmus test of the readiness to support humanitarian action, but also indicates how certain medical specialisms were more receptive. Thus relatively large numbers of psychiatrists arrived because of support from the Maudsley hospital. Biochemistry, physiology and pharmacology were welcoming to medical researchers, thanks to the endeavours of Hill and his colleagues. Supporting the admission of the refugees was a group who wished to modernize British medicine on the basis of science, arguing that the medical refugees possessed a range of research and science-based clinical skills. Some argued (as Hill) that there were areas of social deprivation in which the refugees were needed as practitioners.

The question of refugee medical practitioners in Wales should be seen in a more general context of the United Kingdom. I have identified 4,715 refugee doctors, dental surgeons, nurses (and here numbers were higher), psychoanalysts and medical researchers who came to Britain by 1945.[9] Added to (at least) 1,051 Germans, 607 Austrians and 478 Czechoslovaks, the outbreak of the war saw the arrival of 1,056 Polish medical personnel, who came through Romania and France, and via Iran after the German attack on Russia in 1941. Whereas in 1933 three refugees gained UK medical qualifications, numbers rose to seventy-one in 1934. The opposition of the British Medical Association reduced numbers to thirty-three in 1936, but by 1943 they rose to ninety-six degrees. Most refugee doctors took the

Scottish 'triple qualification', and there was a Polish Medical School in Edinburgh, where 210 Polish students graduated. Substantial numbers moved on – initially to other countries, notably the United States, and it was the policy of refugee assistance organizations that they should do so. It must be emphasized that many of the refugees, notably the Polish cohort, were not Jewish, but the Jewish medical refugees opened up the issue of requalification in 1933–4. After the war, only a minority of the Jewish and Eastern European refugees chose to return to their countries of origin. The relative Scottish openness to refugees attracted some to settle permanently there. By reconstructing as far as possible the total population of medical refugees in the UK between 1930 and the post-war era up to c.1950, individual life-histories can be assessed in a broader context.

During the 1930s the British medical establishment opposed the admission of all but a select few on the basis that Britain was adequately supplied with doctors. Professional obstructionism forced the Scottish universities to rescind a liberal policy on the award of degrees in the mid-1930s. There were also moves to restrict numbers of women entering medical practice, and one might see similar measures of exclusion affecting aliens and refugees as were used against women.[10] Few refugees gained British nationality prior to the war, and so most were insecure as aliens, not knowing whether valuable concessions like the recognition of all foreign degrees, made as an emergency measure in late 1940, might be rescinded.

The trickle of medical refugees in Wales formed part of a broader wave of Jewish refugees from Nazism and other fascist movements. The Board of Deputies of British Jews took a snooty attitude both to Welsh Jews and to the refugees.[11] There were also refugees from the Spanish Civil War, who were warmly received by Welsh socialists. Individual histories show the importance of local support, both Jewish and non-Jewish. The question then arises, how did the medically qualified refugees and medical students fare? In 1933 the Welsh National School of Medicine pleaded that it had no spare places and that it could not afford any financial concessions.[12] The situation was one in which the universities did little, but tolerated a free market of support. In July 1933 Emrys Evans, the Principal of the University College of North Wales at Bangor, expressed general sympathy with the appeal but regretted that the university had no funds for assisting displaced scholars; he felt that individual teaching members were likely to support an appeal which, in the event, was organized by Professor J. L. Simonsen, of the chemistry department. The chemist C. R. Bury of Aberystwyth, W. J. Jones of the University College of South Wales at Cardiff, the Provost of the Welsh National School of Medicine and J. E. Coates of Swansea all responded favourably to supporting appeals for individual teachers to raise funds at their respective institutions.[13]

Voluntary contributions led to problems with the prospective host institution. In November 1933, J. Kenneth Rees the Treasurer of the University of Wales Guild of Graduates collected subscriptions amounting to £60 for a refugee scholar in Swansea. When he attempted to move a resolution at the University Senate in March 1934 in favour of admitting a refugee, Senate resolved: 'that present circumstances do not warrant encouraging any refugees to participate in College life here except as students under ordinary conditions.' The Academic Assistance Council (AAC) responded vigorously that other British universities had offered usual amenities for visiting professors, including staff common-room use. The University Senate then agreed to consider hospitality for a visiting researcher sponsored by the Society for the Protection of Science and Learning (SPSL).[14] At Cardiff, matters went more smoothly, as local support raised funds for the economist Werner Friedrich Bruck for four years.[15] The University of Wales responded to national appeals made by the SPSL very much in line with other universities in 1935 through branches of the Association of University Teachers; but in February 1939 the colleges at Aberystwyth and Swansea considered that an appeals lecture might not be well attended.[16] The Principal of Bangor was willing to host a lecture by a distinguished national figure; here the problem was finding a willing person to travel the distance.[17]

The SPSL took a lead both nationally and internationally. The situation of individual rather than institutional support was sharply illustrated by Thomas Jones, the Secretary of the Pilgrim Trust, and his personal concern for the welfare of refugees. Jones (known as 'T.J.') was from Rhymney, a distinguished civil servant, and founder of Coleg Harlech, where he personally supported a handful of refugees, albeit non-medical. The Trust was founded in 1930 with a £2 million donation from the American philanthropist Edward Harkness. The Trust was based in London, and its activities were not confined to Wales. In May 1933 Abraham Flexner, the author of classic accounts of American and European medical education, pointed out to T.J. that the Rockefeller Foundation might help displaced scholars at the provincial English and Welsh universities.[18] Jones realized this was a great opportunity for the Welsh universities, and forwarded Flexner's letters to Sir William Beveridge, and these contributed to the formation of the AAC.[19] But the Pilgrim Trust, whose trustees included John Buchan the author (and anti-Semite) and MP, declined financial support to the AAC in 1934.[20] Beveridge was also dismayed that the Rockefeller Foundation was grudging in its support.[21] T.J. remained strongly sympathetic at a personal level, while criticizing the British government for not condemning Nazi persecution of Jews.[22] He discussed cases of doctors elsewhere, for example the psychiatrist Erich Guttmann at the Maudsley Hospital in London. He thought that the skills of a woman radiologist might be useful in Wales, but was frustrated by bureaucratic red tape.[23]

The Socialist Medical Association lobbied for refugee doctors and others with relevant skills to take a role in improving health in areas of social deprivation. The Austrian psychologist Marie Jahoda, who came to Cwm Afon, near Pontypool, in 1938 to conduct a study of the unemployed, built on her celebrated study of Marienthal in Austria. Although a significant piece of work, the study was for many years unpublished.[24] Continental exponents of social and industrial medicine, like the industrial diseases expert Ludwig Teleky, the social hygienist Myron Kantorowicz or the sexologist Max Hodann, passed through Britain on the way to the United States (or in Hodann's case to Sweden); a few settled in obscurity in Britain like the social gynaecologist Max Hirsch, but none found their way to Wales. The epidemiologist Major Greenwood, the Treasurer of the SPSL, did not much like these Continental theorists.[25] Welsh Medical Officers of Health did not see that the refugees could make a potential contribution to social medicine. Overall, medical circles in Wales were not easily penetrated by outsiders. Medical refugees encountered the allegation that they were taking jobs away from British graduates. Here, professional protectionism merged with anti-Semitism.[26]

The influx of medical refugees into Wales appears at first sight small by comparison with Scotland. Only the three Austrians, Erich Wellisch, Robert Bauer and Alfred Feiner, gained Welsh degrees. There was nothing quite like the Scottish tradition of offering Jewish medical students, excluded elsewhere, the chance to obtain a medical education, or indeed the possibility of requalifying for practice in the UK. Wales never saw a major initiative like the Polish School of Medicine in Edinburgh during the war.[27] It did, however, offer a 'special scheme of instruction for refugee students'.[28] When the University of Oxford hosted degree ceremonies for thirty-seven Czechoslovak MDs in February and July 1943, five graduates (Ales Dobry, Isidor Leb, Frantisek Stastny, Walter Tausig and Zdenek Urbanek) studied in Cardiff. The Welsh National School of Medicine offered clinical instruction to considerable numbers of medical refugees. Although the refugee students were deemed ineligible for the Welsh degree, and the English Board insisted on two years' clinical experience, it was found that the Scottish Conjoint Board would admit to examination after a year. The situation arose of a generous admissions policy in Wales, and a flexible examination policy in Scotland. The contribution of the Welsh National School of Medicine can easily be overlooked, and it is only by examining committee and individual student records that it becomes clear that relatively high numbers were admitted.

The formal opening of the Welsh National School of Medicine in 1933 coincided with Hitler's takeover in Germany. The Jewish Refugees Committee in London explained in May 1933 the difficulties it was having of placing refugee physicians, so that they might take a recognized UK qualification.[29] In October 1933 six Germans holding medical qualifications were admitted as students, and in January 1934 the overall number of 'German medical men' was fixed at twelve.[30] The Senate heard in January 1934 of how the Jewish refugee students were so satisfactory that 'the School would be well advised to admit a further number of such students'.[31] The Senate heard how 'the four German students who had completed the Final Examinations of the Edinburgh Conjoint Board, viz. Dr Last, Dr Gruenbaum, Dr Abeles and Dr Levy, had personally communicated their very grateful thanks for allowing them to pursue their studies here'.[32] Other German students were Siegfried Cohn, Ilta Wolpert (technically stateless), Peter Salzberg and Ernst Sklarz (admitted in October 1936). The Annual Report of 1934–5 reported that seven German students had obtained a registrable qualification and that: 'They proved very satisfactory students in every respect.'[33]

When it came to the emergency of the Austrian *Anschluss* and the Nazi takeover of Czechoslavakia, the Welsh National School of Medicine showed itself to be more generous than most other British medical schools. There were concessionary schemes to admit fifty Austrian physicians and fifty Czechoslovak physicians with the idea that after two years' study they should be allowed to take a British qualification. While most medical schools took two students, the Welsh National School of Medicine took seven Austrians and fifteen Czechs. One Austrian refugee doctor, nominated by the Refugee Selection Committee in London under the President of the Royal College of Surgeons, was admitted free of all tuition fees for two years to take the Medical Conjoint Board qualifications of England. The concession was extended to a Czech physician.[34] Of the Austrians, Robert Bauer requalified in 1940, Alfred Feiner, Marcell Gang and Rudolph Gottfried in 1941, and Edgar Rhoden was admitted in 1940. This was under the agreement to allow fifty Austrian doctors to requalify in Britain.[35] Marcell Gang was allowed to requalify in Cardiff, but this was on the understanding that he would proceed to Newfoundland, where there was a British government scheme to encourage doctors and dental surgeons to settle. His application to be included on one of the five vacant positions on the quota, which had arisen as a result of emigration, was rejected by the BMA. It meant that he had to apply centrally to the Home Office for permission to practise.[36] His wife Erica Gang did not pursue her medical career.

Six of the Czechs were medical students released from the Czech army to resume their studies and, overall, twelve Czechs can be identified.[37] In May 1940 the School offered similar concessions to Polish students. Only one Pole, Erwin Haberfeld, has left a student record, and the Polish School at Edinburgh acted as a focus for Polish students in Britain.[38] Hynek Rotenstein and Ludwig Neuwirth held MDs from Budapest.[39]

The Cardiff hospitals absorbed the talents of refugee nurses. There was a shortage of nurses in Britain, and while many female refugees arrived under a concessionary scheme to admit refugees as domestic servants, nursing promised independence and occupational fulfilment.[40] It was also a way forward for unemployed refugee doctors. On 6 December 1938 the Matron of Cardiff City Hospital submitted a letter from the Co-ordinating Committee for Refugees Nursing Sub-committee asking if the Recognized Training Schools would accept at least two candidates every year for a period of four consecutive years. It was 'Unanimously decided to recommend that this Hospital is willing to take two suitable candidates as trainees.'[41] Traineeships led to settlement. Alice Elfriede Sebba, an Austrian nurse, was to marry Kurt Gothsmann in Cardiff in 1940.[42] But there were – as in the rest of Britain – wholesale dismissals following the invasion scare in

May and June 1940. Cardiff was declared a 'protected area', so that all Germans and Austrians were to be interned. Heinz (later Henry) Kley was interned while requalifying. Refugee nurses at the Royal Infirmary were also interned.[43] There were limited opportunities in junior clinical appointments. Cardiff City Hospital employed Franz Kellermann, who held a Vienna MD and the Scottish 'triple qualification', as Junior Assistant in the Medical Unit in 1937. When employing H. G. Simchowitz as Radium Registrar in 1941, it made plain that it would follow BMA guidelines that all wartime appointments could only be short-term.[44]

Cardiff's potential as a medical centre was shown by its brain research laboratory, which gained support from the Rockefeller Foundation. Samuel Last, a young Berlin psychiatrist, collaborated with Quastel in 1934. In 1938 Efraim Racker, a newly qualified physician from Austria, joined the highly innovative Department of Brain Research under Juda/Joseph Quastel at the Cardiff City Mental Hospital. There, Racker undertook laboratory research analysing excretion of histidine in patients suffering from mental disorder. Racker regarded his Cardiff period as fundamental in shifting his interests from the clinic to the laboratory. He was interned in 1940, and in 1941 he emigrated to the US, where he had a distinguished career in studying the biochemistry of the brain.[45] Two other refugees left the research group, Michael Tennenbaum and Moritz Michaelis, 'under the new Regulations applying to aliens'. Internment thus broke up a potentially dynamic research group.[46] Even the British-born Quastel was to emigrate to British Columbia, as he was sidelined by English colleagues. Medical research funding had the potential of bringing refugees to Wales, using external resources but, generally, opportunities were few for refugees in medical research in Wales.

Requalification acted as a barrier to refugees becoming GPs in Wales. The list compiled by the refugee assistance worker, Yvonne Kapp, shows the types and distribution of refugees in 1939. The 17 practitioners and doctors listed represent about 1 per cent of the UK total. The total number of 1,626 individuals comprised of 1,359 doctors and 267 dental surgeons (the Austrians being also physicians) on this unique but incomplete list. Despite the small number of students seeking to requalify or to continue disrupted studies at the Welsh School of Medicine, Cardiff, it is interesting to note that in 1950 those who had qualified at Cardiff were in general practice in Wales.

Table 7.1: Yvonne kapp's List, September 1939: 'Refugee doctors and dentists registered with the medical department'

1C	Adler, Eugen	Dent		17 Cathedral Road, Cardiff
3C	Alders, Nikolaus	Gyn		155 Richmond Road, Cardiff
3A	Bauer, Robert			6 Pantmawr Road, Whitchurch, Cardiff
2A	Eisner, Charlotte	Laryng		Pen Pentre, Llandaff, Cardiff
2A	Eisner, Erich	Derm		
2A	Eisner, Georg			Pen Pentre, Llandaff, Cardiff
2Cz	Eisner-Klissmann, Gisela	Child		Domov, Newport Road, Llantarnam, Mon.
2B	Engelberg, Adele	GP		6 Slade Road, Newton, Swansea
3A	Feiner, Alfred			39 Ilton Road, Cardiff
3A	Finsterbusch, Edmund			95 Newport Road, Cardiff
3C	Gang, Marcel			16 The Parade, Cardiff
2B	Haendler, Julius	GP		Gwrych Castle, Abergele, Denbighshire
2B	Racker, Ephraim	GP		Biochemical Laboratory, Mental Hospital, Cardiff
3D	Schaechter, Hans	Dent		194 Cathedral Road, Cardiff
2Cz	Schmidt, Ladislaus	Rheum		Kinmel Hall, Abergele, north Wales
1B	Schnitzler, Paul	GP		Anglesey Infirmary, Bangor
1B	Schwarz, Ernst	GP		North Wales County Hospital, north Wales

Key

1A	Settled specialists	2Ci	Unsettled Italians
1B	Settled general practitioners	2Cz	Unsettled Czechoslovakians
1C	Settled dentists		
		3A	Austrian doctors studying
2A	Unsettled specialists	3B	Czechoslovakian doctors studying
2B	Unsettled general practitioners	3C	Admitted students – miscellaneous
2C	Unsettled dentists	3D	Austrian dentists studying

It was impossible to practice unless one had British (or, curiously) Italian qualifications, as the latter were recognized by the General Medical Council. When Sigmund Freud arrived in Britain in 1939, he insisted that his Viennese cardiologist, Bernard Samet, be permitted to continue as his physician. The Home Office granted an exceptional licence to Samet, who at the time was requalifying at St Thomas's Medical School. Samet was an outstanding cardiologist having trained in the First University Clinic under Wenkebach, where he pioneered the use of the electrocardiograph. He then had a post at the Rothschild Hospital, a large Jewish hospital in Vienna. Samet, aged 44, was appointed to the Ruthin Castle clinic in 1942. This clinic emulated the Mayo Clinic in Minnesota as a research and clinical institution. It was directed by Sir Edmund Spriggs and the pathologist Sidney Patterson, who had been recruited from Melbourne University.[47] Samet's son Paul comments on his father's appointment:

> Was it a challenging environment for him? Probably not in the sense that he was capable of achieving more ... however, the lack of higher qualifications was a hindrance ... he did try to move to other hospitals and enquired about some university lectureships, but by then his age was also against him. So he abandoned the attempt and settled for continuation at Ruthin Castle. If he was unhappy about the choice he never said so.[48]

Despite a genuinely high quality of staff and care, from the mid-1950s the Ruthin clinic experienced financial difficulties and closed in December 1962. Samet remained there until retirement, and Fred Epstein, another refugee, was there briefly from 1945 to 1947. Ruthin served an elite set of patients, mainly from outside Wales. But this refugee medical family also put down roots in Welsh medicine. Samet's wife, Vilma Samet, gained the possibility of being able to practice, when in 1940 all foreign degree holders could register their degrees on an annual basis. She took a post in general medicine at Wrexham. The recognition of degrees was a momentous and far-sighted measure. It at long last provided the majority of the refugees with the opportunity to practise.[49]

The war saw some temporary gains. This can be illustrated by two displaced dental surgeons, both Vienna medical graduates who entered dental surgery as a postgraduate medical specialism. Rudy Schlesinger had requalified in Liverpool, but as an enemy alien could not practise in a restricted area. In 1940 he moved to Mold where he had a surgery until 1946. The RAF appointed him as dental surgeon for their Anglesey base but, as the area was restricted, he saw patients in Prestatyn where he practised until the 1960s.⁵⁰ Jacques Kurer was also a Viennese dental surgeon, who had first qualified in medicine and then had a highly innovative specialist training under Bernhard Gottlieb. Kurer had published a pioneering text on child dentistry as a specialism. He returned to Manchester after the war.⁵¹ In contrast, the dental surgeon Eugen Adler requalified while living in Cardiff, and settled more permanently there.

During the war, substantial numbers of Czech and Polish doctors came to Wales in a military capacity. Two clusters can be identified. Among the Czechs at Penrhos Camp, Pwllheli, were two physicians. Far larger was the Polish No. 3 General Hospital at Penley, Wrexham. The latter was to become a permanency.⁵² Here there were forty-three Polish physicians in 1950; by 1958 sixteen had moved on, and all of these left Wales, although one had an appointment in Chepstow in Monmouthshire. Ruthin Castle, the RAF and Penrhos show that the refugees serviced wartime influxes to Wales.

In the post-war period the refugees were still insecure. Few wanted to return to their countries of origin. The period of the NHS and permanent settlement raises the issue of long-term contributions to health care in Wales and to biomedical research. A scattering of senior academic appointments were filled by former refugees in medicine in Wales.

The life sciences show a similar pattern of resistance and isolated appointments. There was an opening for a geneticist when in 1948 the former Austrian geneticist, Fabius Gross, was appointed Professor of Marine Studies at Bangor. The idea was to study sex determination by studying the effects of different concentrations of salt, and sinking protozoa gametes into different depths of the sea and studying the effects of oxygen absorption. He experimented with nitrates and their effect on fish populations. Here his research was successful in meeting the wartime needs in Britain of an applied biology.⁵³ Tragically, Gross died before he could fully establish the new school at Bangor.

Cardiff provided a few refugees with chances to requalify and to take postgraduate qualifications. The tuberculosis specialist Milosh Sekulich came to Britain in 1942 as a representative of the Yugoslav underground. He came to Wales in 1947 to take qualifications in public health; he was only briefly in general practice in Cardiff and colliery districts between diploma examinations. He remained in academic contact with the Department of Tuberculosis at Cardiff University – in particular, with Frederick Heaf who considered that Sekulich's classification was the best so far.⁵⁴ But he returned to work as a GP in London.

Yet in terms of rank-and-file medicine the refugees contributed to general practice and to hospital medicine. Compared with the 1930s, we see an overwhelming predominance of Polish doctors – in fact twenty-seven out of seventy held Polish qualifications from Polish medical faculties or from the Polish School of Medicine in Edinburgh. This reflects the situation that overall in the UK the Polish refugee cohort was the largest. The more clinically oriented Austrians – of whom there were sixteen – outnumbered the more scientifically minded Germans of whom there were only ten. It meant that Wales took only 0.75 per cent of the overall number of German medical refugees in the UK. By way of contrast the Austrians numbered about 5 per cent of the total of Austrian physicians in the UK. While A. V. Hill's image of the German scientifically minded physician represented an element of the Welsh refugee-influx, it can be seen that the Polish refugees predominated. Interestingly, the Poles often retained their culture, and here perhaps the cultural otherness of Wales provided a favourable background.

The Germans, Czechoslovaks and Austrians were mainly Jewish – ranging from the secular to the orthodox. They tended to shed their previous national identity. The Poles retained a stronger sense of national identity, as exiles rather than as forced emigrants, and the majority were Roman Catholic. The journal *CAJEX*, a Jewish ex-servicemen and women's journal founded in 1950, provides some insight into a scattering of refugees who sustained a Jewish identity, although the community as a whole was dwindling. *CAJEX* included details of the physicians Bernfeld, Feiner and Weis.[55] Some found full satisfaction in their work, but this was not always possible.

Max Weis, a physician from Beuel (a neighbouring town of Bonn), had been arrested the day after the Beuel synagogue was burned down, imprisoned with eighteen other Jewish men, and then dragged off to a concentration camp. The idea of the Germans was to terrorize Jews into emigrating by arresting local notables. He then left Germany with his wife Bella on the infamous ocean liner, the *St Louis* bound for Havana. Cuba and the United States denied landing to some nine hundred passengers. The *St Louis* is a classic case of American aversion to admitting persecuted Jews from Germany, and the ship returned to Antwerp. That Britain, France, Belgium and the Netherlands all offered refuge to the passengers shows the greater sense of an emergency situation as Europe stood on the brink of war.[56] Weis was fortunate in gaining admission to Britain. After he was interned in 1940, he secured a job at the Rookwood Ministry of Pensions hospital at Llandaff from 1942. This was a fulfilling phase of his medical career, when he could devote his time to patient care.[57] There was an eloquent tribute on his death in 1952 by the hospital staff and patients. On the fiftieth anniversary of his death a square was named 'Doktor-Weis-Platz' in Bonn-Beul to commemorate this 'Physician of the Poor' and to mark an initiative against the hate of foreigners.[58]

Refugees and exiles became integrated over time and part of the Welsh medical community. This can be seen particularly well in psychiatry. The Swansea psychiatrist Jerzy Lessovsky decided not to join the Polish Medical Society in Great Britain, and anglicized his name. But an awareness of his past, the loss of family in the Holocaust and his survival, and a determined effort to resettle can be seen in his memoir, *Poles Apart*.[59] The focus was on the professional activities in the present, and the sense of displacement was attenuated into occasional nostalgia and *Sehnsucht* (longing).

How much did the former refugees adapt to the cultural circumstances? The Pontypridd GP Alfred Feiner translated the German nonsense poet, Christian Morgenstern (a sort of German Edward Lear), into English, and was also an accomplished violinist.[60] Runhilt Mayer-von den Steinen had in the 1920s formed part of the aesthetic circle of the poet, Stefan George, but felt her new circumstances to be alien and superficial.[61] But it was possible to plunge into Welsh culture. Vernon (formerly Werner) Bernfeld, originally from Leipzig, was appointed venereologist in Cardiff City Hospital in 1955. Bernfeld was the son of a noted Leipzig dermatologist, and although the University of Leipzig vindictively annulled his degree in his absence in March 1939, it remained the basis for his recognition under the Temporary Registration provisions of 1940. In 1950 he gained his membership qualifications. He was one of the very few refugee venereologists to find a place in British medicine, not least because of the lack of opportunities for independently practising specialists. He played the flute at the National Eisteddfod, and became a 'splendid and inspired' Honorary Secretary of the Cardiff Natural History Society until 1973, developing the Society's civic links while conducting a range of historical investigations.[62] He felt that 'he would not be really Welsh until he had mastered Welsh fluently'.[63] In return came the friendship of 'many interesting and cultural people'.[64] Bernfeld exemplifies a highly fulfilled resettlement.

The cohort of medical refugees who ventured into Wales consisted primarily of rank-and-file GPs and clinicians. The Rhodens in Cardiff were an illustrious medical partnership of husband and wife. Their son Harry qualified in medicine, continuing the practice, while a daughter qualified in natural sciences and then went into cancer research in London.[65] Overall, I can identify sixty-nine former refugees in Wales in 1950. Most were GPs, and most settled permanently.[66] Others like the surgeon Alfred Beck (formerly Czechoslovak), at St David's Hospital Cardiff from 1952 to 1976, and the orthopaedic surgeon Hanus Weisl (who arrived in Britain on a *Kindertransport*), in Cardiff from the 1960s, had distinguished clinical careers. As a result of the upheaval of the war, Wladzmierz Boladz came to Britain only in 1946 after military service and harsh imprisonment in the war. He became a GP at Ystradgynlais from 1949 until 1988 where he was 'a beloved and integral part of the area'.[67]

Overall, the numbers in Wales were sparse, when compared with other areas of the UK. The BMA pursued a policy of dispersal, but on a wholly negative basis by refusing permission to practise in London rather than seeking to open up provincial opportunities. At first the refugees who came to Wales arrived primarily because of individual generosity. The situation changed with the influx of Polish refugee doctors; a few remained at Wrexham, while many sought job opportunities within Wales. That the NHS created positions for specialist physicians in hospital posts, as well as improving the basis of general practice meant that a viable basis was created for long-term careers. A more dynamic approach to developing medical research and social medicine in Wales could have brought in more of the refugee innovators in medical research and clinical medicine. But the collection of life histories suggests that Wales provided a satisfying new homeland for a select number of displaced doctors, and that they in turn contributed substantially to health care in Wales.

Notes

*   I gratefully acknowledge Wellcome Trust support for the research project on medical refugees in the United Kingdom 1930–50. I wish to thank University of Wales, Cardiff Medical School for generous access to its records. I am also grateful to Dr Harry Rhoden for generously responding to my enquiries.

1   Rothschild was possibly employed by a miners' sickness scheme. See Ray Earwicker, 'Miners' medical services before the First World War: the south

THE JEWISH MEDICAL REFUGEE CRISIS AND WALES 197

Wales coalfield', *Llafur*, Vol. 3, no. 2 (1981), 34–52. It is also possible that he was assistant to an established practice. Paul Ludwig Elieser Rothschild is first listed in the *Medical Directory* under London in 1936 and 1937 with an address in Parliament Hill; in 1938 with 'address uncommunicated'. He is listed in 1939–40 as clinical assistant, Fulham Hospital.

[2] Churchill College Archives A.V. Hill Papers LII 5/36 44, 'The good physician'.
[3] Ibid.; R. M. Cooper (ed.), *Refugee Scholars: Conversations with Tess Simpson* (Leeds, 1992), 74–5.
[4] P. J. Weindling, 'The contribution of central European Jews to medical science and practice in Britain, 1930–1960', in W. E. Mosse (ed.), *Second Chance: The History of the German-speaking Jews in the United Kingdom* (Tübingen, 1991), pp. 243–54.
[5] Oxford Brookes University, Medical Refugees Collection, Hill-Blaschko correspondence.
[6] A. J. Sherman, *Island Refuge: Britain and Refugees from the Third Reich 1933–1939* (London, 1973). *Kindertransport* refers generically to organized efforts to bring persecuted Jewish Austrian, German and Czech children to safety.
[7] Louise London, *Whitehall and the Jews 1933–1948: British Immigration Policy and the Holocaust* (Cambridge, 2000).
[8] The controversy is covered in *CAJEX Magazine of the Association of Jewish Ex-Servicemen and Women, Cardiff*, Vol. 29, no. 3 (1979), 26–9; Geoffrey Alderman 'The anti-Jewish riots of August 1911 in south Wales', *Welsh History Review*, Vol. 6, no. 2 (1972), 190–200; Colin Holmes, 'The Tredegar riots of 1911: anti-Jewish disturbances in south Wales', *Welsh History Review*, Vol. 11, no. 2 (1982), 214–25; Colin Holmes, *John Bull's Island: Immigration in British Society, 1871–1971* (London 1988); W. D. Rubinstein, 'The anti-Jewish riots of 1911 in south Wales: a re-examination', *Welsh History Review*, Vol. 18, no. 4 (1997), 667–99.
[9] This figure includes those who remigrated elsewhere after a period of time in the UK, and the small proportion – very low – of Austrians and Germans, and slightly higher, perhaps 5 per cent, of the Czechs and Poles who returned.
[10] Diana Palmer, 'Women, health and politics, 1919–1939', typescript dated 1986 held in Warwick University Library.
[11] Geoffrey Alderman, *Modern British Jewry* (Oxford, 1992), p. 297.
[12] University of Manchester Archives, notes on the refugee situation in 1933.
[13] Bodleian Library Oxford, Society for the Protection of Science and Learning (hereafter SPSL), Box 51/1, f. 17 and 26, Emrys Evans, 6 July 1933.
[14] SPSL 129/1, f. 223–57. The eventual candidate was the historian Dietrich Gerhard.
[15] SPSL 130/3, f. 189, J. F. Rees to Thomson 2 December 1938.
[16] SPSL 130/3, f. 173, Thomson to Laurie 1 February 1939.
[17] SPSL 130/3, f. 177–85.
[18] SPSL 120/4, f. 579–81, Abraham Flexner letters of 12 and 19 May 1933; E. L. Ellis, *T.J.: A Life of Dr Thomas Jones, CH* (Cardiff, 1992), p. 316 on the origins of the friendship between Flexner and 'T.J.'.

[19] SPSL 120/4, f. 583, Beveridge to Flexner; 'T.J.'. Thomas Jones, *A Diary with Letters 1931–1950* (Oxford, 1954), pp. 110–11 on 'German professors', 19 May 1933; cf. p. 426 on the Richborough camp to train Jews as settlers.

[20] SPSL 120/4, f. 602, Jones to Beveridge, 13 April 1934.

[21] Paul Weindling, 'An overloaded ark? The Rockefeller Foundation and refugee medical scientists, 1933–1945', *Studies in the History and Philosophy of Biology and Biomedical Science*, Vol. 31 (2000) 477–89.

[22] Ellis, *T.J.*, pp. 426–7.

[23] National Library of Wales, papers of Thomas Jones, Class M, Vol. 1, Refugees 1937–54, Braun-Lazarus; Vol. 2, Refugees 1933–54, von Metzerradt-Sonnenfeldt f. 17, 15 September 1939 T.J. to Jennifer Williams, Home Office; f. 119, Dr Carl E. W. Lambert to T.J. concerning Dr Erich Guttmann, T.J. to F. A. Newsam, 17 March 1941.

[24] SPSL, Marie Jahoda-Lazarsfeld file. For publication of the report see Christian Fleck (ed.), *Marie Jahoda: Arbeitslose bei der Arbeit: Die Nachfolgeuntersuchung zu 'Marienthal' aus dem Jahr 1938* (Frankfurt am Main, 1989); Marie Jahoda, 'Unemployed men at work', in David Fryer and Phillip Ullah (eds), *Unemployed People: Social and Psychological Perspectives* (Milton Keynes, 1987), pp. 1–73.

[25] For the significance of German social hygiene see my *Health, Race and German Politics 1870–1945* (Cambridge, 1989). Also individuals' SPSL files.

[26] For background see Neil Evans, 'Immigrants and minorities in Wales, 1840–1990', in Charlotte Williams, Neil Evans and Paul O'Leary (eds), *A Tolerant Nation: Exploring Ethnic Diversity in Wales* (Cardiff, 2003), pp. 14–34 – some racial violence as in 1911; Anthony Glaser, 'Jewish refugees and Jewish industries', in Ursula Henriques (ed.), *The Jews of South Wales: Historical Studies* (Cardiff, 1992), pp. 177–205 shows the establishment of modest pharmaceutical and surgical dressing companies; N. H. Saunders, *The Swansea Hebrew Congregation 1730–1980* (Swansea, 1980).

[27] Kenneth Collins, *Go and Learn: The International Story of Jews and Medical Education in Scotland* (Aberdeen 1988); Paul Weindling, 'Czechoslovak medical refugees in Great Britain during and after the Second World War', in Antonin Kostlan and Alice Velkova (eds), *Wissenschaft im Exil. Die Tsechechoslowakai als Kreuzweg 1918–1989* (Prague: Forschungszentrum für Wissenschaftsgeschichte, 2004), 52–64.

[28] Archive for the History of Austrian Sociology, Institute of Sociology, University of Graz, Friedrich, Hertz Collection,Part 7, Welsh National School of Medicine to Edith Hertz, 4 January 1940.

[29] Welsh National School of Medicine (WNSM), Senate 7 July 1933, with attached letter from Jewish Refugees Committee, 28 May 1933.

[30] WNSM, Council Minutes 20 June 1933, 20 July 1933, 17 October 1933, 30 January 1934.

[31] WNSM, Senate 7 February 1934.

[32] Ibid. 7 November 1934; student record cards of Friedrich Moritz Abeles, Max Gruenbaum, Julius Levy, Samuel Siegfried Last.

[33] WNSM, Annual Report 1934–5, p. 5.

THE JEWISH MEDICAL REFUGEE CRISIS AND WALES 199

[34] WNSM, Annual Report 1939–40, p. 7; General Purposes Committee, 19 January 1939; Council, 28 April 1939; University Registrar to Secretary WNSM, 28 February 1939; Senate 7 December 1938, 11 January 1939; Robert Hutchison to Provost WNSM, 10 November 1938; Senate 23 November 1939.
[35] Paul Weindling, 'Austrian medical refugees in Great Britain: from marginal aliens to established professionals', *Wiener klinische Wochenschrift*, Vol. 110 (1998), 158–61; idem, 'Austrian medical refugees in Great Britain 1938–1945' in Sonia Horn and Peter Malina (eds), *Medizin im Nationalsozialismus – Wege der Aufarbeitung* (Vienna, 2001), pp. 289–92; WNSM, student record cards.
[36] BMA Archives, Home Office Medical Advisory Committee BMA Aliens Committee 1939–49, B/12/1/1, ff. 118, 125.
[37] WNSM, Annual Report 1940–41, p. 7; WNSM, student record cards. The Czechs were Maximilian Szinay, Leo Hornung, Izidor Grossman, Marcel Bednar, Egon Lenit, Alfred Goldberger, Josef Varacer, Zdenek Urbanek and at least four (Tausig, Leb, Stastny and Dobry) who gained Czech degrees in Oxford in 1943.
[38] WNSM, Council Minutes 7 May 1940; WNSM, student record cards.
[39] WNSM, student record cards.
[40] Tony Kushner, 'An alien occupation – Jewish refugees and domestic service in Britain, 1933–1948', in Mosse, *Second Chance*, pp. 553–77; John Stewart, 'Angels or aliens? Refugee nurses in Britain, 1938 to 1942', *Medical History*, Vol. 47 (2003), 149–72.
[41] SPSL 120/4 f. 813, meeting 6 December 1938.
[42] University of Cambridge Library, Cambridge Refugee Committee Minutes, biographical notes (1938–40).
[43] Dennis Morgan, *Cardiff: A City at War* (Cardiff, 1998), p. 26.
[44] Glamorgan Record Office, Cardiff City Hospital Minute Books, D/D HC 17 and 18.
[45] SPSL, file of Racker; *International Biographical Dictionary of Central European Emigres 1922–1945* (Munich, 1983), Vol. 2, part 2, p. 935; Cornell University Alumni.
[46] Cf. *City of Cardiff, The Mental Hospital, 32nd Annual Report for the Year 1939, 1940*.
[47] Information from Tom Patterson, Oxford.
[48] Paul Samet, 'My parents in the UK', unpublished MS.
[49] Personal information from Paul Samet, 19 April 2000, and Tom Patterson, who both grew up at Ruthin.
[50] Personal information from Paul Samet, 19 April 2000.
[51] Ibid.; Oxford Brookes Database, Kurer files.
[52] BBC North-East, *Penley Poles* (October 2003), BBC Legacies Project, http://www.bbc.co.uk/wales/northeast/yoursay/askalocal/penley.shtml.
[53] SPSL, Fabius Gross file.
[54] Wellcome Library, MSS, Milosh Sekulich papers.
[55] *CAJEX*, Vol. 1, no. 1 (1950); Maurice Dennis, 'A community in decline?', *CAJEX*, Vol. 22 (1972), 31–4; Alderman, *Modern British Jewry*, p. 323 suggests a decline from 2,300 Jews in Cardiff in 1955 to 1,250 in 1985.

56 John Mendelsohn (ed.), *Jewish Emigration: The S.S. St Louis Affair and Other Cases* (New York, 1982).
57 Henry E. Samuel, 'Dr Max Weis: Jewish doctor who gave his life's services to ex-servicemen', *CAJEX*, Vol. 3 (1952), 66; Registrar General's Office, death certificates of Max and Bella Weis.
58 Anja Blanuscha, 'Platz erinnert jetzt an den "Arzt der Armen"', newsclipping of 26/27 October 2002; 'Signal gegen das Vergessen', *Bonner Rundschau* (26 October 2002); Ruth Schlette, commemorative address on Max Weis.
59 Jeremy Lister, *Poles Apart* (Swansea, 1997).
60 Alfred Feiner, *Selected Poems of Christian Morgenstein*, parallel German text and English translation (Walton on Thames, 1973).
61 When Runhilt was visited by her friend Alice Platen-Hallermund, a former student friend from Heidelberg who was training in group analysis in Britain, Alice recollects that Runhilt felt deeply isolated in what she perceived as an alien and superficial culture. Alice failed to convince her of the merits of *Under Milk Wood*.
62 Glamorgan Record Office, Cardiff Naturalists' Society D/D CNS 7/15–24, Papers of the Secretary Dr W. K. Bernfeld, 1970–76; D/D CNS 7/24/2, President's letter, 31 October 1973. Bernfeld merits inclusion among the refugee historians of medicine. See Paul Weindling, 'Medical refugees and the renaissance of medical history in Great Britain, 1930s–1960s', in W. Eckart (ed.), *Medizinhistoriographie in der Neuzeit* (Paffenweiler, 1999), pp. 139–51.
63 Bernfeld does not conform to the assumption of the refugee as scornful of the Welsh language, Gwyn Thomas, 'Refuge', in Grahame Davies (ed.), *The Chosen People: Wales and the Jews* (Bridgend, 2002), pp. 294–5.
64 Glamorgan Record Office, D/D CNS 7/24/1, Peter Bernfeld to Harmon Bowen, 12 January 1974.
65 I am grateful to Harry Rhoden for information on Cardiff medical refugees, letter of 30 August 2004. Cambridge Refugees Committee, notes on Eva Rhoden, born 1924 who studied at Newnham College, Cambridge.
66 Sources are *The Medical Directory* 1950 and 1958.
67 'To hell and back – Ystrad's adopted "Papa"', undated newspaper cutting from *Brecon and Radnor Express* (1988), deposited in files which are attached to Oxford Brookes Database of Medical Refugees in the UK.

Part I
Dr Julian Tudor Hart: A Profile

PAMELA MICHAEL

Dr Julian Tudor has won international renown for his contribution to the field of primary health care. An articulate and consistent advocate of its central role in modern health-care systems, he has pioneered many of its most progressive developments, from his emphasis on teamwork in community medicine to his insistence on respecting the patient both as citizen and co-health-worker. He framed a seminal concept in health-care theory – the 'inverse care law'. Hart has argued the need for doctors to campaign for social change in order to achieve fairness and equity – and he has led by example. For almost fifty years he has been a central figure in debating the ethical dilemmas of health-care policy. Sir Richard Doll once described Hart as 'the conscience of the medical profession in relation to the provision of medical attention for everybody equally'.[1]

For twenty-six years (1961–87) Dr Julian Tudor Hart served as general practitioner in the upland community of Glyncorrwg in south Wales, a small mining village between Hirwaun and Port Talbot with a population of some 1,700 inhabitants in 1965. Hart witnessed the terminal decline of the coal industry and the concomitant rise of male unemployment in his area. People slowly drifted away in search of work and by 1985 the population of the village had declined to 1,500. The worsening economic conditions were reflected in the health of the people. Although health conditions generally were improving during the second half of the twentieth century, the gap between the health experiences of those in the poorest areas and those in the richest areas was widening. In 1970 in the valleys of Glamorgan the mortality from ischaemic heart-disease of men aged 35–44 was 75 per cent above the rate for England and Wales. Mortality from stroke in men aged 35–64 was 50 per cent above the England and Wales rate.[2] Julian Tudor Hart sought not only to minister to the immediate needs of his patients, but to study their patterns of health and to seek ways of intervening to reduce the levels of mortality and morbidity amongst them.

Born in 1927, Hart studied medicine at Queen's College, Cambridge, and at St George's Hospital, London, graduating in 1952. He took up his first post in general practice in that year in Notting Hill, later vividly recalling the scenes which he then encountered:

> there were still rows of concentrated mixtures for dispensing and a boxed set of post-mortem cutlery on the doctor's desk, long unused. There was no toilet, and horsehair burst out of the chaise longue that served as an examination couch. Everything was covered in dust despite a throughput of 60 patients a day, and the caretaker asked me not to pee in the handbasin like the last doctor.[3]

Such conditions were not untypical and Hart, unsurprisingly, became a staunch advocate of the establishment of modern, well-equipped 'health centres'. He was severely critical of the abandonment of the principle of health centres as the cornerstone of primary care in the political struggle to gain the support of the medical profession for the new National Health Service in 1948.

Hart's determination to remain true to his principles was partly influenced by his parents' strong political commitments and life experiences. After qualifying as a doctor, his father, Alexander Tudor Hart, went to Vienna to study orthopaedic surgery under Professor Boehler. He returned to London and worked as a general practitioner in a working-class district of London. In 1934 he moved to south Wales to take up a salaried post in Llanelli, employed directly by the miners and tinplate union.[4] When the Spanish Civil War broke out in 1936, Alexander Tudor Hart 'offered his services as a surgeon and joined the war against Franco'.[5] He worked as a surgeon in the theatre of war alongside other volunteers such as Dr Reggie Sexton and a young Archie Cochrane, who worked as an anaesthetist (until he was sent back to Britain to continue his medical studies). Dr Tudor Hart was put in charge of the hospital at Huete, which was taken over and supplied with equipment and staff by the British Medical Aid unit.[6] During his service in the Spanish Civil War, Dr Alexander Tudor Hart developed methods for dealing with complex wounds and bone fractures, which 'opened new fields of technique' that helped to save the lives of many soldiers during the Second World War.[7]

After the Second World War the career of Julian Tudor Hart's mother developed, only to be cut short by the onset of chronic illness:

> My mother was crippled by a severe stroke at age 52, at the height of a well-paid career in the pharmaceutical industry. This was a consequence of childhood rheumatic disease, now virtually unknown in the UK, but common in slum-ridden Britain in 1916.[8]

This personal tragedy brought to her son a sense of deep anger and resentment at the social injustice of ill health. 'Premature death, disability and unhappiness are socially selective. They grant their miseries most generously to the poor', he observes. Like his parents, Julian became a member of the Communist Party of Great Britain and in 1963 took part in an election film made by ETV Ltd, alongside Jimmy Reid and Gladys Easton, entitled 'Our Life in Our Hands'. The film was never broadcast because the party was unable to field the required fifty candidates to gain entitlement to television coverage. Julian Tudor Hart admits that his longstanding espousal of Marxism was 'a choice that determined my entire career pathway'. It has certainly influenced his polemical style of writing, and he is as likely to quote Engels, Marx or Gramsci, as to cite clinical authorities in his contributions to academic medical journals.

From his student days Hart took a lively interest in epidemiology and, encouraged by Richard Doll (the leading epidemiologist who was to demonstrate the link between cigarette smoking and lung cancer), he applied for a post in 1960 with the Medical Research Council's Pneumoconiosis Research Unit in Llandough, near Cardiff. Here he was much influenced by the work of Archie Cochrane, who had been working at the unit for the past ten years on the X-ray classification of coal workers' pneumoconiosis. Cochrane had also been conducting one of the first total community surveys, the Rhondda Fach Scheme, a survey of chest diseases among the population of two south Wales mining communities. This was ground-breaking territory. In writing his own obituary Cochrane referred to this period as probably the most productive in his life:

> With an almost obsessional interest in reproducibility, low rates of refusal, and validation he showed that measurements could be made on populations defined geographically with about the same known inaccuracy as measurements made in laboratories. This helped to make epidemiology a quantitative science.[9]

Julian Tudor Hart adopted Cochrane's approach to epidemiological research and assimilated his ideas about evidence-based medicine.

Whilst he was based at the Medical Research Council unit at Llandough, Tudor Hart encountered the ill health of the south Wales mining communities and in 1961 he determined to fulfil an ambition which he had harboured since boyhood of becoming a 'people's doctor' in a deprived coal-mining community of south Wales.[10] He settled in Glyncorrwg, at the upper end of the Afan Valley in Mid Glamorgan, a seemingly unlikely place from which to become a frequent contributor to academic medical journals and a pace-setter in primary-care practice.

At the same time as fielding a full patient caseload, Julian Tudor Hart sustained a programme of epidemiological research spanning a period of over two decades. A Medline search shows that he published over 125 articles and letters in medical journals. One of his first major studies was conducted during 1968 and 1969. This involved reading the blood pressure of all of his patients aged between twenty and sixty-four on two different occasions and taking subsequent readings on all patients exhibiting diastolic pressures warranting treatment. Hart concluded that screening provided the opportunity to treat a lethal condition at a favourable stage, vastly preferable to intervening only after organ damage had occurred.[11] He has been a consistent advocate of the role of the family practitioner and community-health team in carrying out screening and predictive work to identify health problems at an early and treatable stage. Hart has also been willing to interrogate critically his own practice and caseload experiences in order to develop better practice for the future. In collaboration with Cerys Humphreys, a Medical Research Council research registrar, he conducted an analysis of the medical records of 500 patient deaths over the period 1964–85 in order to evaluate medical outcomes and identify possible changes in work practice and organization that would improve outcomes in the future. His findings indicated that most errors made by the general practitioner were the result of 'poor organization and follow up and failure to apply consistent criteria for diagnosis and treatment'. He found that patient behaviour influenced health outcomes in a number of ways. Smoking was an obvious example and Hart's study pointed to the already changing pattern of mortality whereby the proportion of deaths related to smoking amongst men was declining, whereas amongst women it was increasing. He also found that delay or refusal to present symptoms, especially in the case of rectal bleeding, was a critical indicator of poor outcome in cases of bowel cancer. Always a 'reflective practitioner' par excellence, Hart concluded that: 'All 10 delayed cases were essentially failures of the general practitioner to be an effective generalist with personal responsibility to help patients cope both with their own fears and with the pitfalls of referred hospital care.'[12] This and other studies were designed as much to instruct and inform future practice as to ascertain research findings for their own sake. The role of his research was not simply to understand the world, but to change it.

During his student days Julian Tudor Hart began writing about the need to provide general-practice training within standard medical education,[13] and he has continued to campaign for sound general-practice training ever since. In the early days of the National Health Service primary care was viewed as a poor relation, and most aspiring medical students had ambitions to become consultants and to work in hospital-based medicine. There was a deep chasm between the conditions under which doctors were trained and the conditions they found when they moved out into general practice. The general practitioners were largely 'left alone' in 1948, 'to do everything that was either too trivial or too difficult for specialists to do'. At that time, states Hart, GPs 'didn't believe in teams ... they preferred isolation and independence'. Aneurin Bevan, Hart has argued, 'took specialist care in hospitals seriously'. He funded it and gave hospital specialists salaried status. General practice, on the other hand, Bevan 'left undisturbed as a high volume, low cost, apparent solution for all the problems either beneath the notice of specialists, or too difficult for them to solve, adrift from medical science but providing a sheltered home for unmeasurable art'.[14] Hart argues that the compromise adopted in 1948, when general practitioners were allowed to remain independent, self-employed practitioners, delayed the adoption of modern primary-care practice by more than twenty years. Throughout these years Hart was himself practising as a GP and encouraging young doctors to follow suit. He was a strong advocate of primary care as an important site for training and medical education, arguing that it provided an entirely different perspective on the presentation of symptoms: 'Hospital patients are nearly all seen with a degree of hindsight, certainly by the time they see consultants, who seldom appreciate the degree to which their patients have organised their symptoms unless they one day confront the symptom-chaos of primary care.'[15] Hart also believes that primary care provides a good level at which to assimilate fundamental values of the medical profession. Here they can acquire 'formal respect for patients', and appreciate 'the many ways in which doctors must be subordinate to patients', and learn to accept that 'the sick must become the subjects rather than the objects of care'.[16]

Over the years Hart has argued for a much fuller and more proactive role for primary care, where clinical work can achieve real health gain, where health promotion, health improvement and skilled detection work can lead to a real improvement in the quality of people's lives. He has argued too for a programme of research at primary-care level, where not only doctors and other skilled professionals but patients too would participate fully. 'Evidence based primary care', he argues, 'must increasingly recognise patients as equals, bringing their own expertise to the co-productive processes of care.'[17] It is this respect for his patients as fellow-citizens that has been the hallmark of Julian Tudor Hart's career, as general practitioner, writer and socialist.

In promoting primary care Julian Tudor Hart has been strident in his opposition to the continuance of GPs' private contractor status, arguing for a salaried profession. He has been a scathing critic of the United States model of health care and a vociferous opponent of the marketization of the NHS in Britain and of many of the late twentieth-century 'reforms'. At the start of the new millenium he told his audience:

> The commodity approach to NHS care naturally adopted by policy makers using business as their ultimate model is not just inappropriate, it's destructive ... it reduces the space and time within which staff and patients can develop shared responsibilities through continuing anticipatory care and pushes the NHS further toward body repairs and crisis salvage, while making continuing anticipatory care and prevention more difficult and fragmented.[18]

He has advocated a wholly different approach and argued for the transcendence of the provider-consumer model for value production in medical care.[19]

In recent years Julian Tudor Hart has received many accolades. He retired from general practice in 1987 and from the Medical Research Council as senior research fellow in 1992. In 1999 the University of Glasgow conferred on him the honorary degree of D.Sc., the second-such award by the University to a general practitioner, the first being to Sir James Mackenzie.

In 2002 he received the Curtis Hames Research Award. In nominating him for this award, John Frey, III, MD, attested that Hart had not only stayed in practice in an underserved community for his entire medical career, but that:

In doing so, Julian Tudor Hart has used what he has learned from his own patients to change the lives of millions of people, improve the quality of general practice by example as well as exhortation, and create a legacy of research and education that will stand as one of the most important bodies of work in twentieth-century primary care research.[20]

Notes

[1] Dorothy Bonn, 'Julian Tudor Hart: bringing better health to south Wales', *The Lancet*, Vol. 354, 4 September 1999, 842.
[2] J. Tudor Hart, 'Semi-continuous screening of a whole community for hypertension', *The Lancet*, 1 August, 1970, 223–6.
[3] Julian Tudor Hart, 'Soapbox: a new path entirely', *Student BMJ*, Vol. 6 (1998); *http://www.studentbmj.com/back-issues/0798/data/079818.htm*.
[4] He was accompanied by Edith Tudor Hart, to whom he was married at this time, and she took many remarkable photographs of people and living conditions in south Wales during the 1930s. See Wolf Suschitzky, *Edith Tudor Hart: The Eye of Conscience* (London, 1987).
[5] Ibid., p. 14.
[6] John Mahon, *Harry Pollitt: A Biography* (London, 1976), p. 222; W. Rust, *Britons in Spain* (London, 1939), p. 124.
[7] Bill Alexander, *British Volunteers for Liberty* (London, 1982), p. 234.
[8] Julian Tudor Hart, 'In profit driven society, where can justice grow?', Millenium Festival of Medicine Lectures, King's College London, 13 January 2000, *http://www.kcl.ac.uk/depsta/rel/festival/lectures/13012000hart.html*.
[9] Obituary, A. L. Cochrane, *British Medical Journal (BMJ)*, Vol. 297 (2 July 1988).
[10] Julian Tudor Hart, 'My life', *Student BMJ*, Vol. 6 (July 1998).
[11] J. Tudor Hart, 'Semi-continuous screening of a whole community'.
[12] Julian Tudor Hart and Cerys Humphreys, 'Be your own coroner: an audit of 500 consecutive deaths in a general practice', *BMJ*, Vol. 294 (4 April 1987), 871–4, 874.
[13] Julian Tudor Hart, 'General practice today', *The Lancet*, 1950, i, 737–8.
[14] Julian Tudor Hart, 'Our feet set on a new path entirely: to the transformation of primary care and partnership with patients', *BMJ*, Vol. 317 (4 July 1998), 1–2.
[15] Julian Tudor Hart, 'Relation of primary care to undergraduate education', *The Lancet*, 6 October 1973, 778–81, 780.
[16] Ibid.
[17] Hart, 'Our feet set on a new path entirely'.
[18] Hart, 'In profit driven society, where can justice grow?'
[19] Julian Tudor Hart, 'Expectations of health care: promoted, managed and shared?', *Health Expectations*, Vol. 1, no. 1, 3–13.
[20] http://www.stfm.org/awards/bios.html.

Part II
Storming the Citadel: From Romantic Fiction to Effective Reality*

JULIAN TUDOR HART

The Citadel was published by Gollancz in 1937, and since then has never gone out of print. It generated a successful Hollywood film the following year starring Robert Donat and Rosalind Russell, two BBC television series after the war, outraged editorials and shriek-level correspondence in the *British Medical Journal*, and provided a cliché foundation for all levels of public and professional opinion about industrial general practice between the First and Second World Wars. Like Cronin himself, his hero Dr Andrew Manson starts in a professionally isolated mining village in south Wales, moves to the fleshpots of Harley Street, but regains his soul by sticking up for his beliefs in court, rounded off by his wife's death in a random accident. Cronin found his fleshpot not in Harley Street, but in a lifetime of royalties from this winning combination of sentimental pulp fiction with exposure of the private medical trade, with a flawed idealist as hero.

I will not deal with his Harley Street story, though this was the principal cause of contemporary professional anger. I shall concentrate instead on his view of general practice in coal-mining communities, based on a combination of the Lloyd George Insurance Act of 1911 with the older and deeper-rooted miners' prepaid medical-care schemes created throughout the south Wales coalfield before the First World War; and on the extent to which this provided a career model for progressive GPs serving industrial communities.

Cronin's account became the starting point for all views, popular and professional, of pre-NHS medical care for industrial workers and their families. For most progressive people, Cronin's scorn for pompous swindlers in Harley Street legitimized everything else that he wrote, overlooking what I see as an essentially unimaginative and patronizing view of industrial general practice. It was based on only two or three years' experience before he escaped to become an instantly successful novelist. As virtually the only widely read author to write knowledgeably about inter-war industrial general practice, he had immense opportunities to explore lay control and accountability, and its potential for combining primary medical care with public-health objectives. He rejected these, seeking resolution of his doctors' and patients' dilemmas outside the protagonists he had placed as main actors in his social drama. In *The Citadel*, deliverance comes from an American clinical genius without professional qualifications, ostracized by the British medical establishment, but representing none of the social forces actually available in the 1930s to move medical practice away from trade, towards effective service. Cronin did nothing to encourage or support his colleagues who campaigned before the war for a free and universally available National Health Service, or to help them defend and extend the NHS after 1948. Right up to his death in 1981, he devoted himself entirely to production of further sentimental best-sellers and accumulation of royalties.

An incident in *The Citadel* illustrates these limitations. Following an epidemic of typhoid fever, Manson's neighbour Dr Phil Denny enlists him in a plan to compel the local council to replace a leaking sewer by blowing it up. They persuade a young miner to steal sticks of explosive from the colliery. With fuses lit, they float these down the sewer in cocoa tins, exploding a few minutes later. Medical Officer of Health Dr Griffiths is thus compelled to act. Attributing the event to spontaneous combustion of methane, the council finally agrees to spend ratepayers' money on a new sewer, thus taking their constituents from the era of typhoid and cholera into the twentieth century.

Cronin describes Dr Griffiths as 'a lazy, evasive, incompetent, pious swine'. He makes Denny suggest that, to end the typhoid epidemic, boiling the Medical Officer of Health might be more effective than boiling the drinking water. In Cronin's popular 1960s BBC series *Dr Finlay's Casebook*, Griffiths, who was a minor player in *The Citadel*, becomes more fully developed as Dr Snoddy. A major theme common to both is tension between active, accurate, interventionist clinical medicine, personified by Manson and Finlay, and passive, bland, bureaucratic public health, personified by Griffiths and Snoddy.

This chimed with experience for many GPs, myself included. In 1966 I even had a leaking sewer, its existence denied by the Glyncorrwg Urban District Council until I offered them coloured photographs of the leak in action. Even then, when I said that this created huge risks for children swimming in the Corrwg river every summer, the Medical Officer of Health advising our council reproved me for endorsing the illegal acts of children daring to swim in forbidden waters. Many Medical Officers of Health did indeed correspond to this type, wearing out ten seats of trousers for each pair of shoes, but this was a shallow story, in line with the public-health-bashing views of the least thoughtful, least imaginative and least self-critical GPs. Unless general practice accepts public-health objectives, it is powerless to conserve health and becomes ineffective clinical tinkering. Through Manson's dabbling in research, Cronin offers glimpses of the potential for public health within primary care, but never develops it.

Where did Cronin's gunpowder plot come from? In the early 1920s, while Cronin was breaking his teeth as a GP assistant in Treherbert, Dr Bob Roberts served a few miles away both as a GP and as Medical Officer of Health for Mynyddislwyn, a commonly combined function in those days. Dr Roberts was both a clinical and a social activist, but to both roles he brought arrogant assumptions of unaccountability, still common today among the more enterprising NHS GPs still serving the NHS as independent contractors. My knowledge of this comes from his son and my friend, also Bob Roberts, who died in Edinburgh in 2001. Like Manson, Dr Bob faced recurrent outbreaks of typhoid. Like Drineffy, Mynyddislwyn was served by a decayed and leaking sewer. In his capacity as Medical Officer of Health, Dr Bob many times insisted that the old sewer must be replaced, and each time the council treasurer answered that there were no funds available. So Dr Bob enlisted the help of two colliers to blow it up, using precisely the technique described in *The Citadel*. He did not, of course, blow it up himself.

It is hard to believe that Cronin's book did not draw on this real incident of benevolent despotism, in which the GP and public health doctor are combined in one man as both clinical and social activist, moved by experience of care to address causes, rather than to pursue what were then largely futile and ineffective clinical solutions. Evidently it suited Cronin better to divide these functions, making the clinician his hero and demonizing the public-health bureaucrat. He ignored the arrogance of both, in seeking solutions to social problems through individual acts of heroism rather than social solidarity. In those days, local government in south Wales was so impoverished that it could not afford to immunize children against diphtheria, even though central government, then as now, could find money easily enough to wage war in far-off places.[1] Such a book would have demanded more thought from his readers, would have generated smaller royalties and would have repelled Hollywood.

Industrial workers' prepaid medical care was established throughout the south Wales coalfield and metal industries (steel, copper and tin plate) by the end of the nineteenth century, providing unlimited free primary care to workers, and usually to their families, funded by deductions from wages at source. The most developed schemes were in coal-mining communities, including all local citizens by weekly subscription. Terms and conditions of these schemes, generally known as club schemes or contract practice, varied according to the strength and militancy of each lodge of the miners' and metalworkers' trade unions, or the patronage of employers. Through his National Insurance Act of 1911, Lloyd George brought these under government control where they already existed, and created schemes limited only to employed workers everywhere where they did not. He strengthened the role of large insurance companies and weakened, though he did not eliminate, elements of democratic local control.

Poor doctors generally benefited from club schemes, in that their incomes were guaranteed and stabilized. Per capita earnings from patients were small, but with a large list, rapid clinical throughput and full ownership of a practice as a senior partner, some doctors could get rich, though often at the cost of slipshod, cocksure degradation of their skills: 'pile 'em high and sell 'em cheap.' On the other hand, elements of accountability to the laity were threatening, particularly in an era when scientific medicine was more promise than reality, and most medical care depended on hopes sustained by collusive illusion. Throughout the late nineteenth and early twentieth centuries battles raged between the British Medical Association (BMA – the professional union) and the club schemes. The BMA fought bitterly and without reserve to defend two sacred principles, which it saw as mutually dependent: that doctors must be self-employed entrepreneurs rather than salaried employees, and that they must be accountable for the quality of their work only to their professional peers, without any element of lay control.

In *The Citadel*, Dr Manson applies for his second valleys practice to a lodge committee of the miners' trade union. Its secretary is sympathetically portrayed as a man of small education but great enlightenment. He has faith in Manson as a representative of nascent medical science, rather than a small businessman. Such appointments embodied an element of local control that is now totally lost. All NHS appointments of GPs since 1948 have either been through existing business partners or by centrally appointed local bureaucracies, usually dominated by the local professional interest as this is perceived by the most powerful GPs, without effective representation from patients or communities directly involved.

Cronin does little to explore the possibilities latent in this potential partnership between GPs and their communities. Neither trade unions nor elected local councils, either then or now, provide ideal models as employers or directors of medical labour. Progressive doctors who naively imagine this may be so get a rude shock when they meet reality. As I found to my cost, letters written either to trade union secretaries or to colliery managers were uniformly ignored. Professionals serving industrial communities learned either to initiate everything by word of mouth, or to give up any attempt to innovate. It was true then and probably remains true today that if we want lay people to understand the nature of human biology and the inherent uncertainty of clinical interventions, we must impart most of this understanding ourselves, using local customs and idiom rather than trying to impose our own. This meant human speech rather than writing. Local democracy and professional accountability is a learning process for both parties. It has to begin at the beginning, from where we actually are, with the people we actually have.

Cronin was not seriously interested in this. He provided no model for progressive young doctors wanting, like Manson, to lead worthwhile lives and make a real difference to the world, rather than waste medical science on pandering to rich patients with minimal needs. To be fair, this was never Cronin's intention. He just wanted to be rich and comfortable. Having found a way to be popular, he milked it for all it was worth. The popularity of his book rested in large part on a mass hunger for medical care that was effective, affectionate and respectful of personal dignity, but Cronin failed to indicate how primary medical care might become both scientific and humane, tough on disease but gentle with patients, without resort either to miraculous rescue from some wholly external source (*The Citadel*'s maverick American), or to industrializing the care system (the path imposed on British general practice since the late 1980s). Such a unifying model clearly was and still is needed by entrants to primary care who want to understand the world they work in. The gap between the world as it is, and the world as it could be if accumulated human skills and knowledge were fully applied to human needs rather than to expansion of personal property is wider today than ever before. A gap of this kind was the underlying cause of the moral and intellectual explosion set off by the medical students of France in 1968, which suddenly recruited millions of young people the world over to a new generation of would-be revolutionaries. For reasons I cannot explore here, this moral and intellectual revolution lacked a sufficient material base, or sufficient respect for material realities. In profound contrast with the 1930s, when most leaders of scientific thought were firmly on the Left, the intellectual revolution following 1968 sought and found its intellectual allies chiefly from mystical opponents of science. The new wave thus proved more successful in burying the past than in giving birth to the future, and was therefore unsustainable. Having begun among student professionals, it failed to provide them with realist rather than idealist models for professional behaviour.

Superficially, my own life resembled the pre-Harley Street career of Dr Manson. I worked for thirty years in a coal-mining village in south Wales, was a clinical innovator and undertook epidemiological research with my own population in association with the Medical Research Council. I had a real wife beside me, far more intelligent and attractive than Rosalind Russell (who ended as an adornment of the Republican Party, opposing Franklin Roosevelt). I never even thought of going to Harley Street, the red-light district of my profession. Thanks to the NHS, I never had to take a fee from a patient in my entire working life. In these ways I might seem to have followed Manson's footsteps, so many people have asked whether my own career choices were influenced by *The Citadel*. The answer has to be yes, because in the 1950s *The Citadel* was virtually the only model available for progressive, democratically minded GPs entering industrial primary care. But it was and still is a flawed model, offering little help and much confusion to anyone seriously committed to changing even the smallest part of the real world.

Since *The Citadel*, the most influential popular book about British GPs and how they relate to their patients and to society has been John Berger and Jean Mohr's *A Fortunate Man*. It provides a more sophisticated and less sentimental model, and was recently republished with enthusiastic endorsement by the Royal College of General Practitioners. Unlike Cronin, Berger is a Marxist, with a long record of creative criticism of modern and postmodern graphic art, probing close to the causes of our present state of nihilism and despair. However, I have to say that as a model for new generations of pioneers, *A Fortunate Man* fails as much as *The Citadel*, and more so today than when it first appeared in 1967.

On first reading, I wondered if the title was intended to be ironic. This man was surely not fortunate, though in his close relationships with his patients he might appear so compared with other professionals up against an increasingly alienated society. As I recall, his child was mentioned only once in the whole book (when we were told he was in a boarding school). The existence of his wife was merely implied. Initially, the emotional life of this 'fortunate' man seemed built upon the dependence of his patients on their doctor. Later, as he reached more clinical maturity, it was built on their mutual interdependence. *A Fortunate Man* was based on a real person, willing to open his own and his patients' lives to a novelist, a photographer and a multitude of readers. It revealed that there were no biological limits to 'normal' human behaviour, only social limits for which we ourselves had to accept responsibility, hopefully assisted by some saintly GP able to subordinate his own life entirely to service. A couple of years after it was published he killed himself. I was not surprised.

To me, the paternal model presented by *A Fortunate Man* is even less useful than that offered by *The Citadel*, which is at least readily recognizable as in need of drastic revision. We have a magnificent but sadly neglected medical hero in Anton Chekhov, whose devotion to medicine as well as to theatre has been overlooked for far too long.[2] Though his example remains at least as relevant as William Carlos Williams who was born in 1883,[3] they are both now long gone. Today we have many splendid novelists, people like Peter Carey and John Irving, who recognize better than most doctors the equal impossibility either of setting biological limits to normal human behaviour, or of coping without social limits to normal human behaviour – a tension we can only learn to live with. They would recognize that, in a disintegrating society, if social limits were redefined to fit social needs rather than consumer demands we might reach a more humane and more sustainable compromise. And they would probably recognize that for clinical decisions to become truly evidence-based, evidence and expertise from both patients and professionals must be understood as equally essential to good health outcomes.

As scientific knowledge continues to expand exponentially, the gap between the world as it is, and the world as it could be, is becoming ever more intolerable. New generations will enter the caring professions, more conscious of the difference between their aims – to apply this new knowledge fully to meet human needs – and the aims of people who use their power to maximize profit and to kill more efficiently. They need a new professional model. So far as I know, no novelist so far has tackled this subject, but among experienced urban and industrial GPs now in their forties and fifties, are those who will do so. They have abundant material.

Notes

* I thank Charles Webster for helpful comments, and particularly for reminding me of the malign influence of George Bernard Shaw on civic attitudes to immunization against diphtheria. This is paralleled today by Paul Foot in relation to the mumps, measles and rubella vaccine. When socialists return to the understanding of and respect for scientific evidence which Marx and Engels had, their ideas will recover and surpass their former power.

1 Failure to apply existing knowledge for prevention of diphtheria caused about 3,000 deaths a year throughout the 1920s and 1930s. Though fiscal poverty in local government and deference to the trade interests of the BMA in central government were the main factors in this, much responsibility lies with the anti-immunization lobby, above all with George Bernard Shaw. Shaw was rightly held in huge respect by all progressive people, and therefore caused division and confusion exactly where effective action was most possible. In New York this delay never occured, simply because that city implemented a vigorous immunization programme, with a robust attitude both to GPs who wanted to pick up fees but not to organize a programme, and to conscientious objectors to scientific evidence. In the UK, this national disgrace ended in 1940, when arrival of poor evacuees in wealthy households reminded people who mattered that public health is indivisible. This subject is discussed more fully in J. T. Hart, 'The teaching of medical history and education for change', *Social History of Medicine*, Vol. 2 (1989), 391–8.

2 J. Coope, *Doctor Chekhov: A Study in Literature and Medicine* (Chale, Isle of Wight, 1997).

3 William Carlos Williams (1883–1963) was an innovative poet of similar stature to T. S. Eliot and Ezra Pound. He earned his living as a GP serving a poor industrial community in New Jersey from the 1930s to the 1950s. His most accessible work, notably his collected stories *The Farmers' Daughters* (1961), has been an important influence on socially conscious US medical students, and has no British equivalent.

9

What was Wales? Towards a Contextual Approach to Medical History

MARTIN POWELL

The main aim of this chapter is to place Welsh medical history in a broader context. The title derives from Gwyn A. Williams's *When was Wales?*[1] The question of what was Wales involves looking for a 'Welsh effect'.[2] This is based on the social science literature on context and contingency.[3] In simple terms, this involves examining whether the patterning of health and health care in Wales is different from that of England. If so, this may be because of reasons of context or mechanism. To give an example from medical history, as we shall see later, there were fewer hospital beds per capita in Wales than there were in England. This difference in pattern may be a result of different contexts such as a lower level of wealth in Wales. This suggests that less provision is simply a uniform response to different conditions, and that provision in similarly poor parts of England such as the northeast would be equally low. On the other hand, differential provision may be the result of different mechanisms or processes, and in this case similar contexts would produce different outcomes. This may be because of a large number of possible dimensions such as political and cultural factors.[4] For example, a Welsh local authority with a similar level of Labour Party representation might spend more on health care than its counterparts in England because 'Welsh Labour' may have different views from 'English Labour'. In this case, there is a 'Welsh effect' with different mechanisms and processes, and it is reasonable to refer to this as a distinctive 'Welsh medical history' rather than 'medical history in Wales'.

The rest of this chapter briefly outlines some of the historiography of medical history in Wales. It then outlines some of the main features of the context and contingency literature with some examples of its relevance to medical history in Wales. The next section gives a brief outline of the development of health and health care in Wales using three main headings of public health, primary care and hospitals. This is followed by a discussion of patterns and processes, and a conclusion with some indications of a research agenda.

Medical History in Wales

Most studies of medical history and health policy in Britain devote little space to Wales. In his work on the NHS in Scotland, John Stewart notes that it is only with devolution that most texts have paid any real attention to Scottish difference from the English 'norm'.[5] 'Wales' appears in the index of writers such as Ham and Baggott, although details are rather perfunctory.[6] A similar exercise for Allsop and Powell finds that the Welsh cupboard tends to be bare, although the latter refers to the South Wales Hospital Surveys in a number of places.[7] Klein admits a 'Little Englander approach'.[8] Wales does not appear in the index in the book by Jones.[9] Cherry and Berridge have index entries for Scotland, but not for Wales, while Abel-Smith has no entries for either nation.[10] There are a number of mentions of 'Wales' in Hardy[11] but these are usually to note low health status and the effects of the Depression of the 1930s. In other words, Wales is discussed along with Scotland and the north of England as examples of depressed areas, but distinctions between these areas are not really addressed. It is Charles Webster, the official historian of the NHS, who is most alive to the historical nuances of Scotland and Wales, although understandably he devotes more attention to Scotland with its separate legislation.[12]

General histories of Wales tend to say little about health and even less about health care, although they place greater emphasis on housing and education.[13] For example, Davies first mentions hospitals when they were nationalized, writing that in 1948 the hospitals of Wales were in a dire condition.[14] Black simply notes that public health was badly hit and tuberculosis became a major problem.[15] While it is hardly surprising that coverage tends to be thin in books covering vast periods of time from cromlechs to current affairs, texts concentrating on more recent periods do not offer significantly more details. Jenkins notes problems associated with public health.[16] Evans gives some brief coverage of health, housing and welfare services.[17] Smith's *Aneurin Bevan and the World of South Wales* says surprisingly little about Bevan or health.[18] Of the general studies, Morgan gives the greatest level of attention to health issues. He follows the general pattern in giving more attention to health rather than health care. He notes that 'one feature of social life in the valleys in the inter-war period which was consistently alarming was the state of public health', and provides some details of the Welsh National Memorial Association (WNMA) that was set up to deal with tuberculosis.[19]

Until recently there was relatively little specialist literature on health and health care, but very little of this literature has found its way into the more generalist literature examined above. With a few exceptions, very few studies appeared between Stephens's *The Hospitals of Wales* of 1912,[20] and the last decade or so of the twentieth century. In 1987 the editor of *Llafur*, Deian Hopkins, wrote that there were 'far too many empty shelves where studies of demography, migration, standards of living, patterns of consumption, health, welfare and education should sit.' Citing this, Borsay and Porter state that this observation is still valid today.[21] Similarly, in 1995 Griffiths and Law note the dearth of historical writing on medicine and society in south Wales.[22] In the edition of *Llafur* in which my article on 'Wales and the NHS' was published, the editors pointed out that medical history had been neglected in Wales, and hoped that this position would begin to be rectified.[23] As we shall see below, the last few years have seen a significant increase in material on Welsh medical history. While texts on histories of individual hospitals have appeared at fairly regular intervals,[24] there have been relatively few articles and theses on medical history in Wales.[25] It is only in recent years that more local studies have been added to the pioneering work of Gross and Evans.[26] Similarly, there have been recent articles on broader issues of health[27] and, following a long gap after Earwicker, other aspects of provision.[28] A similar pattern applies to theses.[29]

A few general points may be made about this increased volume of recent work. First, work still tends to be fairly piecemeal. While there are valuable studies of individual institutions, localities and elements of health and health care, it is clear that some parts of the system have attracted more attention than others. There is a 'voluntary bias' in that individual hospital histories tend to focus on the glories (or otherwise) of the voluntary hospital system rather than Poor Law and municipal provision that formed the quantitative backbone of provision. We still know relatively little about what the *Lancet* in 1866 termed 'the real hospitals of the land' and which the Majority Report of the Royal Commission on the Poor Laws in 1909 considered had become *de facto*, if not *de jure*, general hospitals.[30] Like contemporary patients, medical historians have been wary of entering the Poor Law and municipal institutions.

Second, there has been a trend to place individual hospital histories in their wider context.[31] For example, Michael examines a hospital within a wider framework of a regional case study in the social history of madness. She concludes by pointing to the importance of social and cultural context in shaping the patient experience of mental illness. However, it is still difficult to see the wood for the trees, or how different pieces of the jigsaw fit together. There is little discussion about to what extent patterns and processes were different within Wales. In other words, a holistic study along the lines of Pickstone for the north-west of England is lacking.[32] Was Wales homogeneous or heterogeneous? Can it be considered in terms of medical history as one entity or were there two or three quite different nations? Were the quarrymens' hospitals in the north different from the coal miners' hospitals in the south? To what extent was Pontypridd distinctive from Tredegar?[33]

The third point compares Wales with other areas. If Wales can be considered a suitable unit for comparison, then how does it compare with England or Scotland, or with depressed regions such as the north-east of England? This links with recent work that advocates comparative history such as Berger's comparison of the south Wales and Ruhr coalfields. As he notes, few historians have attempted to put the south Wales experience into a comparative context. Comparative history is highly problematic and difficult, with issues such as units of comparison, contexts and variables. However, it is a vital counterpoint to the views of local historians along the lines of 'but in Senghennydd things are different'.[34]

The fourth point is that there is relatively little material on the possibly distinctive elements of Welsh medical history, such as the Medical Aid Societies, the national coordination of the WNMA and the Welsh Board of Health, and early municipal effort in Barry.[35]

Context and Contingency

Donaldson writes that contingency theory should be distinguished from universalistic theories.[36] He explains that, at the most abstract level, the contingency approach says that the effect of one variable on another depends upon some third variable, W. Thus the effect of X on Y when W is low differs from the effect of X on Y when W is high. We cannot state what the effect of X on Y is, without knowing whether W is low or high: no valid bivariate relationship between X and Y can be stated. Boyne discusses the differences between universalistic and contingency arguments.[37] In the former, one variable is related to another in a uniform, definite and predictable way, regardless of the context or configuration of other variables. On the other hand, the latter suggests that there are no uniform relationships with variables. The particular relevance of Boyne's argument for medical history relates to the use of case studies. He argues that case-study research cannot examine the net effect of an explanatory variable while controlling for the influence of others, except through the subjective impressions of researchers. Recent work in evaluation research stresses the importance of context, as Pawson and Tilley sum this up in the equation of 'mechanism + context = outcome'.[38] Rose sets out a useful framework for analysing the territorial dimension in UK politics.[39] He argues that there are three different groups of policies. Uniform policies are measures that are the same in law and in the same organizational hands in all parts of the UK, such as defence policies. Concurrent policies are programmes with the same function throughout the UK but delivered by different institutions in different parts. Responsibility is shared between a functional, UK ministry and a territorial ministry such as the Welsh Office. Most social policies are seen to be concurrent. Exceptional policies are adopted and administered by one nation of the UK without involving concurrent action elsewhere, and usually derive from distinctive historical or cultural circumstances of a nation. Rose gives the example of government policy about religion as there are four different policies for four nations and, in Wales, language provides the chief ground for exceptional policies. In Scotland, cultural distinctiveness is not as marked as in Wales, but the existence of a separate Scottish legal system and of a then well-entrenched Scottish Office provides an institutional basis for exceptional policies. Rose goes on to examine the distribution of public policy resources in terms of laws, money and the services of public employees.

In short, these different frameworks all examine whether there is anything distinctive about patterns and processes within a territorial unit. Sharpe and Newton point to a 'Welsh effect' based on regional, historical, cultural, educational or religious factors, arguing that location in Wales had an independent and positive influence on local authority expenditure of the pre-1974 local government system.[40] Boyne provides a conceptual and empirical critique of Sharpe and Newton's thesis.[41] He points to two possible Welsh effects. An additive effect suggests that spending is higher in Wales than in England, even when other variables are taken into account. A mediative effect suggests that the relationship between other variables and spending differs between England and Wales. Boyne concludes that Welsh-county spending in the 1980s was higher than English-county spending because of a need effect, a grant effect and a political-party effect. In this case, there was no Welsh effect, either additive or mediative. However, he suggests that even if there was no regional effect on spending levels, it may be that regional location has an impact on policy content. In other words, there may be a Welsh effect for other variables, times and contexts.

Although not generally using the concepts or terminology of contingency theory, some of these issues have recently been discussed in works of history and devolution. Borsay and Porter discuss the Welsh dimension. They write that until devolution and the National Assembly for Wales, medicine and health care operated within the British polity, and the areas of policy reviewed in this volume shared a legislative framework with their English counterparts. However, nineteenth- and twentieth-century Wales provided a particular social and political milieu for the transaction of medicine and health. The rapid industrialization of the south Wales valleys nurtured the kind of proleterian 'public sphere' that was able to support a network of Medical Aid Societies which, whilst not unique to Wales, was more advanced compared with other localities. They conclude that secondary legislative powers that accompanied devolution are now allowing distinctively Welsh policies to flourish.[42] Michael notes the diversity of experience in patterns of institutional provision for the insane in Britain.[43] She writes that, until recently, England was taken to be the norm, but now research on Ireland and Scotland has pointed out that, within the wider historiography of insanity, England offers but one example. Whilst Wales was subject to the same legislative and administrative directives as England, this did not preclude some measure of difference (for example the Welsh language). She concludes that whilst it would be wrong to speak of a distinctively 'Welsh system' of provision for the insane, there were recognizable differences from the pattern in England. Similarly, Stewart asks whether the National Health Service in Scotland was Scottish or British.[44] He cites Ross who argues that Scotland's system 'stands on its own ground as an independently constituted Service' and that it was 'not a mere variant ' of that in England and Wales. Differences were attributable to, *inter alia*, differences in medical practice, local government, topography and 'certain equally marked characteristics of the Scottish mind and character'.[45] Ross has a separate section (chapters 28–30) on the NHS in Scotland, but no separate section on Wales. The index contains a significant number of entries for Scotland, but only one for Wales. The relevant page contains one paragraph where it is noted that the 1946 NHS Act as a whole relates to Wales equally with England, but points out the existence since 1919 of the Welsh Board of Health (see Chapter 10). In structural terms, Scotland had a number of committees on health issues and the Scottish Secretary of State introduced different legislation from that of England.[46]

Patterns and Processes of Health and Health Care in Wales

As suggested above, the history of health and health care in Wales has tended to be neglected, although there is more on the former than the latter. This section briefly outlines some of the patterns and processes associated with medical history in Wales under three headings: public health, primary care and hospitals.[47]

Public Health
The late nineteenth century saw the development of urban Wales, with rapid population increases in the main coastal towns and the growth of the valley settlements based on heavy industry. Some industrialization in the north left mid-Wales largely agricultural. It is generally agreed that social and economic conditions in both rural and urban areas compared poorly with England. This produced a clear effect in terms of health. Most counties and county boroughs had levels of deprivation and mortality levels well above the English average. This

was most notable in the Depression of the 1930s. For example, Welsh counties were the seven highest in England and Wales for tuberculosis mortality. The extraordinary conditions of an area like Merthyr should be noted: its adjusted death rate was one and a half times the England and Wales average, while its unemployed rate was almost three times the national average. Special Inquiries were set up to examine the high rates of maternal mortality and tuberculosis.[48] In short, Wales provided a textbook example of the links between poverty, unemployment, poor housing and working conditions and poor health.

Primary Care

Many working men belonged to Friendly Societies that have been termed by David Green 'the most important providers of social welfare during the nineteenth and early twentieth century'.[49] These societies, in return for contributions, provided the services of a doctor and sick pay. In his National Health Insurance (NHI) scheme of 1911, Lloyd George effectively nationalized this arrangement for all workers earning less than £160 a year. This scheme excluded hospital treatment (except for tuberculosis) and dependants. The 'panel' system is generally said to have provided rudimentary and perfunctory care, with isolated and overworked doctors in many areas, particularly industrial areas.[50] According to Cronin, in fictional 'Drineffy' the local doctor stated that 'There's no hospital, no ambulance, no x-rays, no anything. If you want to operate you use the kitchen table ... The sanitation won't bear looking at. In a dry summer the kids die like flies with infantile cholera ... I drink like a fish.'[51] Certainly, Wales had fewer doctors than England. According to the 1931 Census, Wales had 0.59 doctors per 1,000 population compared with 0.73 in England and Wales. While counties such as Denbighshire, Merioneth, Flintshire and Caernarfonshire were in the ten best-provided areas in England and Wales, Monmouthshire was in the bottom ten, while at a finer spatial scale Abersychan with 0.08 (2 doctors for 25,000 population) was in the bottom twenty-five areas. Generally, doctors were positively correlated with wealth and negatively correlated with the infant mortality effect. In other words, richer areas – the so-called 'watering holes' such as Eastbourne and Bath – had more doctors than deprived areas such as Merthyr Tydfil.

On the other hand, it has been claimed that the Medical Aid Societies (MAS) provided integrated care for dependants as well as workers. According to the Political and Economic Planning (PEP) Report of 1937, medical institutes were embyro health centres. It described the Llanelli and District Medical Service as a comprehensive service 'which should be the model of any national system of medical services'.[52] David Green points out that the South Wales and Monmouthshire Alliance of Medical Aid Societies (SWMA) was assured by Minister of Health Henry Willink that: 'their pioneering work is fully appreciated', while Bevan stated that: 'I know the valuable services rendered by associations ... You have shown us the way and by your very efficiency you have brought about your own cessation.'[53] For Green, this 'worker control' or lay control as opposed to medical control is a great advantage of such a civil-society model but the degree of worker control achieved in practice is difficult to assess.[54] Moroever, the leading MAS may have been unrepresentative. Generally the government files contain a great deal of adverse comment on the MAS, where it was concluded that virtually none were suitable for development into health centres.[55] It seems strange that there appears to have been little serious and sustained work by Welsh medical historians on such distinctive organizations as MAS.[56] Consequently, the fictional account of Cronin and the polemical account of Green tend to hold the field in secondary and popular accounts.

Hospitals

Hospitals before the NHS were composed of the voluntary and municipal sectors. The voluntary sector, financed by philanthropy, originates mainly from the eighteenth century in England, but from later periods in Wales (see Table 9.1), resulting in lower levels of provision. Early voluntary hospitals were opened in towns as diverse as Denbigh, Swansea, Brecon, Cardiff and Aberystwyth. Many hospitals in the rural areas and mining valleys mainly dated from the late nineteenth century and early twentieth centuries. In the rural areas, the hospitals were generally of the 'cottage' type, but in the mining valleys, a number were restricted to those in a particular occupation or company. Examples of this type included the Caerphilly Miners' Hospital and the Powell Duffryn Workmen's Hospital, Aberbargoed. Aneurin Bevan claimed that it was a travesty to call such hospitals 'voluntary' as some hospitals in south Wales owed as much as 97.5 per cent of their revenue to the workers in the locality.[57]

According to Davies, between 1700 and 1825 154 dispensaries and infirmaries (in roughly a ratio of 3:1) were established in England and

Wales.[58] However, at the end of this period, Swansea had the only infirmary in Wales although dispensaries had been formed in other Welsh towns at earlier dates. Precise details are in conflict with other sources that claim that the Denbighshire Infirmary opened in 1807,[59] but it is clear that the development of voluntary hospitals in Wales tended to lag behind England.

Table 9.1 compares the foundation dates for hospitals and dispensaries in Wales as compared with the border counties of England to give a very crude comparison of the 'border' effect. While, on the limited information available, there does not appear to be a clear time-gap between the foundation of dispensaries in England and Wales, there was a clear lag for hospitals. English hospitals tended to be founded earlier, with relatively few towns waiting until the twentieth century. The Welsh foundations suggest some puzzles. One may be the relatively late foundation of a hospital in Newport (1867). Another is the early foundation of a dispensary in Crickhowell in 1820. Finally, while some towns such as Swansea (1814–17) and Wrexham (1833–41) moved quickly from dispensaries to hospitals, others such as Abergavenny (1828–90) and Holywell (1824–1908) took much longer.

The municipal hospital system was more complex as local authorities were given powers to deal with different issues at different times. Much of the municipal hospital accommodation started life as workhouses. Medical care for 'sick paupers' was extremely rudimentary: few aspects of workhouse life escaped the touch of 'less eligibility'. Although several of the municipal hospitals date from the period 1835–45,[60] it appears that the separation of the mixed workhouse into a separate infirmary also tended to arrive late in Wales. *Burdett's* gives the dates as 1896 for Cardiff, 1897 for Merthyr, 1910 for Swansea and 1915 for Ruthin.[61]

Under permissive legislation, many local authorities provided 'hospitals' that were often little more than isolated shacks for infectious disease. However, in south Wales, the first real effort to provide a hospital for infectious disease was voluntary and dates from 1866, when the people of Cardiff and Penarth procured an old man-of-war, *HMS Hamadryad*, from the Admiralty to serve as a hospital ship during a cholera epidemic.

Tuberculosis had long been thought to be an incurable disease, and little provision was made apart from the 'last resort' of the workhouse. Towards the end of the nineteenth century, the claim that tuberculosis was curable led to the construction of sanatoria. In 1911, this effort

Table 9.1: Foundations of Hospitals and Dispensaries in Wales and the counties of the English border (before 1850; 1850–1900; after 1900)

Hospitals		Dispensaries	
Wales	Borders of England	Wales	Borders of England
Denbigh 1807	Bristol (G) 1735	Monmouth 1810	Stockport (C) 1792
Swansea 1817	Shrewsbury (S) 1745	Swansea 1814	Ledbury (H) 1824
Brecon 1832	Chester (C) 1755	Crickhowell 1820	Ross (H) 1825
Cardiff 1837	Gloucester (G) 1755	Aberystwyth 1821	Wellington (S) 1834
Aberystwyth 1838	Hereford (H) 1776	Holywell 1824	
Wrexham 1841	Stroud (G) 1790	Welshpool 1827	
Bangor 1845	Birkenhead (C) 1828	Abergavenny 1828	
Carmarthen 1847	Stockport (C) 1833	Wrexham 1833	
	Bridgnorth (S)1835	Newport 1839	
	Cheltenham (G) 1839		
Dinorwic 1850	Bourton (G) 1861		
Haverfordwest 1859	Tewkesbury (G) 1863		
Pembroke 1862	Wallasey (C) 1865		
Monmouth 1863	Congleton (C) 1866		
Llanelli 1867	Oswestry (S) 1866		
Newtown 1868	Fairford (G) 1867		
Ruarbon 1870	Hambrook (G) 1867		
Holyhead 1871	Tetbury (G) 1868		
Tenby 1871	Ledbury (H) 1871		
Mold 1877	Moreton (G) 1872		
Caernarfon 1888	Ross (H) 1872		
Llandrindod 1880	Macclesfield (C) 1873		
Merthyr 1887	Berkeley (G) 1877		
Porth 1895	Cirencester (G) 1877		
Bridgend 1896	Lydney (G) 1882		
Builth Wells 1897	Ludlow (S) 1884		
Pembroke Dock 1897	Whitchurch (S) 1886		
Colwyn Bay 1899	Kington (H) 1887		
	Northwich (C) 1887		
	Market Drayton (S) 1892		
	Clun (S) 1893		
	Winsford (C) 1898		
	Leominster (H) 1899		
Pontypool 1903	Much Wenlock (S) 1903		
Rhymney 1903	Hoylake (C) 1906		
Tredegar 1904	Broseley (S) 1907		
Mountain Ash 1910	Port Sunlight (C) 1907		
Pontypridd 1911	Nantwich (C) 1911		
Port Talbot 1913	Ellesmere Port (C) 1919		
Oakdale 1914	Sale (C) 1921		
Maesteg 1916	Knutsford, (C) 1922		
Aberdare 1917	Alderley Edge (C) 1924		
Caerphilly 1917			
Dolgellau 1920			
Towyn 1920			
Chirk 1921			
Aberbeeg 1922			
Rhyl 1924			
Blaenau Festiniog 1925			

Notes
Data from Burdett's *Hospitals and Charities*.[62] The dates in Burdett's may conflict with other sources.
Dates given for voluntary general hospitals (for instance excluding Barry as municipal and Rhyl Children's Hospital, 1872)
Dates for dispensaries are given only when they opened before a hospital in the town.
Borders refer to 'comparator' border administrative counties (including county boroughs) of Gloucestershire (G), Herefordshire (H), Salop (S) and Cheshire (C), although some hospitals in these counties may be at some distance from the Welsh border.

was financially encouraged when tuberculosis was included in Lloyd George's National Health Insurance scheme. In 1921, responsibility for treatment was transferred completely to local authorities. In Wales, the decision to organize a campaign to eradicate tuberculosis pre-dated Lloyd George's initiative. In 1910, a public meeting unanimously decided that a national memorial to the recently deceased King Edward VII should be the Welsh National Memorial Association (WNMA), a voluntary association that essentially was the counterpart of the local authorities in England.[63] Institutions were set up by purchasing existing buildings such as Craig-y-nos, the former home of opera singer Adelina Patti, and building sanatoria such as the South Wales Sanatorium, Bronllys.

There is relatively little literature on municipal health provision compared with the much larger literature on education,[64] but it is marked by a curious dualism between progress and apathy. On the one hand, there is an emphasis on political agency. For example, Stephens wrote that to Wales (Barry UDC) belongs the credit for being the first to take advantage of the 1875 Public Health Act in providing rate-aided hospital accommodation for cases other than infectious disease.[65] In the rural areas, he pointed out that counties such as Denbighshire, Caernarfonshire and Flintshire seem to have been under the control of authorities that realized the value to the community of adequate hospital provision. To the credit of Brecknockshire and Radnorshire, their ratio of rate-aided to voluntary beds compares favourably with the rest of Wales.[66] It is surprising to record that some twenty-five years later a number of new municipal hospitals were built during the Depression years of the 1930s, including Llandough Hospital and Sully Sanitorium by Cardiff County Borough Council, and Church Village Hospital by Glamorgan County Council. These progressive moves are often explained with reference to the socialist tradition of 'Red Wales'.[67] Some 'Old Labour' Welsh local authorities made great efforts to produce 'local welfare states' providing from the 'cradle to the grave', with some Labour councillors being the 'unsung heroes and heroines of South Wales during the depression years'.[68] Labour leaders in local councils include people such as Aneurin Bevan who claimed that he cut his milk teeth in local government.[69] As Foot put it, historians of twentieth-century Britain should not forget that some of the great industrial centres of the nation, with south Wales in the vanguard, voted first through their unions and next at the ballot box for a revolution in British society in the 1920s.[70]

On the other hand, Stephens noted the utter inadequacy of rate-aided (Poor Law) hospital provision in Newport, while the Poor Law institution in Neath was regarded as a positive disgrace.[71] Some years later, the negligence of rural authorities in responding to tuberculosis was stated in blunt terms to the members of Caernarfonshire County Council by the main author of the Clement Davies Report on TB: 'Gentleman, are you not ashamed of yourselves?'[72] The dominant line in the literature stresses that councils tended to be poor because of low rateable value in their areas.[73] However, this was clearly not the only factor. In some areas councillors and municipal officials were not of the best. Cronin gives the example of a District Medical Officer who is not available because: 'He do go to the golf at Swansea afternoons mostly.'[74] Jones writes that councillors in some places were villains rather than heroes, with some Labour groups being corrupt and unscrupulous.[75]

It is clearly the interaction between economic and political factors that shapes municipal activity,[76] and accounts for a mixed picture of provision. Morgan writes that 'social duty came before concern for the financial protection of ratepayers'. Labour-led local authorities in South Wales taxed heavily on a low rateable value to maintain a reasonable level of expenditure upon health, housing, education and other necessities.[77] For example, in the 1930s the Glamorgan rate for public-assistance purposes was more than the total county rate of Surrey and Middlesex.[78] As the south Wales hospital surveyors put it: 'although the standard of service in local authority institutions and hospitals has materially improved in many areas, it still falls short of requirements.'[79] However, without more detailed comparative study, it is difficult to say why some areas might 'underspend' or 'overspend' given their political and economic structure.[80] Similarly, some councils might have been high spenders on education but low spenders on health. As outlined above, some of the processes were somewhat different from England, but did this have any impact on the resulting pattern of hospital provision in the region? In other words, was the hospital system of Wales different from that of England and, more importantly, was it adequate to meet the needs of the region? From Table 9.2 it is clear that voluntary provision in Wales lagged behind England in terms of beds and in-patients over many years. Since the turn of the twentieth century, even the best-provided Welsh county was inferior to the English average.

Table 9.2: Voluntary beds and in-patients (per 1,000 population)

Per 1,000 population	England	Wales	Wales (maximum)	Wales (minimum)
Beds 1871	0.6	0.2	0.7 (Denbigh)	0.0
In-patients 1871	4.3	1.1	3.3	0.0
Beds 1881	1.1	0.2	0.6 (Denbigh)	0.0
In-patients 1881	7.7	1.2	22.9	0.0
Beds 1891	1.1	0.6	0.7 (Flint)	0.2 (Anglesey)
In-patients 1891	9.9	3.2	11.2	0.0
Beds 1901	1.3	0.5	0.7 (Denbigh)	0.2 (Merioneth)
In-patients 1901	13.1	2.1	4.1	0.4
Beds 1911	1.4	0.6	1.0 (Radnor)	0.2 (Merioneth)
In-patients 1911	15.3	5.1	11.6	0.3
Beds 1931	2.3	1.2	2.0 (Glamorgan)	0.3 (Carmarthen)
In-patients 1931	33.8	14.6	25.6	0.6

Source: *Burdett's Hospitals and Charities* (annual).

Table 9.3 shows that Wales generally had fewer beds per 1,000 population than England. Indeed, south Wales had fewer total beds (4.86/1,000) than any of the nine English survey regions, with the lowest English region being Berkshire, Buckinghamshire and Oxfordshire with 5.36 beds per 1,000. In Table 9.4 the total number of beds is separated into municipal and voluntary categories. It is generally the case that England had more beds than Wales for both types of area and hospital. For acute beds, the clear deficiency in Wales may be seen in the municipal sector. This is particularly true for the county councils. Indeed, only two of the seven county councils (Cardiganshire and Glamorgan) had any such beds. The higher

Table 9.3: Total beds per 1,000 population for England and south Wales in 1938.

	South Wales			England		
	All	County Borough	County Council	All	County Borough	County Council
Acute	2.16	3.90	1.47	3.32	4.56	1.88
Chronic	1.11	1.72	0.88	1.28	1.31	1.28
Maternity	0.18	0.23	0.15	0.27	0.38	0.16
Infectious disease	0.66	0.81	0.60	1.00	1.00	0.79
Tuberculosis	0.76	0.62	0.82	0.71	0.76	0.62
Total	4.86	7.28	3.92	6.58	7.97	4.73

Source: MOH/NPHT Hospital Surveys.

number of chronic beds in the Welsh county boroughs is probably accounted for by their slow progress in improving their hospitals and in turning chronic beds into acute beds: a mark of failure rather than success.[81] The same pattern of greater provision in England for both types of authorities is again evident for maternity and for infectious disease. In England, provision for tuberculosis was shared between the municipal and voluntary sectors but in Wales, provision was totally in the hands of the WNMA, which the Surveyors classified as municipal provision. Too much stress should not be put on the fact that the county councils had more beds than the county boroughs, as this merely indicated that sanatoria tended to be located in rural areas because this was considered a more suitable environment.[82] The WNMA sanatoria were open to individuals from a wider area than the local authority in which they were situated. For example, the South Wales Sanatorium in Brecknockshire contained some 300 young men from all parts of the region. Overall, it is clear that South Wales had far fewer beds than England. The only situation where per capita provision in south Wales matched England was the relatively unimportant categories of voluntary provision of chronic beds and maternity beds in the county council areas.

Shortage of facilities in Wales as compared with England persisted until the period leading to the Second World War. Contemporary accounts are clear that the 'Special Areas' tended to lack services. The view of the South Wales District Commissioner, Captain Crawshay, that hospital services in his area were 'the equal of similar services in

Table 9.4: Ownership of beds per 1,000 population for England and south Wales in 1938.

	South Wales						England					
	Municipal			Voluntary			Municipal			Voluntary		
	All	County Borough	County Council	All	County Borough	County Council	All	County Borough	County Council	All	County Borough	County Council
Acute	0.69	1.64	0.32	1.46	2.27	1.15	1.66	2.46	0.70	1.67	2.10	1.17
Chronic	1.10	1.72	0.86	0.01	0.00	0.02	1.24	1.27	1.26	0.04	0.04	0.02
Maternity	0.12	0.18	0.10	0.05	0.05	0.05	0.18	0.26	0.12	0.09	0.12	0.05
Infectious disease	0.66	0.81	0.60	–	–	–	1.00	1.00	0.79	–	–	–
Tuberculosis	0.76	0.62	0.82	–	–	–	0.54	0.71	0.39	0.17	0.05	0.23
Total	3.34	4.97	2.70	1.53	2.31	1.22	4.62	5.69	3.26	1.97	2.31	1.47

any part of Great Britain' was not widely held. Indeed, the Ministry of Health considered that their surveys of services showed that only in Merthyr Tydfil was the position 'satisfactory.'[83] Moreover, the Nuffield Surveyors considered the region deficient in qualitative as well as quantitative terms. Many of the hospitals were small, with limited equipment and facilities, and few resident medical staff or visiting consultants.[84]

Discussion

It is clear that the patterns of health status and health-care provision were different from those of England, with Wales having worse health status and, in many respects, inferior provision. It is now time to revisit the question posed earlier as to whether this different pattern was associated with different contexts or different mechanisms. This discussion is inevitably speculative, but a number of points may be made. First, it is clear that part of the explanation relates to the different context. As a whole, England was more affluent than Wales. Much of the south Wales valleys and parts of north Wales were similar in socio-economic terms to depressed areas of England such as the north-east, with similar themes of poor health, inadequate voluntary hospitals and poor local authorities struggling to fill the gaps.[85] Similarly, large tracts of Wales were poor and rural, with few large and rich towns to support hospital development. It seems reasonable, then, that at least part of the explanation for different patterns between England and Wales can be accounted for by basic socio-economic factors. However, there are some patterns that are difficult to explain in terms of poverty or sparsity. For example, there were higher levels of tuberculosis and lower levels of provision in the rural Welsh counties as compared with their English counterparts.[86] In 1912 Stephens considered that the death rate from consumption was 'nothing short of disgraceful'.[87] Even today, Wales tends to have 'excess' mortality over and above its 'expected' level, given its social class structure,[88] with some of this excess mortality associated with occupational factors such as mining.[89] Moreover, some of the processes or mechanisms appear to be different between England and Wales. For example, both voluntary and more arguably Poor Law/municipal hospitals tended to develop later. Evans points to a diffusion effect. He writes that in England, fashion, urban growth and the development of the provincial medical profession spread hospitals into the provinces in the later eighteenth century. The development of the Cardiff Infirmary was part of the pattern of the diffusion of an innovation to the provinces.[90] However, as we have seen, these diffusion processes appeared to have been delayed at the border. Again, the small size of many Welsh towns and their poverty probably provide a partial explanation for this delay,[91] but it is possible that factors of class structure, culture and religion also played a part. Davies considers that no existing interpretation such as new philanthropic attitudes, religious obligations, economic investment or prestige satisfactorily explains all the known facts about the development of voluntary hospitals in south Wales.[92] Turning to municipal hospitals, it was Liberal Progressive Barry rather than any of the socialist strongholds that first set up a rate-aided hospital.[93]

Some writers argue that the Medical Aid Societies gave the Welsh medical landscape a distinctive element. Earwicker discusses their monopoly situation in medical employment based on geographical and occupational factors: 'It is these conditions that marked out the difference between the South Wales miners medical services and those of Lancashire and Cheshire for example, where in a mixed industrial community, their role was much more akin to an orthodox friendly society.'[94]

Finally, Wales had some national institutions such as the Welsh Board of Health and the Welsh National Memorial Association that differentiated it from English regions of comparable size and socioeconomic conditions. However, there is relatively little work on the efficacy of these national institutions. Morgan claims that the Welsh Board of Health aroused little enthusiasm. At first it was to have so slight a measure of authority that it could not even appoint charwomen without the approval of Whitehall.[95] However, these institutions may have set a model for the NHS in Wales, in that Wales as a whole was made a 'Region' rather than dividing the nation according to the rationality of transport links and existing patient-flows that may have seen mid-Wales in the Birmingham Region and north Wales in the Liverpool Region.

Conclusion: Medical History in Wales or Welsh Medical History?

The conclusions to this chapter may be divided into three main areas. The first relates to the study of medical history in Wales. Although there have been advances in recent years, and many good studies, the whole is still less than the sum of the parts. Although we are beginning to piece together the pieces of the jigsaw, the overall picture still remains unclear.

The second point relates to context. It is important to discover whether health and health care varied within Wales and between Wales and the other nations of Britain with respect to patterns and/or processes. Were any differences in Welsh medical history due simply to differences in variables such as wealth, sparsity, religion and politics? Or were different processes – a Welsh effect – in operation to produce distinctive results? Particular attention needs to be paid to potentially distinctive institutions such as the MAS, the WNMA, the Welsh Board of Health as well as factors such as geography, class structure, culture, language and politics that might make up a distinctive milieu.

This brings us to the final point that concerns methods. Borsay and Porter claim that in the past thirty years the historical study of medicine and health has undergone a revolution, with links to social and cultural history, and has pulled in concepts from the social sciences to become a seedbed for interdisciplinary research. However, they argue that Welsh historiography has been slow to respond to this new subdiscipline. Most research is contained in theses, and published work is typically written in the heroic or antiquarian tradition.[96] My feeling is that their first claim overstates, while their second claim understates the case. However, this chapter has argued for greater attention to be paid to context and contingency. It is necessary to supplement the traditional use of case studies and archive work with methods that place such studies in a broader context. Work is needed both to compare Wales with other nations, and to compare different localities within Wales. Only with progress on these fronts can we move towards a study of Welsh medical history.

Notes

[1] Gwyn A. Williams, *When Was Wales?* (London, 1985).
[2] L. J. Sharpe and K. Newton, *Does Politics Matter?* (Oxford, 1984), but see

George Boyne, 'Regional influences on local politics: the case of the Welsh effect', *Regional Studies*, Vol. 26, no. 6 (1992), 569–80.
[3] For example L. Donaldson, *The Contingency Theory of Organizations* (London, 2001).
[4] For a general discussion, see Boyne, 'The Welsh Effect'. For Wales, see Williams, *When was Wales?*; Dai Smith, *Aneurin Bevan and the World of South Wales* (Cardiff, 1993); Dai Smith, *Wales, A Question for History* (Bridgend, 1999); R. Pope, *Building Jerusalem, Nonconformity, Labour and the Social Question in Wales, 1906–1939* (Cardiff, 1998); on medical history, see John Pickstone, *Medicine and Industrial Society* (Manchester, 1985); Neil Evans, '"The first charity in Wales": Cardiff Infirmary and South Wales society 1837–1914', *Welsh History Review*, Vol. 9, no. 3 (1979), 319–46; Steven Thompson, 'Hospital provision, charity and public responsibility in Edwardian Pontypridd', *Llafur*, Vol. 8, no. 3 (2002), 53–65; idem, 'To relieve the sufferings of humanity, irrespective of party, politics or creed?: conflict, consensus and voluntary hospital provision in Edwardian south Wales', *Social History of Medicine*, Vol. 16, no. 2 (2003), 247–62.
[5] John Stewart, 'The National Health Service in Scotland, 1947–1974: Scottish or British?', *Historical Research*, Vol. 76, no. 193 (2003), 389–410.
[6] Christopher Ham, *Health Policy in Britain* (Basingstoke, 1985); Rob Baggott, *Health and Health Care in Britain* (Basingstoke, 1994).
[7] Judith Allsop, *Health Policy and the NHS* (Harlow, 1995); Alan Trevor-Jones, J. Nixon and R. Picken, *Hospital Survey: The Hospital Services of South Wales and Monmouthshire* (London, 1945); Martin Powell, *Evaluating the National Health Service* (Buckingham, 1997).
[8] Rudolf Klein, *The New Politics of the NHS* (Harlow, 4th edn., 2001).
[9] Helen Jones, *Health and Society in Twentieth-Century Britain* (Harlow, 1994).
[10] Steven Cherry, *Medical Services and the Hospitals in Britain, 1860–1939* (Cambridge, 1996); Virginia Berridge, *Health and Society in Britain since 1939* (Cambridge, 1999); Brian Abel-Smith, *The Hospitals 1800–1948* (London, 1964).
[11] Anne Hardy, *Health and Medicine in Britain since 1860* (Basingstoke, 2001).
[12] Charles Webster, *The Health Services Since the War*, I: *Problems of Health Care: The National Health Service before 1957* (London, 1988) and *The Health Services since the War*, II: *Government and Health Care: The British National Health Service, 1958–79* (London, 1996); idem, *The National Health Service: A Political History* (Oxford, 2nd edn., 2002).
[13] Stewart, 'The NHS in Scotland', 392, similarly notes that historians of Scotland have had little to say about post-war health care, a surprising omission given the nation's poor health record.
[14] John Davies, *A History of Wales* (Harmondsworth, 1993), pp. 615, 621.
[15] J. Black, *A New History of Wales* (Stroud, 2000), p. 197.
[16] P. Jenkins, *A History of Modern Wales, 1536–1990* (London, 1992), pp. 249–54.
[17] D. Gareth Evans, *A History of Wales* (Cardiff, 2000), pp. 47–53.
[18] Smith, *Aneurin Bevan*.
[19] Kenneth Morgan, *Rebirth of a Nation: Wales 1880–1980* (Oxford, 1981).

20 G. Arbour Stephens, *The Hospitals of Wales* (Swansea, 1912).
21 Deian Hopkins, 'Reflections of an editor, 1972–1987', *Llafur*, Vol. 4, no. 7 (1987); Anne Borsay and Dorothy Porter, 'Health and medicine: historical and contemporary perspectives' in Anne Borsay (ed.), *Medicine in Wales c.1800–2000: Public Service or Private Commodity?* (Cardiff, 2003).
22 R. Griffiths and J. Law, *An Introduction to the Sources for the History of Medicine in South Wales* (Swansea, 1995), p. 3.
23 *Llafur*, Vol. 8, no. 1 (2000), 3–4; Martin Powell, 'Wales and the NHS', ibid., 33–43.
24 These include A. Aldis, *Cardiff Royal Infirmary 1883–1983* (Cardiff, 1984); O. V. Jones, *The Progress of Medicine: A History of the Caernarfon and Anglesey Infirmary 1809–1948* (Llandysul, 1984); T. G. Davies, *Deeds not Words: A History of the Swansea General and Eye Hospital, 1817–1948* (Cardiff, 1988); G. Jones, *The Aneurin Bevan Inheritance: The Story of the Nevill Hall and District NHS Trust* (Abertillery, 1998); Pamela Michael, *Care and Treatment of the Mentally Ill in North Wales, 1800–2000* (Cardiff, 2002); E. Davies, *The North Wales Quarry Hospitals* (Caernarfon, 2003).
25 This impression is supported by the relative dearth of writing on health in articles and theses reported in the relevant sections of the *Welsh History Review*.
26 For example, Joseph Gross, 'Hospitals in Merthyr, 1850–1974', *Merthyr Historian*, Vol. 2 (1978), 78–92; Evans, '"The first charity in Wales"'; Thompson, 'Public responsibility in Edwardian Pontypridd'; idem, 'To relieve the sufferings of humanity'.
27 David Lee Williams, 'A healthy place to be? The Wrexham coalfield in the interwar period', *Llafur*, Vol. 7, no. 1 (1996), 87–95; N. Woodward, 'Why did south Wales miners have high mortality? Evidence from the mid-twentieth century', *Welsh History Review*, Vol. 20, no. 1 (2000), 116–42; Steven Thompson, '"That beautiful summer of severe austerity": health, diet and the working-class economy in south Wales in 1926', *Welsh History Review*, Vol. 21, no. 1 (2003), 552–74.
28 Ray Earwicker, 'Miners' medical services before the First World War: the south Wales coalfield', *Llafur*, Vol. 3, no. 1 (1981), 39–52; Linda Bryder, 'The King Edward VII Welsh national memorial association and its policy towards tuberculosis 1910–1848', *Welsh History Review*, Vol. 13, no. 2 (1986), 194–216; Linda Bryder, 'Tuberculosis, silicosis and the slate industry in north Wales 1927–1939' in Paul Weindling (ed.), *The Social History of Occupational Health* (London, 1985); Kate Fisher, 'Cleaning up misconceptions: the campaign to set up birth control clinics in south Wales between the wars', *Welsh History Review*, Vol. 19, no. 1 (1998), 103–29.
29 There have been relatively few theses between Geraint Dean Fielder, 'Public health and hospital administration in Swansea since the end of the eighteenth century to 1914' (unpublished MA thesis, University of Wales, 1962) and J. King, 'Midwives, infant and maternal health in Monmouthshire, 1900–1938' (unpublished Ph.D. thesis, University of Glamorgan, 1999) and Steven Thompson, 'A social history of medicine in inter-war South Wales' (unpublished Ph.D. thesis, University of Wales, 2001).

30 Powell, *Evaluating the NHS*, p. 19.
31 For example Davies, *Deeds not Words*; Jones, *Aneurin Bevan Inheritance*; Michael, *Care and Treatment*.
32 Pickstone, *Medicine and Industrial Society*.
33 Thompson, 'To relieve the sufferings of humanity'.
34 Stefan Berger, 'Working-class culture and the Labour movement in the south Wales and the Ruhr coalfields, 1850–2000: a comparison', *Llafur*, Vol. 8, no. 2 (2001), 5–40; Berger, 'And what should they know of Wales?: why Welsh history needs comparison', *Llafur*, Vol. 8, no. 3 (2002), 131–9.
35 See pp. 223–4, 227 for more details on these issues.
36 Donaldson, *Contingency Theory*, p. 5.
37 Boyne, 'The Welsh effect'.
38 R. Pawson and N. Tilley, *Realistic Evaluation* (London, 1997); J. Connell and A. Kubisch, *Applying a Theories of Change Approach to the Evaluation of Comprehensive Community Initiatives* (Washington, DC, 1996); H.-T. Chen, *Theory-Driven Evaluations* (Newbury Park, CA, 1990).
39 Richard Rose, *Understanding the United Kingdom: The Territorial Dimension in Government* (Harlow, 1982); see also Peter Madgwick and Richard Rose (eds.), *The Territorial Dimension in United Kingdom Politics* (London, 1982).
40 Sharpe and Newton, *Does Politics Matter?*, pp. 152, 162.
41 Boyne, 'The Welsh effect', 569–80.
42 Borsay and Porter, 'Health and medicine', pp. 16–17; see also Steven Thompson, 'A proletarian public sphere: working-class provision of medical services and care in south Wales, c.1900–1948' in Borsay (ed.), *Medicine in Wales*, pp. 86–107.
43 Michael, *Care and Treatment*, pp. 2, 5.
44 Stewart, 'The NHS in Scotland'.
45 Ibid., 391; J. S. Ross, *The National Health Service in Great Britain* (London, 1952), pp. 335–6.
46 Ross, *The NHS in Great Britain*, Chs 28–30 (p. 103); see also Webster, *Problems of Health Care*.
47 This section draws on Powell, 'How adequate? was hospital provision before the NHS? An examination of the 1945 South Wales Hospital Survey', *Local Population Studies*, Vol. 48 (1992), 22–32, and Powell, 'Wales and the NHS', where the more detailed sources and footnotes may be found.
48 *Report on an Investigation into Maternal Mortality in Wales* (London, 1937); *Report of the Committee of Inquiry into the Anti-Tuberculosis Services in Wales and Monmouthshire* (London, 1939).
49 David Green, *Reinventing Civil Society* (London, 1993), p. 30; idem, *Working Class Patients and the Medical Establishment* (Aldershot, 1985), but see John Mohan, *Planning, Markets and Hospitals* (London, 2002), and John Mohan and Martin Gorsky, *Don't Look Back?* (London, 2001) for a critique.
50 Anne Digby and Nick Bosanquet, 'Doctors and patients in an era of national health insurance and private practice', *Economic History Review*, Vol. 41, no. 1 (1988), pp. 74–94.
51 A. J. Cronin, *The Citadel* (London, 1983; first published 1937), p. 17. This is

based on Cronin's experiences as a young doctor in the south Wales valleys before he became famous as a novelist.

[52] Political and Economic Planning, *The British Health Services* (London, 1937), pp. 151–2.

[53] Green, *Reinventing Civil Society*, pp. 110–11, 114–15.

[54] Steven Cherry, 'Accountability, entitlement and control issues and voluntary hospital funding *c*.1860–1939', *Social History of Medicine*, Vol. 9, no. 2 (1996), 215–33; Martin Gorsky, Martin Powell and John Mohan, 'British voluntary hospitals and the public sphere' in Steve Sturdy (ed.), *Medicine, Health and the Public Sphere in Britain, 1600–2000* (London, 2002); Mohan and Gorsky, *Don't Look Back?*; Earwicker, 'Miners' medical services'; Thompson, 'A proletarian public sphere'.

[55] Webster, *Problems of Health Care*, p. 382.

[56] But see for example Earwicker, 'Miners' medical services'; Thompson, 'A proleterian public sphere'; Jones, *Aneurin Bevan Inheritance*.

[57] Hansard HC (series 5), Vol. 422, col. 47 (30 April 1946).

[58] Davies, *Deeds not Words*, p. 12.

[59] *Burdett's Hospitals and Charities 1929* (London, 1929).

[60] Trevor-Jones et al., *Hospital Survey*.

[61] *Burdett's*; cf. Abel-Smith, *Hospitals*.

[62] *Burdett's Hospitals and Charities 1929* (London, 1929).

[63] Bryder, 'The King Edward VII WNMA'.

[64] For a recent study see Robert Smith, *Schools, Politics and Society: Elementary Education in Wales, 1870–1902* (Cardiff, 1999).

[65] Arbour Stephens, *The Hospitals of Wales*, p. 14; B. Luxton, 'Ambition, vice and virtue: social life, 1884–1914' in D. Moore (ed.), *Barry: The Centenary Book* (Barry, 1984); P. Stead, 'The town that had come of age: Barry 1918–1939' in Moore (ed.), *Barry*.

[66] Arbour Stephens, *The Hospitals of Wales*, pp. 54–6.

[67] Jenkins, *History of Modern Wales*, ch. 17.

[68] Morgan, *Rebirth of a Nation*, pp. 235–6, 292–3. For a wider view of health care in the depressed areas, see John Mohan, 'Neglected roots of regionalism? The commissioners for the special areas and grants to hospitals in England', *Social History of Medicine*, Vol. 10 (1997), 243–62.

[69] T. Mervyn Jones, *Going Public* (Cowbridge, 1987), p. 106.

[70] Michael Foot, *Aneurin Bevan: A Biography. Volume One* (London, 1962), p. 85.

[71] Arbour Stephens, *The Hospitals of Wales*, pp. 50.

[72] Davies, *History of Wales*, p. 588.

[73] Evans, *History of Wales*, p. 52; Black, *New History of Wales*, p. 196; Jenkins, *History of Modern Wales*, ch. 17; Robert Smith, 'The reform of local government finance 1928–1937: a study of south Wales', *Welsh History Review*, Vol. 21, no. 1 (2002), 149–79.

[74] Cronin, *The Citadel*, p. 22.

[75] Jones, *Going Public*, pp. 106–8.

[76] Martin Powell, 'Did politics matter?', *Urban History*, Vol. 22 (1995), 360–79;

idem, 'An expanding service: municipal public health expenditure in the 1930s', *Twentieth Century British History*, Vol. 8 (1997), 334–57.
77 Morgan, *Rebirth of a Nation*, pp. 235–6.
78 Stead, 'The town that had come of age', 426 fn; Robert Smith, 'The reform of local government finance'.
79 Trevor-Jones et al., *Hospital Survey*, p. 3.
80 See Thompson, 'To relieve the sufferings of humanity' for discussion of the debates between the 'rate-aiders' and the 'voluntarists' in different south Wales towns.
81 Powell, 'An expanding service'.
82 Linda Bryder, *Below the Magic Mountain: A Social History of Tuberculosis in Twentieth-Century Britain* (Oxford, 1988); F. B. Smith, *The Retreat of Tuberculosis 1850–1950* (London, 1988).
83 Mohan, 'Neglected roots'.
84 Powell, 'How adequate'. These comments refer to the south Wales region, as north Wales and mid-Wales were covered by the north-west of England Surveyors.
85 Mohan, *Planning, Markets and Hospitals*; Mohan, 'Neglected Roots'.
86 Morgan, *Rebirth of a Nation*; Evans, *History of Wales*.
87 Arbour Stephens, *The Hospitals of Wales*.
88 P. Townsend and N. Davidson (eds), *Inequalities in Health* (Harmondsworth, 1982).
89 Williams, 'A healthy place to be?'
90 Evans, 'The first charity', 320–1.
91 For example, the 1801 Census records the population of Cardiff as 4,672, Swansea as 6,420 and Merthyr as 8,945, Aldis, *Cardiff Royal Infirmary*, p. 2
92 Davies, *Deeds not Words*, p. 13.
93 Luxton, 'Ambition, vice and virtue'; Stead, 'The town that had come of age'; compare Thompson, 'To relieve the sufferings of humanity'.
94 Earwicker, 'Miners' medical services', p. 49.
95 Morgan, *Rebirth of a Nation*, 205, and Bryder, 'The King Edward VII WNMA' and Jones, *Going Public*, pp. 73–9 on the WNMA.
96 Borsay and Porter, 'Health and medicine', p. 1; cf. Thompson, 'To relieve the sufferings of humanity', 247.

10

Devolution and the Health Service in Wales, 1919–1969*

CHARLES WEBSTER

In modern times the publicly provided services associated with health have expanded until collectively they now constitute one of the most important sectors of the United Kingdom economy. As a consequence the departments of state associated with health have assumed great importance. Both the Ministry of Health, established in 1919, and its modern successor, the Department of Health, are counted among the largest departments in Whitehall. Consequently, the question of the location of health administration has assumed central importance in the debate on devolution. It is no exaggeration to say that comprehensive command over services relating to health was regarded as essential for the viability and parity of status of the Welsh Office when this department was established in 1964. Of all the transfers to the new Welsh Office in the first years of its existence, health was the biggest gain. At the date of change, in 1969, the NHS accounted for exactly two-thirds of the spending of the Welsh Office and in due course this massive bonus was handed down to the Welsh Assembly. The complex story of events between 1964 and 1969 is worth setting in context and recounting in full, not only to clarify a situation that is easily and often misunderstood, but also to draw attention to the obstacles impeding the realization of devoluntionary policies.

The importance of the health services was not lost on either the friends or enemies of devolution. The intransigence of the Ministry of Health and its successors over the prospect of relinquishing its Welsh colonial possessions constitutes a significant part of the explanation for the slow pace of moves towards Welsh devolution. When the Welsh Office was eventually established by the Wilson Labour government, it took a further five years of acrimonious debate before Labour belatedly honoured its manifesto commitment to include health in the portfolio of the new department and its Secretary of State. The following review of the problem of devolution from the angle of health care demonstrates the difficulties experienced by the Labour government in coming to terms with its recent conversion to Welsh devolution. In practice, it proved more difficult than was evident on the surface to bury the ingrained prejudices inherited from the past. Immediately the Welsh Office became a reality, recidivists within the Cabinet and Whitehall mobilized their forces to undermine fulfilment of electoral commitments and they determined that every devolutionary concession became mired down in labyrinthine consultations. In the wider context, this process throws light on the painful contortions experienced by Harold Wilson's ministers in responding to the rising tide of nationalist sentiment. As a case study, this narrative counts as a victory for the devolutionists. However, it also points to the existence of structural characteristics that were not eliminated in 1969 and were liable to impede Wales from attaining real independence of action in the fields of health policy and administration.

The Legacy of the First World War

The intensive debate conducted between 1964 and 1969 constituted a crucial phase in a long campaign to wrest the control of the health services in Wales from the Ministry of Health and the Minister of Health in London. Although the Ministry and Minister were responsible for both England and Wales, Welsh opinion was increasingly convinced that the English interest was paramount and that Wales received nothing like a proportionate degree of consideration. The objective of the devolutionists was to convert the Welsh Board of Health into a health department of a Welsh Office located in Cardiff and answerable to a Secretary of State for Wales, who would represent the Welsh interest at Cabinet level.

The disadvantageous position of Wales with respect to control over affairs relating to health is underlined by comparison with Scotland. Under a well-developed board system, devolution in Scotland was well advanced by 1900. The pace of change further accelerated after the First World War. The Secretary for Scotland was upgraded into a full Secretary of State in 1926. Scottish health administration was reorganized in 1919, when miscellaneous board functions were assimilated under the Scottish Board of Health. This proved to be a temporary arrangement. In 1929, the Department of Health for Scotland, conforming to the standard civil service pattern, replaced the nominated Board of Health.[1] Although this change was controversial at the time and was suspected of undermining Scottish administrative autonomy, in practice the Department of Health gained in authority when it became a constituent part of the Scottish Office.[2] As discussions concerning the development of a national health service indicated, the Department of Health in Edinburgh was well equipped to negotiate from a position of strength with the Ministry of Health in London.[3]

Compared with the situation of Scotland, Wales occupied an inferior status in all spheres of administration. Periodically minor concessions to Welsh sentiment were offered, often in order to preserve some degree of parity with Scotland. For instance, in 1912 both Scotland and Wales were granted separate Commissions to administer the new system of National Health Insurance, while in 1919 Boards of Health were established in both Scotland and Wales. In Wales this was represented as a significant concession to nationalist sentiment. Section 5 of the Ministry of Health Act 1919 established a Welsh Board of Health to operate in tandem with the new Ministry of Health. This produced an appearance of symmetry with Scotland, but the comparison was deceptive. The Scottish Board of Health represented a further development of a long-established board system and a staging post on the path to further administrative modernization undertaken within the course of the next decade. The Board of Health in Wales was entirely dissimilar. It arose less from the desire to establish greater autonomy in health affairs in Wales, but more out of a need to find a satisfactory means of continuing the work of the Welsh National Insurance Commission. Since in Wales there was no existing body to take on this function, a Board of Health was established for this purpose. The Welsh Board of Health was in essence a reincarnation of the Welsh Insurance Commission and the three members of the latter were appointed officers of the new Board. Granted, the Board of Health assumed additional duties, especially after the 1929 Local Government Act, but its terms of reference were drawn as restrictively as possible to prevent deviation from instructions emanating from London. The Welsh Board of Health was therefore not conceived as an evolutionary stage in the process of devolution or administrative modernization, but as a regional outpost of the Ministry of Health. Furthermore, entrusting health to a board of the type established in Wales possessed symbolic importance as a self-evidently conservative gesture. Before 1919, both the Royal Commission on the Civil Service and the Haldane Committee on the Machinery of Government attacked the system of administrative boards and called for their replacement by departments in which full responsibility was laid upon ministers and their civil servants.[4] The Insurance Commissions were thought to typify the weakness of the board system. Consequently, while administration by boards was being phased out in England and Scotland, the obsolete board system was not only freshly introduced in Wales, but also its scope was progressively extended from National Health Insurance to many other services relating to health.

In the course of its fifty-year history, the Welsh Board of Health exemplified the deficiencies of the board mechanism. In general, the Board of Health performed its duties precisely in the spirit intended by its designers. As such the Board served as a useful instrument for London, but it was not an appropriate basis for furthering the cause of devolution. The Welsh Board of Health was therefore a constitutional dead end, a fossilised relic, representing an administrative device inappropriate to the twentieth century.

Underlining the weakness of the Welsh Board of Health was the continuing existence of an entirely separate national body, the King Edward VII Welsh National Memorial Association. This was not a creature of Whitehall, but in 1910 it arose as a specifically Welsh initiative, conceived as a campaign to combat tuberculosis. In 1912 this body was linked with the new tuberculosis arrangements developed in conjunction with National Health Insurance.[5] Next, in 1921 the Memorial Association took over delegated responsibility for the enhanced tuberculosis services, the counterparts of which in England were controlled by separate local authorities. The integrated national tuberculosis service was unique to Wales and was a source of national pride. The National Memorial Association therefore became cited as a successful devolutionary model, suitable for extension to the health service as a whole. However, as noted below, shortcomings of the Welsh tuberculosis system were exploited by the critics of devolution to urge the dangers of Welsh autonomy.

Given the inbuilt limitations of the Welsh Board of Health and the Welsh National Memorial Association, the best realistic opportunity for developing the case for health devolution resided with the Welsh Consultative Council on Medical and Allied Services. This advisory body was a further product of the 1919 legislation and it was a counterpart to similar consultative councils formed in England and Scotland. Advisory bodies of this kind were the brainchild of the Haldane Committee.[6] Consultative councils were supposed to provide a permanent source of expert advice to ministers. This worked well in education, but the councils were soon allowed to atrophy in the health departments.[7] Best remembered is the English Consultative Council on account of its association with the Dawson Report, which contained ambitious proposals for a comprehensive health service.[8] The Scottish Consultative Council produced a similar plan for Scotland.[9]

Although little noticed by modern scholarship, the Welsh Consultative Council also came up with proposals for a comprehensive health service. Like Dawson's Council it advocated a hierarchical organization of services and it was notable for its emphasis on primary care. The Council was responsible for two published reports, while two further reports remained unpublished after its abolition. The Welsh Consultative Council was conspicuous for its commitment to devolution. In its second report the Council proposed that the development of health services in Wales should be entrusted to a 'Welsh National Council of Health'.[10] It noted that there was not yet support in England for devolving administration to the provincial or regional level. The Council was no doubt alert to the advocacy of the provincial system by figures like Sir Halford Mackinder and C. B. Fawcett. The latter's influential *Provinces of England* had only recently been published.[11]

Despite advocacy of regional schemes for cooperation among local government experts, this idea failed to catch on in government. Regional administration in the public sector of health care was limited to a handful of special cases. The idea was not applied more generally, even though such arrangements might have resulted in economy and improvement in services.[12]

The Welsh Council detected a strong 'sentiment of nationality ... deeply embedded in their consciousness' in Wales.[13] A Welsh National Council of Health seemed an appropriate response to this national feeling. This council might assume some degree of control over the services provided by local government and National Health Insurance. In practice, the Consultative Council fell back on its 'Alternative I', under which all health services would be provided by existing public authorities and funded by rates and taxes. Such modest reforms, like the proposals contained in the Dawson Report, were unwelcome to the Ministry of Health and the Welsh Board of Health. As a consequence the English and Welsh Consultative Councils were first quietly suppressed and then in 1926 formally abolished. The Scottish Council produced no report of its own after July 1921, although its meetings staggered on until 1924.[14] As Spurr drily observes, officials in the health departments never invested confidence in the consultative councils, which they saw as irritants to be removed at the first opportunity.[15]

The Welsh Consultative Council was all but forgotten, but one witness portrayed this as a 'tragic and untimely end', which was greeted in Wales with 'disappointment, disillusionment and utter frustration'.[16] Negative experiences of this kind after the First World War created consternation and, in some circles, strengthened the argument for home rule. This environment contributed in 1925 to the birth of Plaid Cymru. Health service issues played an increasing part in the programme of Plaid Cymru.[17] Notwithstanding the economic crisis, the argument for greater autonomy for Wales continued to gather support and gain in sophistication. Periodically, attempts were made in Parliament to secure a Secretary of State for Wales, a Welsh equivalent to the Scottish Office, as well as other more specific demands like a National Council for Education.[18] Health invariably featured as a candidate for autonomy, although inevitably education and the economy took precedence in the devolutionist argument. The emergence of effective advocacy from MPs such as Clement Davies, later leader of the Liberal Party, increased the impact of the devolutionist case. The report on tuberculosis in Wales, produced under the chairmanship of Clement Davies, greatly added to his political reputation; it also made an impact as a contribution to the health devolution debate.[19] More effectively than any other document produced during the inter-war period, the Clement Davies report publicized the impoverished state of health and health services in Wales. The tuberculosis report fuelled the consternation of Welsh patriots and on this occasion their sense of grievance became echoed in Westminster and in the UK press.[20] James Griffiths described the tuberculosis report as 'a call to action by the people of Wales'.[21] The threat of war reduced the impact of this new demand for reform, but it was by no means extinguished.

Welsh Reconstruction during the Second World War

In the event, the cataclysm of a Second World War had the effect of further galvanizing the campaign for devolution.[22] As part of its confidence-building initiatives, the government immediately became committed to planning for post-war reconstruction, which inevitably involved attention to the special needs of Scotland and Wales. When the Secretary of State for Scotland established a Council on Post-War Problems, a dozen MPs demanded a similar advisory council for Wales. At a meeting in November 1941 Arthur Greenwood conceded the need for such a committee. This tied the hands of Greenwood's senior colleagues, who were palpably annoyed by the Welsh demand for parity of treatment with Scotland, but reluctantly they agreed to form the Welsh Reconstruction Advisory Council.[23] Another minor gain for the devolutionists was the granting of an annual 'Welsh Day' for debates, the first of which took place in 1944.

The Scottish Council was important for guiding policy on the NHS. The Welsh equivalent exercised no comparable influence, although it was helpful in reinforcing the argument for further administrative devolution. Although the first Welsh Day debate took place in October 1944 at the height of discussions on the future NHS in England and Wales, the health service was not mentioned by any speaker. The debate was dominated by economic issues. Wales received only negligible special consideration during planning for the NHS. Wales was indeed fortunate to emerge as a unified region under the new health service. Some alarm was caused when the Second World War hospital surveys failed to adopt Wales as a single region for survey purposes. In addition the cancer scheme launched in 1939, which was the first of the government's regional planning initiatives, proposed linking north Wales with Liverpool. This set the tone for the wartime official surveys, which anticipated continuing linkage of north Wales with hospital services in Liverpool. In response, the advocates of devolution produced a report on hospital services making the case for a united hospital service for Wales.[24]

The regional issue was central in planning for the future health service. This involved examination of the performance of all existing regional planning bodies, some of the main examples of which existed in Wales. The results were not encouraging. By contrast with its anodyne public statements, the Ministry of Health's confidential verdict on regional bodies was unflattering about most of the existing regional machinery, including the Welsh National Memorial Association.[25] The Ministry's praise for interventions in south Wales by the Special Areas Commissioner for England and Wales served to underline the ineffectiveness of the National Memorial Association and the Welsh Board of Health.[26]

Confidential soundings supported negative conclusions about Welsh health administration. Sir John Maude, Permanent Secretary to the Ministry of Health, was influenced by a devastating indictment of the engineering services of the Welsh Board of Health. On this basis Maude concluded that it would be disastrous to increase the influence of any 'Welsh speaking, Welsh educated, or local men' on the Board of Health.[27] This negative assessment was decisively confirmed by Thomas Jones, one of the most influential Welshmen of the day, who was consulted on the latest devolution memorandum signed by thirty-six MPs, which restated the argument for a Secretary of State for Wales and a Welsh Office. Jones wrote with authority founded on direct experience of the Welsh National Memorial Association and the Welsh Insurance Commission. Notwithstanding its grandiose building in Cathays Park and large staff, he regarded the Welsh Board of Health in Cardiff as a failure, its senior staff being characterized by second-rate quality. Jones was known to have reservations about Sir John Rowland, the recently retired Chairman of the Board; he was no more sanguine about the likelihood of improvement under Frederick Armer, who had recently taken over this office. Jones concluded that the Welsh Board of Health represented the wrong model; instead he supported the approach adopted in education, with a Welsh Department located in London as part of the Board of Education. A Secretary for Wales might be appointed, but again this office should be located in London and limited to advisory functions.[28] Jones therefore added to the body of testimony suggesting that devolution would be subversive to the improvement of public services and that home rule was being exploited as a mechanism for personal aggrandisement by careerists lacking in basic competence.

The Devolution Debate from 1945 to 1964

For Whitehall departments already predisposed against further devolution, support from Jones was cherished as an invaluable asset. His advice echoed through documents produced over the following two decades. During the war, coalition ministers were advised in preparing for the post-war settlement to resist anything other than minor extension of administrative devolution; if that proved insufficient, the existing Advisory Council might be strengthened by placing a Secretary for Wales in charge of its activities.[29]

Despite positive encouragement at the beginning of the war, by 1945 it was evident that the supporters of devolution were making little progress. The government even failed to respond to the case for devolution presented in 1943. The advocates of devolution therefore entered the post-war period with a sense of apprehension. It seemed possible that fresh concessions would be less than those achieved after the First World War.

On the health front the omens were not positive. Aneurin Bevan, Attlee's Minister of Health, made no secret of his antipathy to devolution. During the inaugural Welsh Day debate he was the sole speaker to break with the generally harmonious tone and dismiss the proceedings with contempt.[30] This intervention exposed a split among Welsh Labour MPs, especially obvious because, in the debate, Bevan was followed by his friend James Griffiths, who made the most convincing speech in favour of devolution.[31] Griffiths was appointed Minister of National Insurance in Attlee's government. Bevan and Griffiths found themselves on the Machinery of Government Committee, which inherited responsibility for policy on devolution. The records of this Committee and the Cabinet indicate that Labour ministers were overwhelmingly hostile to devolution. They calculated that only token further concessions were required. Their little package comprised: exhortation to government departments to consolidate recent changes that had already been made in the distribution of business to departments in Wales, quarterly departmental liaison meetings and production of a regular White Paper drawing together information relating to Wales. These trivial proposals represented the fruits of ministerial deliberations stretching over a whole year.[32] The response was naturally greeted with dismay by Welsh MPs, who regarded it as total repudiation of 'the claims of Wales as a nation'.[33] It took a further two years of lobbying before they were in a position to secure further concessions.[34]

In the meantime Bevan proceeded with his plans for the great new health service without paying heed to Welsh national sentiment. The appeal from the mining valleys to convert their Medical Aid Society clinics into health centres was rejected and, indeed, it was not supported by Bevan, despite his personal links with the Medical Aid Societies.[35] There was also hesitation about adopting Wales as a single entity in the new regional hospital system. Liverpool demanded inclusion of north Wales in its region, citing support in north Wales, especially among doctors.[36] The University of Liverpool complained of the 'amputation of North Wales from Liverpool, which flagrantly ignores all existing practice'. The University added that 'this exclusion of North Wales from the Liverpool region is a virtual denial of the functional conception of a region'.[37] Other representations favoured a single Welsh region. For instance, Captain Geoffrey Crawshay, Chairman of the Welsh Board of Health, argued that the Board would be inconvenienced by having to deal with two separate regions. The Welsh National Memorial Association was invoked in support of an all-Wales region. Officials in London were swayed by the demands of Welsh MPs for attention to 'national sentiment'. This factor effectively secured a single Welsh Region for the hospital service. However, officials also noted that Bevan was only reluctantly converted to this alternative.[38] The Welsh National Memorial Association was now dissolved, but the Welsh Board of Health continued, although with diminished functions.

The coexistence of two national bodies, the Welsh Board of Health and the Welsh Regional Hospital Board (later Welsh Hospital Board) brought few advantages to Wales. For instance, whereas the Scottish Department of Health secured favourable treatment over the distribution of resources, Wales slid to near the bottom of the league table of the fourteen regions controlled by the Ministry of Health. In the drafting of official reports and policy documents scant attention was paid to Wales. This contrasted with Scotland, which issued its own Hospital Plan in 1962 and its own Green Paper at the start of the health service reorganization process in 1967. Scotland also possessed a complete range of Standing Advisory Committees, which actively addressed planning issues in the Scottish health service. The equivalent committees in London nominally related to England and Wales, but only scant attention was paid to the specific needs of Wales.

The only opportunity for devoting specific attention to the Welsh health service came about through the channel of the Council for

Wales and Monmouthshire, which was something of an unwanted stepchild of the Attlee government. When in 1948 the Secretary of State for Scotland established his Scottish Economic Conference, the government was forced to consider a counterpart for Wales. The Council for Wales and Monmouthshire represented a further minimal and reluctant concession to Welsh national feeling on the part of the Labour government.[39] As Kenneth Morgan indicates, this body never exerted much influence and in the end became the 'dead letter' that sceptics among Labour ministers predicted and wanted.[40] Reflecting the sense of betrayal among devolutionists, they mounted fresh campaigns, including for a parliament for Wales.[41]

The Council for Wales and Monmouthshire soon faced a changed political situation. From 1951 until 1964 the Council operated under Conservative administrations. The Conservatives were a recent convert to the Welsh cause; they made some minor concessions, including placing a Cabinet Minister in charge of Wales as an addition to his main departmental responsibilities. In practice this Welsh role was exercised by a junior minister in the relevant department.

During its early years, under the chairmanship of Huw Edwards, the north Wales trade unionist, the Council made some constructive interventions. Prominent among these was the report published in 1957 by its Government Administration Panel on the machinery of government in Wales. This was deferential in tone, but firmly devolutionist in its conclusions. The Panel recommended that the government offices in Cardiff relating to housing and local government, education, health and agriculture should be reconstituted as four departments of a Welsh Office headed by a Secretary of State.[42] The Panel reviewed the work of the Welsh Board of Health. The relevant paragraphs indicate difficulties over striking the right note concerning the Board. It was injudicious to criticize the Board, since this would imply the incompetence of Welsh officials; whereas, if the Board was judged a success, it might be argued that there were no grounds for further change. In the event the report gave full credit to the Board of Health, the success of which was taken as a vindication of the ability of Wales to handle routine administration. The Board was therefore presented as the logical penultimate step in an evolutionary process, the final stage of which was full devolution.[43] This blueprint for devolution was decisively rejected by the government. Prime Minister Macmillan delivered a terse response to the devolutionist argument, rejecting any further measure of devolution to

Wales and suggesting that in this case the evolution had already reached its natural conclusion.[44]

The Wilson Administration and Welsh Devolution 1964–1968

After much vacillation the Labour opposition adopted the recommendations of the Council for Wales and Monmouthshire. This major shift of policy owed much to the diplomatic skills and personal influence of James Griffiths, who was one of the few consistent devolutionists within the Labour leadership.[45] The 1959 general election manifesto committed Labour to appointing a Secretary of State for Wales with full departmental responsibilities. The Labour Party pamphlets, *Forward with Labour: Labour's Plan for Wales* (1959), *Signposts for the Sixties* and *Signposts to the New Wales* (1962), and finally the 1964 general election manifesto, also came out firmly in favour of devolution. Other proposals for devolution were also in the air at this time in Labour circles. For instance, the Welsh Council for Labour committed itself to establishing an elected Council for Wales, possessing executive powers over health functions such as the ambulance service, community care and health centres, also with the duty to nominate the members of all hospital authorities. Such changes were consistent with the philosophy of regionalism that took root among the Labour avant-garde during the 1960s.[46]

In 1964 James Griffiths was appointed Secretary of State for Wales in Harold Wilson's Labour administration. To Griffith's disappointment, the functions initially transferred to his control were considerably narrower than those suggested in *Signposts to the New Wales*. Initially the Secretary of State was given direct control over roads, housing, local government, environmental planning, forestry and water and sewage, as well as specific provincial issues such as the Welsh language, but not agriculture and fisheries, education or health. In statements clarifying the role of the new office, the Prime Minister assured disappointed devolutionists that the Secretary of State would be given 'real powers to oversee the activity of all government departments in Wales and to see that they co-ordinate'.[47] The huge shortfall in responsibilities transferred to the Welsh Office represented a humiliation for Griffiths and indicated that the change of policy signified by Labour had not reflected a genuine change of heart within the Labour leadership or within Whitehall. Signifying this survival of old instincts, even the inveterate progressive Richard Crossman described the policies for Wales as a 'silly election pledge'.[48]

Griffiths preserved his characteristic statesmanship, but he naturally resented the limitations imposed on his department. In particular he pressed for the immediate transfer of the Board of Health to the Welsh Office. This was particularly easy since it occupied the same building as housing and local government, which were now placed under Welsh Office control. However the Ministry of Health refused to countenance further incursion into its territory. Just before his retirement in April 1966 Griffiths returned to the issue and wrote to the Prime Minister asking for an extension of the powers of the Secretary of State to include the departments specified in Labour policy statements. Sir Goronwy Daniel, his Permanent Under-Secretary, keenly supported this plea. A few days later the same appeal emanated from Cledwyn Hughes, who replaced Griffiths as Secretary of State. Hughes was fully committed to devolution and he was a supporter of an elected Council for Wales.[49] Griffiths and Hughes pointed out that devolution was already a proven success in the fields where they were given full command, but arrangements were much less satisfactory in areas such as health, where the situation of Wales still compared unfavourably with that in Scotland. Also, with only limited powers, the Welsh Office was too small to deal with other departments as an equal. The Welsh ministers realized that other Whitehall departments were unsympathetic to releasing their hold on agriculture, education and health, but they urged that this change was justifiable on efficiency grounds and that it was increasingly demanded by the political situation.[50] Moving forward along the lines recommended by Griffiths and Hughes presented few practical problems. Considering the smoothness of the initial operation to establish the Welsh Office, it was entirely logical to implement the rest of Labour's election pledge. But this was far from the Prime Minster's intentions. Harold Wilson was slow to appreciate the growing threat of nationalism and when the danger materialized, he failed to take command of the situation. As a consequence, concessions to Wales were wrung out of the government only after a battle of attrition among Wilson's ministers as they painfully came to terms with the reality of the nationalist threat to Labour.

Indicative of his disregard for the views of his Welsh ministers and the political sensitivity of the issues involved, the Prime Minister entrusted a review of Welsh devolution to Sir Laurence Helsby, Joint Permanent Secretary to the Treasury and head of the Home Civil Service. In the course of a short exercise conducted in the spring of 1966, Helsby treated his commission as a matter of routine. His final memorandum was drafted to reflect the full antagonism to devolution of relevant Ministers, the Treasury and all departments threatened with loss of functions. The Permanent Secretaries involved cited support from high-placed Welshmen, such as Sir Archie Lush, Chairman of the Welsh Hospital Board, and Dr Elwyn Davies, Secretary for Welsh Education in the Department of Education and Science. Helsby's memorandum argued that a further transfer of powers to Wales would add to costs and bureaucracy without increasing the efficiency of services.[51]

As already noted, Harold Wilson was no enthusiast for devolution. Crossman claims that the Prime Minister rejected his initial pleas for a policy review on devolution.[52] The Prime Minister was perhaps slightly more alert to the nationalist threat than Crossman appreciated. After the Carmarthen by-election in July 1966, in which a Labour seat recently won by Megan Lloyd George with a majority of 10,000 was taken by Plaid Cymru, Wilson appreciated that it was politically inexpedient to grant the final say on Welsh devolution to an official. He therefore proposed that a small committee of ministers under James Callaghan, the Chancellor of the Exchequer, should reconsider the functions of the Welsh Office.[53] This was of course not a radical concession to devolutionary feeling. Wilson may well have been more concerned with pacifying the Secretary of State for Wales than in achieving an outcome different from that advocated by Helsby. The Prime Minister must have known that he was placing this assignment in the hands of a senior minister and Welsh MP known for his rooted opposition to devolution. Also, the input from officials was likely to emanate from precisely those individuals responsible for the adverse verdict of the Helsby Report.

In the event, Callaghan failed to undertake this commission, with the result that the same assignment passed to Patrick Gordon Walker. The latter had, in January 1967, just returned to the Cabinet as Minister without Portfolio, among other things charged with overseeing a review of the social services, ineffectively begun by Douglas Houghton.[54] Gordon Walker therefore had direct links with health and education, two of the main candidates for devolution in Wales. Before the completion of his report on Welsh devolution Gordon

Walker was promoted to the Department of Education and Science, thereby losing any right to be regarded as a disinterested party.

In May 1967 Gordon Walker met Hughes and his officials in Cardiff. Hughes offered a compromise involving the phased transfer of education and health, while deferring action over agriculture. Hughes's main priority was the transfer of the Board of Health to the Welsh Office, which he proposed should take place in April 1968.[55]

Hughes thought that his case would be assisted by a further impressive by-election performance of Plaid Cymru in March 1967, this time in the Labour heartland of Rhondda West. However, Gordon Walker was not swayed by what he saw as an ephemeral setback. As in the case of the Helsby review, Gordon Walker took the majority of his evidence from the opponents of devolution, led by Helsby himself. Kenneth Robinson, the Minister of Health, and Sir Arnold France, his Permanent Secretary, saw no merit in further devolution. France warned that strengthening the Welsh Office in the manner intended by Hughes would lead to demands in Wales for parity of treatment with Scotland on funding. He argued against treating Wales as a natural unit; devolution would stand in the way of developing closer links between north Wales and Liverpool. Robinson believed that it was necessary to treat all regional claims on their merits and to resist all 'undue concession to nationalistic arguments'. He therefore not only opposed health devolution in Wales, but he also believed that the firmly established Scottish system of devolution represented a step in the wrong direction. Robinson warned that 'nationalism fed on itself and, now that parliamentary pressure for Welsh independent administration seemed to have eased, we should be cautious about reviving it and inviting a new round'.[56] Gordon Walker's interview with members of the Welsh Board of Health confirmed Robinson's assertion that the Board was satisfied with existing arrangements, but it evinced no strong opposition to change. On the other hand, Councillor W. R. Jeffcott, Chairman of the Board of Governors of the United Cardiff Hospitals, was vehemently opposed to further devolution.[57] Callaghan recommended Jeffcott and Sir Archie Lush of the Welsh Hospital Board as reliable witnesses, no doubt because he hoped that they were both opponents of devolution.[58]

Gordon Walker also discovered that James Callaghan was an uncompromising opponent of devolution.[59] At this date Callaghan opposed all concessions on the grounds that any advance would be used by the nationalists as a lever for further demands. He also saw no electoral advantage in making concessions and even opposed Hughes's proposals for a nominated Council for Wales, suspecting that the Welsh Secretary wanted to establish a Welsh parliament.[60] Consistent with this attitude, Callaghan signified his agreement with the draft report and indeed he encouraged Gordon Walker to cite this support in communications with the Prime Minister.[61] Callaghan was then caught up in the turmoil of the devaluation crisis, as a consequence of which he resigned his office as Chancellor. This no doubt accounted for his decision not to comment in detail on the draft report, but it is less clear why he also elected not to comment on the Gordon Walker Report upon his transfer to the Home Office.[62] As indicated below, in his new capacity Callaghan experienced a distinct change of heart over devolution.

Ministerial exchanges over the Gordon Walker report continued through the autumn of 1967. Much of the debate was concerned with the staffing implications of devolution. On broader issues, the surviving documentation shows little support for Hughes. Among the ministers, Robinson was especially uncompromising.[63]

Gordon Walker submitted his final report on the functions of the Welsh Office to the Prime Minister on 18 December 1967.[64] If anything, the Gordon Walker Report was even more negative than the Helsby Report. Gordon Walker believed that there was no objective evidence that the proposed extension of the functions of the Welsh Office would contribute to efficiency or improved services. Neither was he convinced that there was widespread political or public demand for such a change. As far as he was concerned, Hughes's proposals were a misguided concession to extreme nationalism. He acknowledged that the least objectionable proposal was transfer of the Welsh Board of Health to the Welsh Office. This raised no technical problems and involved only an insignificant increase in staff. He was nevertheless opposed to such a change since it was likely to stimulate demand for further concession, including establishment of a Welsh parliament. In particular, it would stir up memories of policy commitments in *Signposts to the New Wales* and place the government on the defensive concerning the transfer of agriculture and education.[65]

Naturally, Hughes was dismayed by the Gordon Walker report, which was inconsistent with the declared policy of the Labour Party and with the thinking that motivated establishment of the Welsh Office. If it was unacceptable to transfer health to the Welsh Office, it had been no more defensible to adopt its existing functions. The success of the

Welsh Office within its existing remit suggested that health could be transferred without risk. Gordon Walker's report therefore implied that the policy implemented in 1964 was a mistake. Hughes was adamant that the draft report represented a political miscalculation. By rejecting Hughes's moderate proposals, Labour was spurning the opportunity to bring administration closer to the people and develop policies in keeping with their aspirations. Hughes warned that only the devolutionist path would enable Labour to retain political leadership in Wales and its appeal among the younger generation.[66]

Hughes complained to the Prime Minister about the wider implications of the Gordon Walker report, which he took as a vote of no confidence in himself and the Welsh Office. By asking the government to honour its election commitments, Hughes and his department had exposed themselves to a trial that Hughes believed had been conducted in a biased and incompetent manner. He warned that the Gordon Walker report would play into the hands of the Welsh Nationalists, with politically disastrous consequences for Labour. Instead of this negative approach, he called for constructive policies acceptable to the Welsh people. Hughes offered to make further compromises on the grounds that Welsh pubic opinion might be palliated by the immediate transfer of one important function to the Welsh Office. Health was self-evidently the most suitable candidate; even Gordon Walker conceded that no harm would be incurred by this measure. Hughes again proposed 1 April 1968 as the date for this extension in the functions of the Welsh Office.[67]

Gordon Walker remained intransigent. He accused Hughes of taking his remarks out of context, insisting that harmlessness related only to the numbers of staff involved.[68] The robustness of Gordon Walker's antagonism to devolution derived from his own political disposition, but also no doubt it reflected backing from his colleagues ranging from Callaghan to Robinson. Naturally, any further steps towards devolution were opposed by ministers connected with departments faced with diminution of their powers and by Treasury ministers on grounds of efficiency. Griffiths and Hughes were committed to devolution, but Willie Ross, their counterpart in Scotland, was notorious for his antipathy to nationalism. As one analyst puts it: 'Ross prevailed on his Scottish henchmen and Wilson not to budge an inch in opposing nationalism.'[69] It is therefore evident that, notwithstanding its explicit devolutionist policy commitments,

Wilson's ministerial team was only marginally more favourable to devolution than Attlee's notoriously centrist Cabinet.

The Wilson Administration and its Devolution Committee 1968–1969

On the basis of the decisive judgements of Helsby and Gordon Walker, Harold Wilson decided that the issue of Welsh devolution was resolved. It was minuted that the Prime Minister 'inclined to accept Mr Gordon Walker's report but he has asked whether the Chancellor would wish to make any comments, particularly from the staffing point of view'.[70] Once again his political instincts suggested that such an uncompromising rejection of stated government policy required the backing of more formal ministerial deliberations than had yet taken place.

This further review was urged by Richard Crossman. As already noted, in 1964 Crossman was sceptical about Welsh home rule, but his attitude rapidly shifted. He confronted the devolution issue in his capacity as Minister of Housing and Local Government. Afterwards, as Lord President of the Council, he assumed formal responsibility for questions relating to the constitution. The continuing by-election successes of the Welsh and Scottish nationalists convinced him that 'devolution is now in the air'. On grounds of both political expediency and principle he called for Labour to adopt a more conciliatory attitude; he even told Wilson that he was unwilling to speak in the House of Commons against a parliament for Wales. Even before the officially sanctioned review of devolution policy, in his capacity as Lord President, Crossman kept in touch with the work of Cledwyn Hughes; he also encouraged a group of younger MPs to study devolution. The leading lights among his protégés became junior Ministers in relevant departments and soon found their way into the Devolution Committee.[71]

Even before Gordon Walker had finalized his report, in November 1967 Crossman made the case for devolution to be re-examined as a matter of urgency.[72] This fuller review of policy was easily justified, not only because of the growing threat from the nationalists, but also on account of the need to brief the Home Affairs Committee and the Cabinet in advance of the reports of the two Royal Commissions on Local Government in England and Scotland, which were expected imminently. Also a recent White Paper on local government in Wales was relevant since it had made recommendations in favour of a nominated and advisory Welsh Council.[73] Wilson was swayed by Crossman's argument; indeed he immediately began thinking about parliaments for Edinburgh and Cardiff. Wilson's advisers remarked on Crossman's 'unconventional approach', but they sanctioned his proposal for a committee comprising hand-picked junior ministers chaired by Crossman himself.[74] On 16 February 1968 the Prime Minister invited Crossman to chair this Ministerial Committee on Devolution for Scotland and Wales.[75]

The Devolution Committee went over the ground covered by the Helsby and Gordon Walker Reports, but with a remit for both Scotland and Wales. The Prime Minister asked the Committee to pronounce on the 'practicality and political desirability' of further devolution. Crossman's Devolution Committee conducted its work within the space of a few months and it has never attracted much comment. Understandably Kenneth Morgan concludes that 'it yielded nothing'.[76] As indicated below, the exercise was scarcely the dramatic success that Crossman intended, but it marked the beginning of a more constructive approach to devolution and produced a workable plan for immediate extension of the functions of the Welsh Office. However, these goals were reached by the most tortuous route.

Crossman's Committee granted Cledwyn Hughes a third platform in two years to make the case for expanding the powers of the Welsh Office. Welsh devolution was the subject of the first substantive paper discussed by the Committee.[77] Faced with this perhaps unexpected opportunity and broader platform, Hughes expanded his thinking to consider the merits of a separate parliament for Wales and an elected Council for Wales, as well as the well-worn arguments for extending the powers of the Secretary of State. The elected Council for Wales favoured by Hughes would have exercised executive functions, the most ambitious of which was taking over the Welsh Hospital Board. The Devolution Committee was sympathetic to neither a Welsh parliament nor an elected Council for Wales. However it agreed to consider devolution of further powers to both the Scottish and Welsh Offices. Hughes now urged the transfer of health on 1 April 1969, together with an agreement to take over agriculture and education at a later date.[78]

On 6 April 1968 Cledwyn Hughes was transferred to Agriculture; George Thomas succeeded him at the Welsh Office. Crossman

DEVOLUTION AND THE HEALTH SERVICE IN WALES 259

commented grumpily on this change, which he regarded as the 'sacking' of a devolutionist and his replacement by 'an avowed UK man'. Hughes remained on the Devolution Committee, but departmental policy forced him to temporize his support for devolution. Crossman lamented that other ministerial changes made at this date, especially the appointment of Fred Peart as Lord Privy Seal, strengthened the anti-devolutionist camp on his Committee.[79]
Crossman's pessimism proved to be well founded. He looked on with alarm as the Committee realigned itself to concur with the Helsby and Gordon Walker Reports. Although during his active political career George Thomas was never more than a reluctant supporter of devolution, as Welsh Secretary he robustly defended the line established by Hughes. He repeated the case for a strengthened Council for Wales and for the expansion in powers of the Welsh Office. As a compromise, he offered to reduce the executive capacities specified for the Council for Wales to such modest items as the Wales Tourist Board and the Welsh Arts Council rather than major functions like the Welsh Hospital Board. He repeated his predecessor's bid to transfer the Welsh Board of Health to the Welsh Office, still maintaining 1 April 1969 as the target date, with Agriculture to follow on 1 April 1970. It was evident at this stage that education was no longer regarded as a serious candidate for transfer in the immediate future. The committee remained sceptical about strengthening the Council for Wales. More worrying to Crossman, they imported the arguments of Helsby and Gordon Walker against any major strengthening of the Welsh Office. Indeed, the Gordon Walker Report was unearthed and adopted as the basis for discussion during the final stages of the Committee's deliberations. In retaliation, George Thomas circulated Cledwyn Hughes's rebuttal of the Gordon Walker Report.[80] Indicative of the recidivist tide overtaking the Devolution Committee, it decided that further strengthening of the Welsh Office should be limited to 'those functions which had the most symbolic importance, but which could produce the least additional administrative cost or inefficiency'. At this stage it seemed likely that the Committee would recommend against the transfer of any significant departmental function.[81]
Final papers circulated to the Devolution Committee indicated a widening gulf between the combatants. The anti-devolutionists were evidently in command. The draft report completely rejected home rule parliaments and it expressed scepticism about an elected Council for Wales. It recommended only minor strengthening of the Welsh Office.

With respect to health, it was concluded that 'there was an even balance between the political advantages and administrative disadvantages'. On agriculture, the Committee supported the compromise proposed by Hughes.[82] Education was not even mentioned. The main concessions contained in the report related to ancient monuments and tourism, both of which were recommended for transfer to the Welsh Office, with the blessing of the central departments concerned. The draft report insisted that the current sense of alienation in Scotland and Wales was a reflection of economic problems, which were being addressed by means other than devolution. Concerning the 'vague demand for a greater Scottish and Welsh say in their own affairs', the draft report concluded that Scottish and Welsh opinion could be won over by a 'vigorous and sustained campaign of public education'. The Committee was confident that its modest concessions represented a sufficient response to any reasonable aspiration to self-government.[83]

In his dissenting memorandum Thomas warned that if the committee 'think these proposals will favourably impress Welsh opinion they are mistaken'. Indeed he predicted that adverse reaction to the package would drive Labour supporters into the ranks of the nationalists. He reiterated the case for strengthening the Welsh Council and for transferring agriculture, education, health and children's services to the Welsh Office.[84] At the final meeting of the Committee Thomas was supported by Peter Shore, who argued that the Committee had underestimated the strength of the nationalist threat. He unsuccessfully urged that their report should express openness to all alternatives, including home rule. The meeting agreed to only minor amendments of the draft report. With respect to the transfer of health to the Welsh Office, it was agreed to set out the arguments of the Secretary of State for Wales in favour of this proposition, followed by the arguments of the majority of the committee against this change.[85]

Crossman shared Thomas's dismay concerning the draft report of the Devolution Committee. His blame extended to Peter Shore, who had throughout allowed Edmund Dell, 'a fanatical unionist', to attend as his substitute. Crossman labelled the draft report a 'pretty hopeless document'. 'All the little devices' contained in the report might have been appropriate two years earlier, but he agreed with Shore that it lacked realism in current circumstances. A much-publicized speech made by Edward Heath, leader of the opposition, on 18 May 1968, known at the time as the 'Declaration of Perth' calling for a more positive approach to devolution in Scotland, made the draft report seem all the more inadequate.[86] The Lord President was also alarmed by the continuing electoral successes of the nationalists, which he believed threatened Labour with the loss of half its seats in Scotland in the next general election. The Devolution Committee seemed oblivious to the reality of this threat. Crossman decided in effect to circumvent his Committee and commission further work on the report, although he doubted whether it could be improved sufficiently to appease nationalist feeling.[87] Crossman's audacious intervention rendered the report distinctly more friendly to devolution. Members of the Devolution Committee were given a few days to make representations, but any complaints were of no avail. The report was not amended again before its submission to the Parliamentary Committee.

The final report contained a paragraph outlining the majority sceptical stance on the Council for Wales, but it added a paragraph stating the contrary views of the Secretary of State for Wales. The section dealing with the powers of the Welsh Office was significantly redrafted. In its final form, this section began by reminding readers of the policy statements to which Labour was committed. This reintroduced the possibility of full transfer of agriculture, education and health to the Welsh Office. As already noted, education was not even mentioned in the draft report. The final report also entirely changed its line on health. The draft report concluded that there was 'an even balance between the political advantages and administrative disadvantages' of this transfer. The final report baldly stated that the Committee was in favour of the transfer of health, although the Minister of Health remained opposed. With respect to agriculture, the compromise proposed by Hughes was adopted, while it was agreed to defer consideration of education until after the next general election. The final report left untouched all the other minor recommendations contained in the previous draft.[88] It is evident that without the eleventh-hour revision of the decision on health – an action only possible by virtue of Crossman's direct ministerial superiority over Robinson – this package of 'little' devices would indeed have been portrayed as a humiliation by devolutionists.[89] Crossman himself was still alert to the limitations of the final paper, which he variously described as 'cold, calculated', 'the lowest common denominator of consensus', or 'minor suggestions about bashing the nationalists and fiddling with Grand Committee meetings'.[90]

The Devolution Committee represented an important stage in the political battle over devolution in Wales, but its report was by no means the end of the story. The judgement of Crossman concerning the need for a more positive approach to devolution was soon and strikingly confirmed by the result of the Caerphilly by-election in July 1968, where the massive Labour majority was cut to under 2,000. Crossman described this result as a 'disaster'.[91]

The Caerphilly by-election came too late to affect the first deliberations of the Parliamentary Committee, which discussed devolution on 24 June. The Parliamentary Committee, chaired by the Prime Minister, was the high court of senior ministers, among other things concerned with constitutional issues. Introducing his report Crossman made no secret of the committee's opposition to concessions to nationalist feeling. He nevertheless insisted that a majority ought to support the package of devolutionary measures recommended in the report. He urged that modest concessions together with a sustained campaign of public education were the minimum requirement for protecting the government's credibility. Once again Crossman and his allies faced hostile criticism. It was argued that nothing was needed other than the government's current economic policies and more determined efforts to 'hammer home' the case against devolution. Given disarray among his ministers, Wilson agreed to work with Crossman and the territorial Secretaries of State to prepare yet a further variant of the Devolution Committee report.[92]

This small committee of ministers chaired by the Prime Minister considered this problem over the summer of 1968. Ironically, their first meeting was held on 18 July, the day of the Caerphilly by-election. For the short term, these ministers backed the recommendations of Crossman's report and they sanctioned further papers on detailed implementation. A brief consideration of longer-term policy raised for the first time the possibility of establishing a Royal Commission on the Constitution.[93] Especially in the light of Thomas's repeated predictions that the Caerphilly seat would be lost to Labour, Crossman urged that the government's response was inadequate.[94] Thomas similarly informed his colleagues that he did not believe that 'the package of proposals now in mind will be of net political benefit to us in Wales'.[95]

Active discussion of what Crossman was now calling 'the eternal problem of devolution' resumed in the autumn of 1968, now with a degree of urgency in view of the need for an announcement of government policy at the beginning of the new session of Parliament.[96] These hurried discussions were resolved at two further meetings of the ad hoc Committee and two meetings of the Cabinet. These exchanges confirmed that Wilson's ministers were no nearer to achieving consensus. However, owing to last-minute horse-trading the lines of division changed to yield an unexpected result. Crossman and his allies were completely outmanoeuvred. Crossman argued for substantial strengthening of the Devolution Committee package, with the aim of publishing in the spring of 1969 a coherent and comprehensive policy on devolution. In the meantime he recommended suspending action on piecemeal measures, the main item of which was of course the devolving of health administration to Wales. This retreat by Crossman on immediate measures of devolution was an acute disappointment to George Thomas and it had the perverse result of throwing Thomas into the arms of the anti-devolutionists, Callaghan and Ross. Crossman had particularly little liking for Ross, whom he attacked repeatedly, among other things for treating 'nationalism as a mere emotional attitude, which can be cured by economic policies alone'.[97] Callaghan built up an alliance of disparate elements around an ingenious compromise. He now favoured conceding immediate implementation of the reform package contained in Crossman's report, together with the establishment of a longer-term review of constitutional aspects of devolution. Devolution would be just one aspect of the work of a 'Commission on the Constitution appointed by the Queen', a variant of a Royal Commission that would be given a virtually unlimited remit on matters relating to the UK constitution. For Thomas, Callaghan's scheme had the merit of guaranteeing the immediate transfer to the Welsh Office of the Board of Health along with many other smaller and less contentious accretions. For anti-devolutionists such as Ross, Callaghan's proposal had the attraction of virtually no changes in Scotland in the short term, and a good prospect that the Constitution Committee would be a route to the graveyard for the more ambitious devolutionist programme. Crossman and his allies sniped at the Callaghan solution, which they regarded as disingenuous, but their position was weakened by the new alliance between Callaghan and the Secretaries of State for Scotland and Wales, who could argue that they were implementing the package of reforms advocated in Crossman's own report.[98]

On account of the last-minute character of the above compromises, the government's announcement of a high-profile devolution initiative contained in the Queen's Speech on 30 October 1968 came as a surprise to the media. Consequently, for the moment, devolution rather than the economic crisis captured the headlines. Media comment was largely oblivious to the underlying turmoil and discord among Wilson's ministers over this issue. Most attention was attracted by the proposal for a constitutional commission, but the media also highlighted the specific measures relating to Wales. *The Times* described the latter as an 'immediate concession to Welsh nationalism'.[99] It was hardly noticed that these reforms were much less than had been promised in 1964. While the health transfer represented belated implementation of the 1964 election pledge, it was noticeable that no prospect was offered of honouring the similar pledge on education.[100]

On 1 April 1969 the Secretary of State for Wales assumed full executive responsibility for health and welfare services in Wales. The new arrangements brought an end to the fifty-year existence of the Board of Health. This was recast as the Health Division of the Welsh Office. In the eyes of the Welsh people this outcome saved the Secretary of State for Wales and the Welsh Office from humiliation. The transfer of health was of definitive importance. The Secretary of State for Wales could now legitimately claim that his department merited a rank among the major departments of Whitehall. This claim would have entirely lacked credibility without the inclusion of services relating to health in the orbit of the Welsh Office. The transfer of health was therefore a major victory for the devolutionists and an important stepping stone towards home rule. However the tangled route by which this success was achieved constituted an omen, suggesting that the attainment of meaningful independence of action on policy and administration in health and the social services was likely to require further protracted struggles. Subsequent events have amply borne out this prognosis from history.

Notes

* The author would like to express his thanks for the advice given on this subject and comments on the draft of this paper particularly from Lord Gwilym Prys-Davies, also from my other friends and colleagues, the late Professor Sir Rees Davies, the late Lord Cledwyn Hughes and Professor Kenneth Morgan (Lord Morgan of Aberdyfi).

[1] H. J. Hanham, 'The development of the Scottish Office', in J. N. Wolfe (ed.), *Government and Nationalism in Scotland* (Edinburgh, 1969), pp. 51–70; Sir

David Milne, *The Scottish Office and other Scottish Government Departments* (London, 1957); L. Paterson, *The Autonomy of Modern Scotland* (Edinburgh, 1994).
2. J. Jenkinson, *Scotland's Health 1919–1948* (Oxford, 2002), pp. 99–111.
3. C. Webster, *The Health Services since the War, Volume One: Problems of Health Care: The National Health Service before 1957* (London, 1988), pp. 17–79; Jenkinson, *Scotland's Health 1919–1948*, pp. 393–448.
4. *Royal Commission on the Civil Service, Fourth Report* (London, 1914), Cd. 7338, ch. 9, and paras. 68, 69, 72; *Report of the Machinery of Government Committee* (London, 1918), Cd. 9230, para. 31. In his review of the impact of the Haldane Commission, Street erroneously states that the three Insurance Commissions were wound up and replaced by Departments in 1919, Sir A. Street, 'Quasi-government Bodies since 1918', in Gilbert F. M. Campion (ed.), *British Government since 1918* (London, 1950), p. 159. The anomalous character of the Welsh Board of Health was recognized in the Geddes Report in 1922, which recommended that the Board should be abolished.
5. L. Bryder, 'The King Edward VII Welsh National Memorial Association and its policy towards tuberculosis, 1910–48', *Welsh History Review*, Vol. 13, no. 2 (1986), 196–216. For tuberculosis in Wales, also see the chapters by Steven Thompson and H. Glynne Roberts in this volume.
6. *Report of the Machinery of Government Committee*, paras 34–7; S. Stacey, 'The Ministry of Health 1919–1929' (unpublished D.Phil. thesis, Oxford University, 1984), 87–9; R. V. Vernon and N. Mansergh (eds), *Advisory Bodies: A Study of Their Uses in Relation to Central Government 1919–1939* (London, 1940).
7. J. Graves, 'The use of advisory bodies by the Board of Education', in Vernon and Mansergh, *Advisory Bodies*, pp. 176–226; R. N. Spann, 'The use of advisory bodies by the Ministry of Health', in Vernon and Mansergh, *Advisory Bodies*, pp. 227–81.
8. Ministry of Health, *Interim Report of the Consultative Council. The Future Provision of Medical and Allied Services* (London, 1920), Cmd. 693.
9. Jenkinson, *Scotland's Health 1919–1948*, pp. 79–81.
10. *Medical and Allied Services in Wales. Welsh Consultative Council. First Report* (London, 1920), Cmd. 703; *Second Report* (London, 1921), Cmd. 1448.
11. C. B. Fawcett, *Provinces of England: A Study of Some Geographical Aspects of Devolution* (London, 1919).
12. W. A. Robson, *The Development of Local Government* (London, 1931).
13. *Welsh Consultative Council, Second Report*, para. 80.
14. Jenkinson, *Scotland's Health 1919–1948*, p. 84.
15. Spann, 'The use of advisory bodies by the Ministry of Health', p. 231.
16. Ramiah Dorawwanmy Aiyar, *Blueprint of a Welsh Hospital Service* (Cardiff, 1945), p. 32. This included forewords by Clement Davies MP, and H. J. K. Bamfield of the Indian Medical Service.
17. D. J. Davies and N. Davies, *Can Wales Afford Self-Government?* (Cardiff, 1939); R. E. Jones, *Wales after the War* (Cardiff, 1939 – an English-language version of a collection of articles by Saunders Lewis, formerly published in Welsh as *Cymru wedi'r Rhyfel*).

18 Sir Reginald Coupland, *Welsh and Scottish Nationalism: A Study* (London, 1954), pp. 336–80; J. Graham Jones, 'Early campaigns to secure a Secretary of State for Wales, 1890–1939', *Transactions of the Honourable Society of Cymmrodorion* (1988), 153–76; K. O. Morgan, *Rebirth of a Nation: Wales 1880–1980* (Oxford, 1980), pp. 203–5.
19 Clement Davies chaired the important *Report of Inquiry into the Anti-Tuberculosis Service in Wales and Monmouthshire* (London, 1939). Lord Prys-Davies informs me that the Clement Davies Report made a lasting impression on Jim Griffiths.
20 Lord Prys-Davies draws my attention to the Editorial Notes, inspired by the Davies Report, perhaps contributed by Professor W. J. Gruffydd, later MP for the University of Wales, in *Y Llenor*, Vol. 18 (1939), 1–3. The tuberculosis report was highly praised and described as a 'terrible indictment' and 'formidable indictment' by *The Economist* and *The Times* respectively (*The Economist*, 18 March 1939, p. 556, *The Times*, 14 March 1939, Editorial, p. 15). The tuberculosis report was debated in the House of Commons on 22 March 1939, opening with a powerful speech by James Griffiths. A further discussion titled 'Wales and health' and chaired by Clement Davies was convened by the Honourable Society of Cymmrodorion on 31 March 1939. This was broadcast on the BBC and featured in the Society's *Transactions*. All of these interventions highlighted the incompetence of local government in the handling of health in Wales.
21 *House of Commons Debates*, Vol. 345, col. 1340, 22 March 1939.
22 J. Graham Jones, 'Socialism, devolution and a Secretary of State for Wales, 1940–1964', *Transactions of the Honourable Society of Cymmrodorion* (1989), 135–60.
23 Public Record Office (PRO), CAB 117/254.
24 Aiyar, *Blueprint of a Welsh Hospital Service*.
25 Ministry of Health, 'Some notes on regionalism', April 1941, PRO, CAB 117/214.
26 J. Mohan, 'Neglected roots of regionalism? The commissioners for the special areas and grants to hospitals in England', *Social History of Medicine*, Vol. 10 (1997), 243–62. For praise by Maude and colleagues for the Special Area Commissioner's work in south Wales, see Oral Evidence of Meeting on the Machinery of Local Government, 16 April 1941, PRO, CAB 117/219.
27 Maude to Sir George Chrystal, 21 May 1941, PRO, CAB 117/214.
28 Thomas Jones memorandum, 6 May 1944, PRO, CAB 87/42. For background on Jones, E. L. Ellis, *T.J.: A life of Dr Thomas Jones, CH* (Cardiff, 1992), especially pp. 137–50.
29 MGO 64, 22 January 1945, PRO, CAB 87/75. For fuller consideration of the post-war period, J. G. Evans, 'British governments and devolution in Wales: attitudes and policies, 1944–1979' (unpublished MA thesis, University of Wales, 1987); Morgan, *Rebirth of a Nation*, pp. 377–94.
30 *House of Commons Debates*, Vol. 403, cols 3211–14, 17 October 1944.
31 Ibid., Vol. 403, cols 3214–18, 17 October 1944.
32 PRO, CAB 87/75; CAB 134/504.

33 D. R. Grenfell MP and W. H. Mainwaring MP to Clement Attlee, 14 August 1946, PRO, CAB 134/504.
34 Jones, 'Socialism, devolution and a Secretary of State for Wales', 143–5.
35 PRO, MH 77/93–4.
36 Sir A. Webb-Johnson to Sir Wilson Jameson, 2 December 1946, PRO, MH 90/4.
37 University of Liverpool, 'Memorandum on the Areas of Regional Hospital Boards', 15 November 1946, PRO, MH 90/2.
38 'NHS in Wales', PRO, MH 77/104. Crawshay served during the war as Deputy Regional Commissioner and afterwards as Controller for Wales, Aircraft Production.
39 K. O. Morgan, *Labour in Power 1945–1951* (Oxford, 1984), pp. 309–12; Jones, 'Socialism, devolution and a Secretary of State for Wales', 145–6.
40 Morgan, *Rebirth of a Nation*, p. 378. For a fuller account of the work of the Council, Evans, 'British Government and devolution', 92–9.
41 J. Graham Jones, 'The Parliament for Wales Campaign, 1950–56', *Welsh History Review*, Vol. 17 (1955), 411–51.
42 *The Council for Wales and Monmouthshire. Third Memorandum* (London, 1957), Cmd. 53.
43 Ibid., paras. 50–61, 217–23.
44 Letter from Prime Minister to Chairman of the Council for Wales, 11 December 1957, published as *Administration in Wales* (London, 1957), Cmd. 334.
45 James Griffiths, *Pages from Memory* (London, 1969), p. 166; Jones, 'Socialism, devolution and a Secretary of State for Wales', 156–7; Morgan, *Rebirth of a Nation*, pp. 377–8.
46 J. P. Mackintosh, *The Devolution of Power: Local Democracy, Regionalism and Nationalism* (Harmondsworth, 1968).
47 Harold Wilson, speech in Montgomery, 14 July 1965, *Western Mail*, 15 July 1965.
48 Richard Crossman, *The Diaries of a Cabinet Minister, Volume One: Minister of Housing 1964–65* (London, 1975), p. 117.
49 Morgan, *Rebirth of a Nation*, pp. 390–1.
50 Griffiths to Wilson, 5 April 1966; Hughes to Wilson, 19 April 1966; memorandum by Daniel, 12 May 1966, Cabinet Office, CAB 2MS 25/56/01C.
51 For supporting correspondence and Helsby, 'Responsibilities of the Welsh Office', 1 July 1966, Cabinet Office, CAB 2MS 25/56/01C. Lord Prys-Davies points out that Sir Archie Lush was in other contexts favourable to devolution.
52 Richard Crossman, *The Diaries of a Cabinet Minister, Volume Two: Lord President of the Council and Leader of the House of Commons 1966–68* (London, 1976), pp. 610–11, 19 December 1967; idem, *The Diaries of a Cabinet Minister, Volume Three: Secretary of State for Social Services 1968–70* (London, 1977), p. 69, 19 May 1968.
53 10 Downing Street minute, 18 October 1966, PRO, CAB 35/10 Part I.
54 Wilson to Gordon Walker, 28 February 1967, PRO, CAB 35/10 Part I.
55 Meeting of Cledwyn Hughes, Gordon Walker and officials, 4 May 1967, PRO, CAB 35/10 Part I.

56 Meeting of Robinson, Gordon Walker and France, c.10 June 1967, PRO, CAB 35/10 Part I.
57 Meeting of Gordon Walker with Welsh Board of Health and Councillor W. R. Jeffcott, 19–20 June 1967, PRO, CAB 35/10 Part I.
58 Meeting of Callaghan and Gordon Walker, 12 June 1967, Cabinet Office, CAB 2MS 25/56/01E.
59 K. O. Morgan, *Callaghan: A Life* (Oxford, 1997), p. 361.
60 Meeting of Callaghan and Gordon Walker, 12 June 1967, Cabinet Office, CAB 2MS 25/56/01E.
61 Brief for Callaghan and draft letter, c.10 October 1967, Cabinet Office, CAB 2MS 25/56/01E.
62 Gordon Walker to Wilson, 18 December 1967, PRO, CAB 35/10 Part I.
63 Robinson to Wilson, 7 November 1967, PRO, CAB 35/10 Part I.
64 Gordon Walker to Wilson, 18 December 1967, PRO, CAB 35/10 Part I.
65 Gordon Walker, 'Functions of the Welsh Office', 18 December 1967, PRO, CAB 35/10 Part I.
66 Hughes to Gordon Walker, 11 August 1967, PRO, CAB 35/10 Part I.
67 Hughes to Wilson, 11 October 1967, PRO, CAB 35/10 Part I.
68 Gordon Walker to Wilson, 8 January 1968, PRO, CAB 35/10 Part I.
69 J. G. Kellas, *The Scottish Political System* (Cambidge, 2nd edn., 1975), p. 41.
70 Minute by Prime Minister, 4 January 1968, Cabinet Office, 2MS 25/56/01G.
71 Crossman, *Diaries, Volume Two*, pp. 610–11, 19 December 1967; *Diaries, Volume Three*, p. 69, 19 May 1968.
72 Crossman to Wilson, 13 November 1967, PRO, CAB 164/658.
73 Welsh Office, *White Paper on Local Government in Wales* (Cardiff, 1967), Cmnd. 3840.
74 Burke-Trend to Prime Minister, 17 January 1968, PRO, CAB 164/658.
75 Minute by Prime Minister, 16 February 1968, Cabinet Office, 2MS 25/56/01G.
76 Morgan, *Rebirth of a Nation*, p. 391.
77 Cledwyn Hughes, 'Further constitutional changes in Wales', 22 February 1968, DS(68)2, PRO, CAB 134/2697.
78 DS(68) 5th mtg, 3 April 1968, PRO, CAB 134/2697.
79 Crossman, *Diaries, Volume Three*, p. 69, 19 May 1968.
80 Secretariat, 'Functions of the Welsh Office', 26 April 1968, DS(68)14; George Thomas, 'The strengthening of the Welsh Office', 2 May 1968, DS(68)15, PRO, CAB 134/2697.
81 DS(68) 7th mtg, 24 April 1968, PRO, CAB 134/2697.
82 Robinson, 'Strengthening of the Welsh Office', 8 May 1968, DS(68)16; Hughes, 'Strengthening of the Welsh Office', 8 May 1968, DS(68)17, PRO, CAB 134/2697. Crossman, 'Revised draft conclusions of the Ministerial Committee on devolution for Scotland and Wales', 20 May 1968, DS(68)20, PRO, CAB 134/2697.
83 DS(68)20, para. 17.
84 Thomas, 'How adequate are the proposals in DS(68)20?', 23 May 1968, DS(68)22, PRO, CAB 134/2697. Thomas made similar representations direct to the Prime Minister, Thomas to Wilson, 28 June 1968, PRO, CAB 164/658,

DEVOLUTION AND THE HEALTH SERVICE IN WALES 269

expressing the hope that Wilson would use his speech in Newtown on 6 July to advocate the devolution policy.

[85] DS(68) 10th mtg, 27 May 1968, PRO, CAB 134/2697.
[86] Mackintosh, *The Devolution of Power*, p. 169.
[87] Crossman, *Diaries, Volume Three*, pp. 82–3, 27 May 1968.
[88] Crossman, 'Draft Conclusions ... Second Revise', 30 May 1968, DS(68)23, PRO, CAB 134/2697.
[89] From the date that Crossman became Chairman of the Social Services Committee in April 1968 he challenged Robinson on many issues of health policy. Then, in November 1968 Crossman took over Robinson's department completely and Robinson was removed.
[90] Crossman, *Diaries, Volume Three*, p. 106, 24 June 1968.
[91] Ibid., p. 145, 18–19 July 1968.
[92] P(68)8, Crossman 'Conclusions of the Ministerial Committee on Devolution for Scotland and Wales', 18 June 1968, P(68) 8th mtg, 24 June 1968, PRO, CAB 134/3031.
[93] MISC 215(68) 1st mtg, 18 July 1968, PRO, CAB 130/390.
[94] Crossman, *Diaries, Volume Three*, pp. 144–5, 18 July 1968.
[95] Thomas to Peart, 9 August 1968, PRO, CAB 164/658.
[96] Crossman, *Diaries Volume Three*, p. 235, 23 October 1968.
[97] Ibid., p. 106, 24 June 1968.
[98] MISC 215(68) 2nd and 3rd mtgs, 23 and 28 October 1968, CAB 130/390; Cabinet Conclusions CC(68) 43rd and 44th mtgs, 24 and 29 October 1968, CAB 128/43. For Crossman's caustic commentary, *Diaries, Volume Three*, pp. 234–5, 23–4 October 1968. Harold Wilson's *The Labour Government 1964–1970* (London, 1971) is silent on these controversies, except for mentioning that the idea of a constitutional commission emanated from Callaghan (p. 725).
[99] *The Times*, 31 October 1968, editorial, p. 11.
[100] *House of Commons Debates*, Vol. 772, col. 38, 30 October 1968.

11

Change the Welsh Way: Health and the NHS, 1984–1994

JOHN WYN OWEN

'Change the Welsh Way' deals with the ten-year period 1984–94 during which I held post as first Director (CEO) of the NHS in Wales.[1] At the turn of the twenty-first century there was much discussion about the role and function of the director of the NHS in England and, following the resignation of Sir Alan Langlands in February 2000, health ministers came under pressure to review the wide-ranging responsibilities of the post. Jimmy Burnes, writing in the *Financial Times*, claimed that 'people in the NHS describe Sir Alan's job as impossible. The chief executive is required to act both as key policy adviser to ministers and as leader of the NHS. However, as a civil servant, he is not allowed his own agenda.'[2] It is the scale of the English NHS Chief Executive's task that is impossible but the same is not true of the situation in Wales which is an ideal size, not least because it is possible to get key opinion-leaders into one room to secure ownership of principles and strategies, and create partnerships to enable innovation to take place right across the board, even in health and health care.

Highlights

Nicholas Edwards in his autobiography *Wales, Westminster and Water* devotes only two pages to the health service in Wales.[3] I believe that this is an inadequate reflection of the foundation which he laid for some very important and pioneering work in health and in health care, and which was subsequently built on by his successors as Secretary of State for Wales. Some of the highlights – there are too many to include them all – range from the pioneering initiatives in mental handicap, through to rapid progress in the acute sector, including the building of five district general hospitals simultaneously, as well as the beginnings of an innovative programme of community hospital developments. Major developments in the field of health promotion included the Heartbeat Wales scheme, the first regional health promotion project to be adopted in the UK, the launch of Breast Test Wales and of an innovative perinatal initiative, and the establishment of World Health Organization (WHO) collaborating centres in health promotion and regional health strategy. The first 'strategic intent and direction', incorporating both health services and public health, was adopted. The adoption of a comprehensive research and development strategy for Wales was fundamental to the overall strategy. Other initiatives of this period included a pioneer private finance initiative, which successfully established new satellite dialysis units at Bangor and Carmarthen, and brought provision in Wales up to the standard of the best in Europe, and a new emphasis on collaboration with industry and the private sector in general. This collaborative approach facilitated the establishment of the Medicentre in Cardiff and the incubator plant for medical innovations adjacent to Ysbyty Maelor in Wrexham. A new management style placed emphasis on securing benchmarking standards and it set targets to be used as analytic tools for management. The period was also marked by a new awareness of the need to introduce modern information systems and utilize the latest technology to assist the smooth running of the health services. Innovations in this field included the medical records project, the information for health strategy and the implementation of advanced hospital and community health information systems at Ysbyty Glan Clwyd. This period also witnessed the first regional x400 data network,[4] which formed the basis of subsequent developments. Interestingly, Rachel Lomax has said that the officials who computerized and developed the information system for Crickhowell House[5] had learned their skills in NHS Wales Information Technology. New technology was employed to develop community information systems and child health information systems and to facilitate telemedicine and health informatics. Technological innovation was also revolutionizing surgical techniques and new treatment centres were established for hernias, varicose veins, hips and knees. Together with all of these changes, the new-style NHS in Wales sought to involve doctors and nurses in management. A well-trained and motivated workforce was seen to be at the heart of progress and the People Strategy (for supporting personnel), the launch of Project 2000, for modernizing nurse training, and the establishment of an NHS Wales Staff College were key developments in this field.

However, it wasn't all good news. There were problems of overspending and difficult issues regarding the financing of health services in Gwynedd and in Mid Glamorgan. There was also slow progress in implementing the original Hine Report for cancer services in north Wales. Furthermore, there were underlying tensions between policy and management in the Welsh Office; notably, cultural differences between the Civil Service and the NHS and disagreement on how best to develop mental illness provision, whether as a social-care issue or a health matter. But overall this was a period of development, which saw the establishment of an outlook on health services that was simultaneously being adopted in other countries, notably New Zealand and Australia. It was a time too when a number of new principles became enshrined in international policy. The concept of 'health gain' became the currency of the World Bank at this time, and Welsh activities informed the development of the WHO Ljubljana Charter, which formally enshrined the rights of the patient.

The Office of the NHS Director

So what led to the post of Director NHS Wales being established, forty years after the foundation of the NHS? The answer is the Griffiths Inquiry of 1983. Uniquely, the NHS Management Inquiry led by Sir Roy Griffiths was presented in the form of a letter and was not intended to be a major addition to the already considerable library of NHS literature. What Sir Roy found at the time is best summed up by the two following well-known quotes.

> If Florence Nightingale were carrying her lamp through the corridors of the NHS today, she would almost certainly be searching for the people in charge.

> To the outsider it appears that when any change of any kind is required, the NHS is so structured as to resemble a mobile, designed to move with any breath of air but which in fact never changes its position and gives no clear indication of the direction.

His principal recommendation was the introduction of general management at all levels. He proposed that responsibility for planning, implementation and control of performance should be drawn together in one person and that there should be clear accountability. He advocated that strategic intent and direction should be formulated at the national level, that it should manifest concern with the determination of purpose, objectives and direction for the health service, gain approval of the overall budget and make decisions regarding resource allocation, monitor strategic decisions and receive regular reports on performance and other evaluations from within the health service. He recommended that leadership should be provided by chief executives at all levels of the NHS and that clinicians be involved in the management process; that a fully developed management budget should be a primary requisite; that managing the workforce should become a major priority; and that community views should be canvassed and the experience and perceptions of patients taken fully into account. These recommendations are still relevant today and can be regarded as a template of success in health services. 'Change the Welsh Way 1984–1994' reflects significant progress against each of these headings.

The Griffiths recommendations were accepted in full. I was appointed the first Director of NHS Wales and reflected the spirit of the time. I came from the private sector, from a health services company established by the previous Labour administration and privatized in Margaret Thatcher's time. I had previously worked in the NHS – in Carmarthen, Cardiff and at St Thomas's in London – and I had a strong background in planning, education and research, seeing these as the basis for effective management. I saw the priorities for my task, in line with the Griffiths report, as developing strategic direction; a method of accounting for health and health services; an emphasis on quality; resource management; the engagement of clinicians in the management process; sound administration of the estate function, supplies and information technology; a high priority for the management of the people employed in the health service; partnership with organizations related to health services; and development of working arrangements to engage the community in our efforts.

Uniquely the responsibilities in the post of Director incorporated being the Accounting Office for the health service vote (i.e., budget allocation), a member of the Senior Management Group in the Welsh Office and Chairman of the All-Wales Health Common Services Authority. I was accountable as Director of NHS Wales directly to the

Secretary of State for the NHS and to the Permanent Secretary for the management of Welsh Office resources. I was a member of the Health Policy Board for Wales and Chairman of its Executive Committee. Whereas the line responsibilities of the Chief Medical Officer and the Chief Nursing Officer remained to the Secretary of State as his principal advisers, they were coordinated for health service purposes through the Executive Committee. It would be fair to say that there were tensions in respect of all of these responsibilities, particularly between the NHS Director's twin roles as an executive officer and as a principal policy adviser, which had always been the traditional role of the senior civil service. During my time as Director of NHS Wales I served four Secretaries of State, each with their different characteristics (three were avowed European). I worked with three Permanent Secretaries, all of whom had their different styles, with the Minister of State, Lord Wyn Roberts as he became, and with six junior Ministers. These managerial arrangements, particularly the Health Policy Board, sound similar to those mentioned under the headline in *The Times* on Tuesday, 22 February 2000: 'Doctors and nurses drafted in to manage the NHS ... in an attempt to sideline Whitehall bureaucrats and to speed up improvements.'

One very important point to make about the office of the Secretary of State for Wales and the junior Ministers was the wide-ranging portfolios that they carried. The Secretary of State for Wales dealt with health, education, transport, housing, agriculture the environment – everything in fact apart from foreign affairs, defence and some Home Office functions – all the policy areas now devolved to the National Assembly for Wales with its sixty members, subject committees, regional committees, assembly secretaries and a First Secretary. Ministers could not concern themselves with the detailed running of all of these areas; they were also members of the Cabinet or Cabinet committees as well as constituency MPs (three out of four Secretaries of State for Wales had constituencies in England). The important point is that in Wales we had in one office – the office of the Secretary of State with its locations in London and in Cardiff – the capacity to work across departments which would have been impossible in Whitehall and allowed innovation to take place through resource reallocation. The mental handicap strategy is an example of shifting from health to social care.

Griffiths Reforms and Working with Patients

One strong feature of the ten years of my directorship of the Welsh NHS was the continuity between the Griffiths recommendations and the 1990 health reforms. In 1990 the UK government embarked upon a reform of the UK health system to raise standards everywhere to those of the best and to increase choices for patients. The NHS was, however, to continue as a service funded out of taxation and mainly free at the point of use. Purchaser and provider responsibilities were separated; an internal market was created for health care; money was to follow the patient and the patient's voice was to have a greater prominence.

What we were able to do in Wales was to implement the change within a strategic framework of aiming to raise the level of health of the people of Wales to amongst the best in Europe by the turn of the century, by focusing on health gain (adding years to life and life to years), valuing people as individuals and providing a resource-effective health service informed by a focused research and development framework. County health authorities working with general practitioner fundholders were reorganized as small management organizations buying health care on contract from hospital and community trusts and general medical and dental practitioners. Separating planning and provision for better health and health care were the unique features of the Welsh approach.

Though the change that tended to catch the eye was the purchaser-provider split, I would argue that one of the most important long-term initiatives introduced in the UK health system at the turn of the decade was the development of truly ambitious health strategies aligned to a very large extent with the 'Health for All' campaign. In England this drive was taken forward under the Health of the Nation banner. In Wales, and rather earlier than in England, we developed a health strategy of our own – our Strategic Intent and Direction. In fact it was David Hunt's conviction of the benefits of the Strategic Intent and Direction which provided a purpose for the Thatcher reforms and also led the Cabinet to press ahead with the Health of the Nation in England. Both Scotland and Northern Ireland also developed their own health strategies. Though they differ in detail and scope, the various strategies had at their heart an emphasis on tackling the major public-health challenges of the time, including cardiovascular disease and cancer, as well as a heavy emphasis on health promotion and prevention. They highlighted the need for intersectoral action and the development of healthy alliances. It was widely recognized that health services alone cannot deliver health gain; there was a need to bind in other key players in both the private and public sectors, whether in the worlds of education, industry, transport, the environment or housing. In addition to the focus on health gain, the Secretary of State, reflecting the Prime Minister's interest, determined that the NHS must play its full part in pursuing the aims of the Government's Citizens' Charter initiative. The aim was to clarify citizens' rights and citizens' responsibilities for their own health. The objective was to ensure that citizens were placed centre-stage in health planning and the delivery of services. We won a disproportionate number of charter marks in the first round!

Partnership was also a key commitment – with industry, the private sector and the voluntary sector. Wales was the first in the field with a private sector renal dialysis unit – one of the first examples of Private Finance Initiative/Public Private Partnership (PFI/PPP) – and with a clinical service. Key NHS players had been actively involved in projects such as commercial exploitation by the NHS, represented by the Medicentre at the University Hospital in Wales; NHS Wales was also a founder member of the business-oriented Welsh Health Technology Forum. Then there was partnership with local government. One of the biggest successes had been the development during the 1980s of a path-breaking strategy for people with learning disabilities. We also sought partnership with higher education, seeing this as one of the main agents for change and economic prosperity. This partnership was strengthened with the devolution of responsibility for university funding to the Welsh Office and unique to Wales, I think, was the College of Medicine's place on the board of every district health authority. Hence partnership was a long-standing feature of the Welsh approach to business in the area of health, with very close relationships being developed with all key players.

Strategic Management

One of our strongest claims to success during 1984–94 was our pioneering approach in strategic management and ensuring that each tier added value. In 1988 the health service in Wales developed the first corporate management programme of its kind in the United

Kingdom. This introduced the idea – a novel one at the time – that improving health may be one of the goals of a health care system. It also initiated a quality assurance programme, again a first in UK terms. But perhaps the corporate management programme's main claim to fame is found in a footnote to one of its tables which suggested that there would be merit in establishing a health oriented think-tank to advise on strategic planning. In 1989 I established the Welsh Health Planning Forum – a multidisciplinary group drawing on clinical, managerial and consumer expertise both from within and from outside the NHS.

The corporate management programme foreshadowed a number of the 1990 NHS reforms – my point earlier about the continuum between general management and the internal market – but it did need to be brought up to date in light of promoting 'better health' and 'working with patients'. We therefore produced an 'Agenda for Action 1' and an 'Agenda for Action 2' and then extended the breadth of the management strategy to *Caring for the Future*, a consultation paper which was published at Christmas 1992 and *Caring for the Future* which was published definitively in March 1993.

Strategic Intent and Direction

As Director of NHS Wales I placed considerable importance on adopting a strategic management approach to business with a fairly straightforward approach about ensuring a systems and integrated approach to planning, resource allocation, resource management, information, systems for quality, personnel, supplies and the estate. To me it means being clear about who does what, by when and then evaluating performance. I believed that there were four key success factors to this approach in the NHS: first, defining clearly the purpose of the service and what we are there for – the vision. However, having a vision is one thing but it must be owned by as many stakeholders as possible. So sharing the vision and securing the ownership for it are the second and third essentials. Developing a strategy tied to the Health for All principles was the relatively easy part. The hard part – the part requiring real work – was the fourth key to success – to translate that policy into integrated, effective system management and clinical action, and for progress to be monitored.

Best in Europe – Strategic Intent

Our strategic intent – our vision for the NHS – was working in partnership with others, to take the people of Wales into the twenty-first century with a level of health on course to compare with the best in Europe. The intention was to be in the upper quartile of performance in WHO Europe by about 2010.

This was an ambitious programme, much more ambitious than it would appear at first sight. Wales, in common with other parts of the United Kingdom, was making reasonable progress over the 1980s and our ranking in the health league table was higher in all cases than in 1981. However our performance in heart disease and cancer in particular did not put us into the Europe super-league in terms of health and it would require determined effort over years to see progress. But we did see the value of using targets and establishing European benchmarks. The European dimension really was important to us and we were the only part of the United Kingdom to have established such a strategic link. Subsequently, benchmarking was extended in Australia and New Zealand following the Welsh experience.

Strategic Directions

Our strategic direction was health gain, adding years to life and quality life to years; to make our services genuinely people-centred, reflecting the Patients' Charter and sound stewardship of resources (intellectual, estate, money); to make the NHS more resource-effective, making sure that we got the right balance between prevention, promotion, diagnosis, assessment, treatment, care and rehabilitation; between primary and secondary care; and between programmes whether for heart disease, cancer, mental health or learning disabilities, or any other area.

The Welsh Health Planning Forum (having looked at the health needs of the people of Wales and the opportunities for improvement) proposed ten priority areas ranging from cancer and cardiovascular disease through to the neglected sectors of physical disability and distress and learning disability, and broad-ranging areas such as emotional health and health environments. There was a requirement for better targeting of NHS efforts to address issues such as equity, access and effectiveness and for a recognition that the health service needs to assemble a coalition of interest to achieve health gain. The major effort was in ten priority areas, and this was worked up in guidance protocols – investments for health gain – on how the various threads could be pulled together. However we also worked on two client groups, the elderly and children – our attempt to build an effective bridge to the world of social care.

Strategic Cascade

I may have given the impression that we adopted a very top-down approach to business in Wales but nothing could be further from the truth. Though the Welsh Office had a key role in offering strategic leadership and direction, we really saw that action had to take place locally and close to the point of delivery. To reinforce this message from the very beginning of the NHS reforms, we expected our health care commissioners, health authorities and family health services, acting together, to develop local strategies for health covering the period to the year 2002. The long-term local strategies set local goals and the major milestones for service action. They were not to be technical documents but three-year rolling health plans which proposed specific management action to achieve the milestones set in the local strategies. The process of developing and then approving these commissioner plans provided the strategic framework within which NHS Trusts developed their own strategic and business plans. So a very strong feature of the Welsh approach was a strategic approach to both commissioners and providers. This played a major part in managing the internal market as well as encouraging the creation of good working relationships between all the players at local level.

Organizing for Change

Developing the vision was one thing, putting it into effect was the really hard part and, as always, there were tensions. The change process I initiated was based on principles of a learning organization and NHS Wales put a great deal of effort into clarifying the roles and functions of each of the key players and sought to explore the concept of the learning organization and the place of an NHS Staff College.

Organization Development Review and the Role of the NHS Directorate

With Coopers and Lybrand we worked up Organization Development frameworks for the NHS Directorate, health authorities as joint commissioners, GP fundholders, Community Health Councils and NHS Trusts. The frameworks were developed in collaboration with managers, professionals and staff across NHS Wales. We developed organization health-checks to tease out aspects related to culture, systems, processes and structure. As part of the Organization Development Review we identified four interlocking roles for the NHS Directorate:

- first, strategic leadership: setting direction and using strategic management to work towards the achievement of the agreed vision, drawing on planning skills and the ability to influence events through mechanisms such as resource allocation.
- secondly, line management of joint commissioners largely through the endorsement of long- and short-term plans and the individual performance review criteria agreed for top managers.
- thirdly, monitoring of the NHS Trusts and the maintenance of a sound but not intrusive accountability regime for these providers.
- fourthly, the regulation of the market at two levels. At one level was the entire health care system: the outcome of the combined efforts of purchasers' and providers' needs and testing these against the criteria which were developed by Robert Maxwell – equity, access, appropriateness. At the other was a clearer set of rules of engagement between commissioners and providers involving others, including the Audit Commission, in seeing that these were adhered to.

A very important distinguishing feature of the Welsh approach was the development of a Memorandum of Understanding between the Welsh Office and each NHS Trust. The accountability agreement confirmed the Trust's commitment to a number of All-Wales initiatives, including the strategic intent and direction. It also identified the broad criteria for intervention by the NHS Directorate.

A Learning Organization

As I said, one of the hallmarks of implementing change in Wales was the adoption of the concepts of a learning organization. This was an attempt to handle the difficult conceptual issues of pursuing a strong, coherent, national policy and strategy while at the same time promoting further devolution of responsibility, facing the reality of a diffusion of managerial authority and managing the increasing pace of change. Rather than resort to the usual bureaucratic response to change, NHS Wales aimed to embrace a culture of continuous transformation. This recognized the need to engage more fully than in the past the people involved in the management and delivery of services in setting and achieving goals. This demanded a different way of doing business and a different set of relationships. It was against this background that we established the NHS Wales Staff College to play a leading role in the future development of the service. Initially the College was to concentrate on leadership development, supporting existing leaders and identifying and working with the next generation of both professional and management leaders, playing an important role in high-level Organization Development and acting as an agent in bridging some of the management divides between health and the related public and voluntary services. The College was expected to act as a hub for key learning networks and to provide a capacity for problem solving and consultancy activities. One thing about the College was that it was not to be a centralist body. Its success was to come from establishing a track record with its clients in the service and securing their enduring ownership. It is very pleasing to see that the NHS Wales Staff College has continued and expanded its efforts and it should be of interest that it has been followed as an exemplar in Australia and New Zealand and now in Norway.

Health and Social Care 2010

Some of the other work of the Planning Forum is worth a brief mention. The 2010 Project, which identified frameworks for service looking ahead to the year 2010, was piloted in four areas and in two phases. The first phase involved developing a view of what services might be in 2010 and the second phase the setting of a range of benchmark measures for the year 2002, against which the Forum's ideas could be tested for realism. The 2010 Framework assumed that a number of factors – changes in the attitude and circumstances of the population, technical developments and the evolution of policy and funding arrangements – would challenge existing relationships within the health sector and between health and social care. We had anticipated that general care teams would meet most of the basic health and social care needs including health promotion, initial diagnosis, most forms of treatment, antenatal and postnatal care and social support for the elderly, infirm or the disabled. It postulated that the distinctions between health services and social services would become blurred. This work informed the Heathrow Scenarios for Nursing and the UKCC (United Kingdom Central Council) 2010 Commission.

Bringing it all Together

In the face of such a complex agenda I believed that it was essential for us to spell out our priorities and identify key accountabilities, building on our corporate planning experience, as well as resource management – information technology, organization development, involvement of doctors and nurses. At Christmas 1992 we published our first comprehensive management strategy for health, covering the period to the turn of the century. This was a plan for turning strategy into practical action – caring for the future. *Caring for the Future* was not an old-fashioned blueprint, a sterile example of top-down planning, but an effort to present and develop a shared and dynamic agenda for change in Wales. It was produced after exhaustive consultation with hundreds of managers and clinicians throughout Wales. Notwithstanding that, we gave the plan a pathfinder status. In addition to confirming a range of targets of a Health of the Nation type, *Caring for the Future* included what we judged to be the top ten management priorities for the period to the mid-1990s. They included local strategies for health, health promotion, integration of District Health Authorities and Family Health Service Authorities, the development of locality planning, empowering staff, the development of a research and development framework and promoting efficiency, developing more refined methods for resource allocation and developing a system of accountability for NHS Trusts. A distinguishing feature of NHS Wales was the development of a 'Memorandum of Understanding' between each NHS Trust about communications and the development of systems audit. Here we were grateful to the Nuffield Provincial Hospitals Trust for support with our work on the 2010 vision and some of the developments on community hospitals.

In 1995 the National Audit Office undertook a major review of our strategic intent and direction concluding that 'the Strategic Intent and Direction was a pioneering response to the World Health Organisation's strategy *Health for All by 2000*'.[6] The National Audit Office found that health authorities, through the process of developing their local strategies for health, identified those changes to NHS services and the activities of other agencies which are necessary to make progress in improving the health of the population.

Wales in Europe

'Wales in Europe' was very much the slogan of the time, as we were faced in the early 1980s with the demise of the coal and steel industries and had urgently to find ways of improving the Welsh economy. The Welsh Office was indeed successful with its programme of inward investment. We also considered that the health of the people was an important asset in economic development and that ideas and innovation in health services had good prospects for exploitation and contributing to the economy of Wales. We undertook a number of projects involving commercial exploitation by NHS Wales, such as the development of the Medicentre at the University Hospital Wales, the incubation unit at Ysbyty Maelor, Wrexham, the estates services and the Welsh Health Common Services Authority (WHCSA) and Welsh Health Development International at WHCSA.

Our relationships both ways with the WHO were very significant. These were initiated as part of Heartbeat Wales which introduced the concept of target setting, measuring progress and comparing performance. Wales became host to WHO Collaborating Centres, in health promotion and in regional strategies, and eventually they became founder members of the 'European Regions for Health Network'. The Welsh model – Strategic Intent and Direction – was also of health policy interest to a number of countries as Europe was transformed following the demise of the Soviet Union. Wales as a case study, with input from the Welsh Health Planning Forum, was used to inform the deliberations of WHO, the EU, the World Bank, the European Investment Bank, and eventually led to the Copenhagen

Declaration and also the Ljubljana Charter. Morton Warner[7] and I attended an initial meeting in Madrid in 1993 and the Welsh Office Strategic Intent and Direction was used to inform the planning of the next stages of policy work in WHO Europe. Based on Welsh experience there was a general recognition that most successful health systems are those which have learned to get their strategy right. The Ljubljana Charter reflects aspects of Wales's Strategic Intent and Direction in advocating that health care systems should be:

- Driven by values of human dignity, equity, solidarity and professional ethics.
- Targeted at protecting and promoting health.
- Centred on people, allowing citizens to influence health services and take responsibility for their own health.
- Focused on quality, including cost effectiveness.
- Based on sustainable finance to allow universal coverage and equitable access.
- Oriented towards primary care.

Impact in Wales and Beyond

So, what was achieved during that period of 'Change the Welsh Way'? Clinical services did improve, as evidenced by the introduction of breast cancer screening, improvement in perinatal mortality, better access to dialysis and team-care valleys. The Strategic Intent and Direction pioneered health planning in the UK and beyond. It helped the Cabinet agree to England's Health of the Nation and gave a purpose for the Thatcher reforms. The currency of health gain became internationally accepted by the World Bank and by the World Health Organization. The Strategic Intent and Direction informed health policy beyond the United Kingdom – Australia, New Zealand, Sweden, Spain. The National Audit Office endorsed the pioneering work of the Welsh Health Planning Forum. At the 1998 St David's Forum, Steven Monaghan[8] indicated that we had indeed closed the gap in the European health league tables. The Welsh approach contributed to informing the deliberations of the WHO Ljubljana Charter. Our concepts of partnership and local health planning have become the norm for the present administration in Wales. The Strategic Intent and Direction has been given new life as part of the new, modern NHS. We placed people at the centre of our developments in line with the Citizens' Charter and this too is very much a reflection of the way things are going today. Our investment protocols for health gain were a new way of linking research, service planning, clinical effectiveness and clinical and management practice and shaped subsequent developments in England and beyond. Project 2000 was launched and laid the basis for the reform of nurse training in Wales, moving it into the higher education sector and preparing nurses for new roles within a changing NHS. The Staff College initiative has yet to be copied by our nearest neighbours but has been replicated in Australia, New Zealand and Norway. Resource management, information technology, the data network, telemedicine, our quality strategies and our estates supplies function were at the forefront of health services management.

Conclusion

Above all, NHS Wales introduced a new concept of corporate strategy. The corporate management programme placed the Welsh Health Service in a unique position by placing all the tiers of the service within a single planning and management framework, including clinicians. The corporate dimension to the programme described the strategic management objectives which had to be integrated at an all-Wales level in order to sustain work that health authorities locally had to undertake themselves. Its inherent strength was that it placed clear responsibility on specific agencies for achieving particular objectives within clearly identified timescales.

'Change the Welsh Way' could be used as a template for what success looks like in any health service. The bottom line for health policy is avoiding premature death, improving the quality of life (years to life and life to years), health gain, people-centred services giving individuals and communities information to make informed choices and, also, sound stewardship of resources. The Strategic Intent together with its extension in the form of the Ljubljana Charter was the product of implementing the Griffiths Inquiry in Wales. Uniquely we integrated better operational management of the NHS, drawing on the Griffiths principles of clear strategic direction, measurable results, effective leadership, clinicians in management, concern for the people who work in the health service and a quality health service that engages the community. These are the tests of success and are still today's challenges.

Notes

1. I would like to acknowledge the help of many people and in particular the substantial support which the Nuffield Trust provided for 'the Welsh way'.
2. *Financial Times*, 22 February 2000.
3. N. Edwards, *Wales, Westminster and Water* (Cardiff, 1998).
4. The 'x400 data network' was a telecommunication network for data telephone and video dedicated to NHS Wales and was at the forefront of information and communication technology and what is now referred to in England as the communication spine and at the heart of the £6 billion health IT strategy.
5. Crickhowell House was the headquarters of the Welsh Health Common Services Authority and brought all the main advisory services for the NHS in Wales under one roof. This centralization of function resulted from an option appraisal, which showed that it made economic sense to do so. It had longer term significance, for it was located in Cardiff Bay and instigated the Cardiff Bay Scheme because roads, power, sewerage etc. had to be put in place. The building currently houses the Welsh Assembly.
6. *Improving Health in Wales*, National Audit Office, HC633 Session 1995–96 (7 August 1996).
7. Morton Warner was Director of the Welsh Health Planning Forum and is now Professor at the University of Glamorgan and Director of the Welsh Institute for Health and Social Care.
8. Steve Monaghan was the author of a report with Jane Davidson and David Bainton on health and health policies in Wales prepared for the Nuffield Trust. S. Monaghan, J. Davidson and D. Bainton, *Freeing the Dragon: New Opportunities to Improve the Health of the Welsh People* (London, 1999).

12

History is What You Live: Understanding Health Inequalities in Wales

GARETH WILLIAMS

Graig level killed a few men, besides silicotics, arthritics, ripped flesh, smashed bones and damaged souls ... Black historied all right, the Graig level, where we slaved in dust and water, where I worked with or in the same headings as Sid Hullen (dust, dead), Jimmy Shanklyn (rheumatic fever, dead), Walt James (dust, dead), Cliff Williams (TB, dead), my father (dust, arthritis, dead) ... Just a small level, the Graig, where lads were punished by grinding toil, and before that weakened by the diet of beggars ... These men were unsung in any chronicle of existence.[1]

Introduction

Ron Berry's vivid autobiographical description of life in 'the greatest coal-producing valley in the world',[2] the Rhondda Fawr, in the first half of the twentieth century has the capacity to shock. History is what you live, and it leaves its mark on how you die. In the original text the names and causes of death continue, movingly, for a whole page: a roll of dead friends and heroes. It conveys a rough-and-ready familiarity with the relationships between life and work, death and loss, which those of us working in secure professional occupations only a couple of generations later can scarcely begin to understand. This is not just a list of deaths and their causes; it is a litany inviting a response.

In writing from his own experience Berry wants us to feel and taste the way in which work affected the men who did it, physically and mentally. While expressing himself autobiographically he endorses an important epidemiological point: 'The social is, literally, embodied; and the body records the past, whether as an ex-officer's duelling scars or an ex-miner's emphysema';[3] social injustices become embodied in the individual as disease.[4] Accidents and diseases injured, impaired and killed coal miners, and did so in the context of relentlessly hard manual labour, poverty and deprivation. The wider context is important. The intensification of coal production was sustained only at the expense of human health and safety.[5] Moreover, the expansionary requirements of capitalism sucked in women's labour as much as that of men.[6] The effects on women's lives and health, where the 'unremitting toil of childbirth and domestic labour killed and debilitated Rhondda women as much as accidents and conditions in the mining industry killed and maimed Rhondda men,[7] were even more devastating.

I have begun with a glance towards an autobiographical account of the life and health of colliers and their families in south Wales in the early twentieth century for three reasons. First, it provides a striking example of the general theme of this chapter: that rates of ill health and death in the population are shaped by the varying social and economic conditions under which people live. Secondly, it is within autobiography that events are turned into meaningful episodes, providing integrative, knowledgeable narratives about social life.[8] Thirdly, an historical sociology of health inequalities is fundamental to a more comprehensive analysis of contemporary health inequalities; and the health status of the population of south Wales today cannot be understood without understanding the history of the region.[9] Berry's words suggest a model of the determinants of health that is, in the language of modern epidemiology, multi-factorial: ill health is partly to do with the dangers of specific aspects of work, in this case of being a coal miner, but it is also an expression of more pervasive features of social structure in a particular time and place. The words make the point powerfully: the relentless, *grinding* nature of the daily *toil*, for men and women, and the *beggarly* quality of the food they ate.

In dealing with the complex science of health inequalities we cannot evade politics and economics, and their refraction through human experience in particular times and places. As Blane argued in an analytical commentary on the celebrated report of Douglas Black's working group on inequalities in health (the Black Report):[10]

> Scattered throughout the literature are the reports of studies that have examined the effects upon health of single factors such as hazardous work, inadequate diet and poor housing. Although it is possible to consider these

factors in isolation, it is important to bear in mind that they can be traced back to the social structure via intermediate level phenomena such as the distribution of income and wealth and the organization of industry.[11] Understanding inequalities in health involves examining the multiple effects on health over time of workplaces, the organization of employment, the housing in which people live, the quality of their relationships, the social organization of neighbourhoods, the availability of shops and services, the impact of policies, and the way in which all of these are framed by wider developments in economy, society and culture. It also means that these multiple effects themselves can be conceptualized in quite different ways with different consequences for political decisions about what is to be done.[12]

In this chapter I want to do three things. First, I want briefly to review the evidence and the debate on inequalities in health. Although this general issue is well understood I want to spend some time thinking about the ways in which the 'problematic' of health inequalities has changed since the publication of Sir Douglas Black's report. I will then go on to say something about health in Wales more specifically, drawing our attention to the intense concentrations of ill health in particular localities within Wales. Finally, I will return to the more general issue of interpretation, and how we need build upon but also move beyond epidemiology to construct an historical sociology of health inequalities. In the conclusion I will touch briefly on the policy and practical responses to health inequalities.

Health inequalities

The systematic nature of the relationship between social class or social deprivation and health has been observed since the middle of the nineteenth century;[13] and the public health movement emerging in the UK between 1830 and 1860 was 'an early instantiation of ideas of equality in relation to health'.[14] Although data on rates of mortality among different groups and in different areas had been available for some time, it was during this period, following the establishment of the Registrar General's Office for England and Wales in 1836, that these data came to be systematically recorded, collated, analysed, published and, dedicated followers of Foucault might say, invented.[15] In a society characterized by rapid industrialization and urban inmigration, and dominated by infectious diseases in childhood and early adulthood, the effects of infant mortality on population life expectancy were of particular concern.[16] Moreover, it was clearly evident from early data that social class (as measured by occupation of the head of household) and area of residence had some ill-understood combined effect on mortality. In 1843 the *Lancet* published data indicating the existence of a mortality gradient between the social classes of 'gentry and professional', 'farmers and tradesmen', and 'labourers and artisans' and, for any one of these, considerable differences between those living in Bath, Bethnal Green, and Manchester. While the average age of death for labourers and artisans in Bath was 25 years, for example, in Manchester it was 17 years.[17]

The overall socio-demographic picture in Britain and elsewhere throughout the twentieth century, as McKeown brilliantly argued, is of improving economic and social conditions leading to increasing life expectancy and population growth, with public health interventions and medical care playing a distinctly supporting role.[18] With improvements in infant and child health, death rates have been halved and life expectancy has risen. In the twenty-first century it is chronic, degenerative conditions such as heart disease, cancer and stroke that dominate the mortality statistics; and these, along with diabetes, musculoskeletal disorders, chronic respiratory diseases and mental health problems, are also responsible for high rates of long-term illness and disability in some population groups. In spite of overall improvements in health, the unequal distribution of ill health is a continuing and growing feature.

One of the crucial arguments to be developed since the Black Report is that inequalities in health in the UK should not be understood as simply being about 'how the poor die' (to echo George Orwell).[19] While inequalities in health can be seen in terms of the disadvantages of simply being poor, they can also be seen in relation to the 'health gap' between rich and poor, or the 'health gradient' that tracks socio-economic position across the population.[20] The concept of the gradient means that there is an increased risk of premature mortality on each step down the class ladder, and this is the case for women as for men.[21] If you take coronary heart disease, the single biggest cause of death in the UK, death rates among men are approximately 40 per cent higher among manual workers than among non-manual workers; and the death rate for wives of manual workers is about twice the rate for wives of non-manual workers.[22]

In economically developed societies the importance of the class gradient, and relative differences between groups, as opposed to absolute poverty or wealth, has been illustrated very powerfully by the work of Marmot and his colleagues on British civil servants working in Whitehall, who were followed up twenty-five years after data collection first began.[23] These workers are all relatively affluent people living in one of the wealthier parts of the UK, and are white-collar, nonindustrial employees with long-term job contracts. In spite of this relative wealth and security, when you compare mortality rates between men (and they were all men) working in different grades it is clear that position within the hierarchy has a strong correlation with mortality risk, not just between top and bottom but across all employment grades.[24] Such findings indicate the complex connections between social structure and health outcomes.

Another body of work that has challenged social scientists to reflect upon what it is about inequality in society that produces inequalities in health are analyses looking cross-nationally at the effect of income, wealth and the distribution of income and wealth on mortality rates.[25] The evidence suggests that, beyond a certain level of economic development, the health of the people in a society has less to do with how absolutely rich or poor those societies are, measured by gross domestic product, and more to do with the equality of the distribution of income, wealth and resources within societies. This, it is argued, can explain the higher life expectancy in Greece, for example, compared with a richer country such as the USA; and why the class gradient of mortality in Sweden is both less marked and consistent than in England and Wales; and why social classes with the worst mortality in Sweden have lower death rates than the best (social class I) in England and Wales.[26]

Within the UK, inequalities in health by social position, whether measured in terms of income and wealth or occupation, or indeed length of education or the quality of housing, are reiterated in regional mortality and morbidity.[27] Maps of regional mortality in the UK show that the spatial patterning of health is repeated at area level,[28] with high mortality in the post-industrial regions of central Scotland (notably Glasgow), Northern Ireland, north-west and north-east England, inner London and the Valleys of south Wales (see figure 12.1).[29] There are huge differences between different kinds of regions and local authority areas, with a ten-year life-expectancy gap being seen between the best (Chiltern, 78.4 years) and the worst (Glasgow City, 68.4 years).[30] And it is not just mortality. There are also clear class gradients in the incidence of disease, long-term illness

Figure 12.1: Standardized mortality ratios (SMRs) in the UK by country and unitary authorities, 1997.

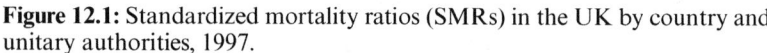

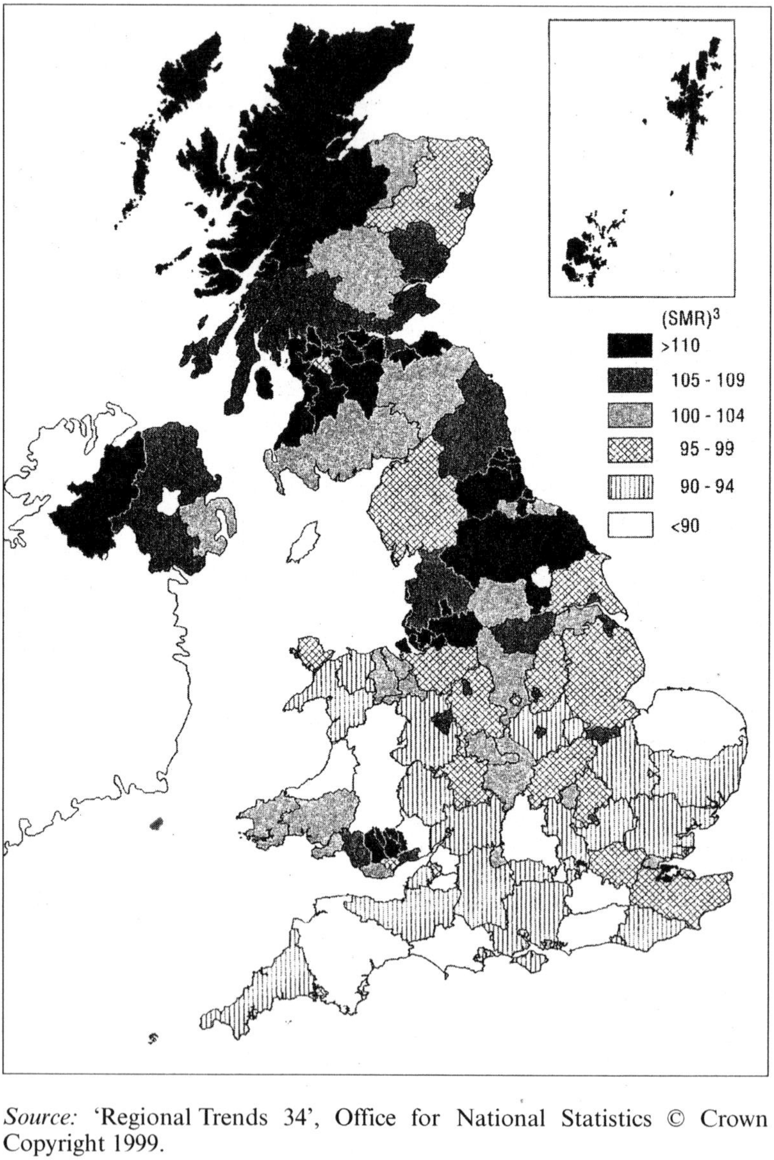

Source: 'Regional Trends 34', Office for National Statistics © Crown Copyright 1999.

and self-rated health.[31] Morbidity from coronary heart disease and most major cancers displays a social class gradient, as do subjective measures of physical and psychosocial health that may be predictive of later mortality. For limiting long-term illness (self-reports of chronic ill health affecting everyday life), prevalence rises from 10 per cent of the population in the prosperous south-east of England, to an average of more than 20 per cent in former coalfields and industrial ports,[32] with parts of north-east England and south Wales recording rates of 30 per cent.[33]

While such differences are a stimulus to both epidemiological and political analysis, part of the sociological interest in all this is that during the last twenty-five years of overall improvements in life expectancy, inequalities in relation to both class and place have widened considerably. In the 1970s death rates were twice as high amongst unskilled manual workers as they were amongst professionals, but by the 1990s they were three times higher.[34] Mortality differences between communities or areas have also polarized since the 1980s. Whereas at the start of the 1980s people aged less than 65 in the poorest areas of Britain were a quarter more likely to die each year than in the population as a whole, by the 1990s this disadvantage had increased to a third.[35] The stark conclusion is that social and spatial inequalities in health are large, and the gaps are now wider than they have ever been since records have been kept.[36]

Health inequalities in Wales

The specific features of health inequalities in Wales have been hidden, perhaps by a continuing tendency to follow the notorious old encyclopedia entry: 'For Wales, see England.' Before looking at health inequalities within Wales it is worth considering how Wales compares with other parts of the United Kingdom.[37] In Wales as elsewhere, mortality has fallen steadily since the 1980s, including mortality from major causes of death such as cancers and circulatory diseases; and men have higher death rates and shorter life expectancy than women.[38] Infant mortality rates fell until the early 1990s but have fluctuated since,[39] with figures for 1999 showing a higher rate in Wales than in Scotland or England. In broad terms, taking age-standardized mortality rates as the measure of overall health in the population, the health of the people of Wales is worse than that in England, but slightly better than Scotland and broadly similar to Northern Ireland. Life expectancy is two or three years shorter than the best in Europe and death rates are relatively high. Figures for 1998 show life expectancy in Wales to be 74.5 years for men and 79.5 years for women, the same as for Northern Ireland.[40]

If you look at age-adjusted mortality rates for a specific major cause of death such as ischaemic heart disease, Wales is worse than England, but better than Scotland and Northern Ireland, and the same is true if you look at death rates from cerebrovascular disease. For other major causes of death however, such as cerebral infarctions, hypertensive disease and hypertensive heart disease, rates in Wales are the highest in the UK;[41] and most strikingly, and intriguingly, as has been indicated, Wales has the highest prevalence of long-term and limiting long-term illness (LLTI) in the UK,[42] with particularly high rates in the former coal and steel areas of south Wales.[43]

In Wales, as elsewhere in the UK, the most striking data emerge from comparisons between localities within the country. These differences are most often defined in relation to local authority boundaries, but it is important to bear in mind there are often 'hidden' differences within such areas that are as great as the visible differences between them. Mortality rates for particular post-industrial communities may be higher than other 'similar' communities a relatively short distance away. In general, however, age-standardized mortality rates overall are higher in the south Wales valley areas of Merthyr Tydfil, Blaenau Gwent, Caerphilly and Rhondda Cynon Taff, and lower in the more rural areas of Ceredigion, Monmouthshire and Powys. Merthyr Tydfil, the unitary authority area with the highest rates, has mortality rates 50 per cent higher than the area with the lowest rates, Ceredigion. Life expectancy is 71.1 years in Merthyr Tydfil and 76.1 years in Ceredigion. While the mortality figures in the worst parts of Wales are not quite as bad as those of the worst Scottish areas, nonetheless the life expectancy figures in the worst local authority areas in Wales in the period 1995–7 had not reached the UK average for 1986.[44] If you look at potential years of life lost, rural areas with high injury rates (often related to agricultural work) such as Denbighshire have high rates of potential years lost, but Merthyr Tydfil remains the worst on this measure too, with rates in Monmouthshire being about 50 per cent lower. This kind of poor health in particular localities is not new, with Merthyr Tydfil and Rhondda, for example, often being cited in historical accounts.[45]

If you take the two major causes of death, circulatory disease and cancer, mortality rates[46] for circulatory disease range from 227 per 100,000 population in Ceredigion through 254 in Cardiff to 332 in Caerphilly and 350 in Merthyr Tydfil. Mortality rates for all cancers range from 168 in Monmouthshire to 201 in Wrexham, 220 in Torfaen and 227 in Merthyr Tydfil. Looking at potential years of life lost for all causes of death to the age of 75 (per 100,000 potential years of life), they range from 135 in Monmouthshire to 197 in Merthyr Tydfil.[47] Taking area-based measures of deprivation and applying them on a ward-by-ward basis, mortality rates in the most deprived quintile of electoral wards in Wales are 25 per cent higher than in the least deprived quintile. Using the European age-standardized mortality rate per 100,000 population,[48] the figures range from 734 in the least deprived quintile, to 926 in the worst.[49]

As I have indicated, Wales has very high rates of limiting long-term illness (LLTI) compared with the rest of the UK, higher even than Scotland, in spite of the higher mortality rates in Scotland, and this is true across all age groups. Prevalence of limiting long-term illness is particularly high in coalfield areas everywhere, higher than in inner London areas and rivalled only by old port and industrial areas.[50] However, the rates of long-term and limiting long-term illness in Wales are higher than you would predict on the basis of mortality rates. The LLTI rates are particularly high in the post-industrial world of the south Wales valleys. At a county/regional level, Mid Glamorgan, West Glamorgan and Gwent have the highest rates of LLTI in Britain. At the level of district authorities, based on 1991 data, seven of the ten highest scoring districts are in south Wales. When the 1991 data are analysed at the level of wards and 'pseudo postcode sectors', fifteen of the top twenty areas are in Wales (fourteen in south Wales and one in Wrexham in north-east Wales), with communities such as Maerdy (Rhondda), Betws (Ogwr), Pen-y-Waun (Cynon Valley) and Gurnos (Merthyr Tydfil) scoring particularly highly. Analysis of the 2001 Census indicates broadly the same league table, with the only challenge to this undesirable Welsh dominance coming from Easington in County Durham, a former coal-mining area in north-east England (see Table 12.1). The lowest rates are in Guildford, Chichester and other towns in southern England.[51]

As can be seen from table 12.1, six of the ten worst areas for LLTI in 2001 are in south Wales, with Merthyr Tydfil, along with Easington, recording 30 per cent or more of the population having some kind of

Table 12.1: Health (2001 Census)

Limiting long-term illness		General health – not good	
Local authority	Percentage	Local authority	Percentage
Easington	30.8	Merthyr Tydfil	18.1
Merthyr Tydfil	30.0	Easington	17.3
Neath–Port Talbot	29.4	Blaenau Gwent	16.5
Blaenau Gwent	28.3	Neath–Port Talbot	16.4
Rhondda Cynon Taf	27.2	Rhondda Cynon Taf	15.7
Caerphilly	26.3	Caerphilly	15.0
Carmarthenshire	26.3	Barnsley	14.1
Bolsover	25.8	Carmarthenshire	13.9
Blackpool	25.4	Torfaen	13.9
Barnsley	25.2	Blackpool	13.9

LLTI. Reports of LLTI are more likely amongst people with heart disease, respiratory illness, mental illness, back pain or arthritis.[52] While rates of LLTI are high across Wales compared with elsewhere in the UK, within Wales there is a difference of more than ten percentage points between the worst and the best local authority areas.[53] These very high rates of LLTI in Wales are repeated for other measures (see Table 12.1), with 15 per cent or more of the populations of Merthyr Tydfil, Blaenau Gwent, Neath–Port Talbot, Rhondda Cynon Taf, Caerphilly and Carmarthenshire reporting their general health as 'not good', and the same areas getting higher scores (worse health) on the SF-36 health status questions.[54] As the table shows, the same six Welsh local authority districts rank in the top ten for self-reports of general health not being good. Furthermore, in view of the fact that those with long-term illness are more than twice as likely to be economically inactive,[55] it is perhaps not surprising that the 2001 Census records the same six local authorities in the top ten areas for those of working age who are unable to work and are claiming benefit for permanent sickness or disability.

Social determinants: explaining health inequalities

Although inequalities in the rates of disease and death have been observed in the population of the UK since the great reform movements of the nineteenth century, the modern debate on health inequalities dates from the 'publication' of what became known as 'the

Black Report', after the chairman of the committee of inquiry, Sir Douglas Black, President of the Royal College of Physicians.[56] What the report showed in one volume for the first time were the huge disparities in the chances of long life and good health for different groups in the population of the UK. Data displaying the social class gradient in such a comprehensive form were powerful enough, though the cross-sectional nature of the data on which it was based opened Black's report to criticism as it attempted to explain the differences observed and suggest policies for action. What was important about the Black Report was that it took the debate beyond singular explanations for differential health risks, such as smoking or employment, and tried to build different categories of explanation, focusing on how the consistent class gradient could be explained. Black and his colleagues identified four possible types of explanation of social inequalities in health: measurement artefact; natural or social selection; materialist-structuralist; and cultural-behavioural. Black's committee, and other commentators, came down firmly in favour of explanations of the materialist-structuralist type. Only these explanations, it was argued, could simultaneously account for the improvements in the general health of the population and the maintenance of class differences in health. The primacy of some kind of materialist-structuralist framework was later reviewed and supported by Whitehead.[57] While the possibility that the size of the class gradient was an artefact of the measurement process itself was a real one at the time Black reported, more recent evidence indicates that socio-economic differences in health and the class gradient are very real indeed.[58] The social selection explanations – that social position is in some way determined by health, rather than vice versa – have been similarly refuted, except as components in an overall analysis of life-course effects.[59]

While there is clear evidence that smoking is a risk factor for early death, neither smoking nor other individual risks such as cholesterol or blood pressure explain the differences in mortality in different employment grades among the Whitehall civil servants.[60] Lifestyles have continued to be the focus for national strategies of health improvement, but they explain a relatively small proportion of the health inequalities between different socio-economic groups.[61] Moreover, in Wales there is only a 1 per cent difference in smoking prevalence between 'unhealthy' Merthyr Tydfil and 'healthy' Ceredigion, though there are more striking differences between the two in the consumption of fresh fruit and green vegetables (CMO).[62] Whatever statistical significance may emerge from analysis of the relationships between these factors, they do little to move forward a more satisfactory and meaningful social scientific understanding of dietary and other consumption behaviours, their relationship to social structures and their impact on health outcomes.

Notwithstanding the prima facie plausibility of cultural and behavioural factors, the key to explaining differences in both behaviour and health outcomes does seem to lie in what are referred to as structural or material factors, primarily those associated with poverty and deprivation arising from socio-economic position. These factors may be understood both as hazards inherent in society which have a direct impact on health, and as the conditions that create unhealthy behaviours, and make behaviour-change in response to public health advice less likely. Material factors include the physical environment in the home, neighbourhood and workplace, and the living standards secured through earnings, benefits and other sources of income.

Perhaps because of the overwhelming evidence that only materialist explanations appear to have the power to explain health inequalities, there have been few advances in analysis of this area since Black.[63] In recent times, however, the availability of new data sources and new techniques, as well as the development of new theoretical perspectives on the relationships between individual lives and social structures, have opened new ways of thinking about these questions. Social class remains a key concept in understanding the relationship between social structure and health but:

> 'social class', at any given point is but a very partial indicator of a whole sequence, a 'probabilistic cascade' of events which need to be seen in combination if the effects of social environment on health are to be understood.[64]

The concept of a probabilistic cascade is a suggestive one, expressing the way in which things can build up over time, exposing people to different kinds of risks and benefits at different points in the cycle or course of life – the way in which: 'advantages and disadvantages tend to cluster cross-sectionally and accumulate longitudinally'.[65] At an individual level the cross-generational and cumulative effects of poverty and disadvantage have been shown in the effects of maternal malnourishment and low birth-weight over time.[66] These processes clearly involve complex interaction between socio-economic, biological and behavioural factors over the life course.[67] The cumulative effects of area histories have been less well explored, but given the increasing evidence of dramatic area variations in mortality and morbidity that appear to be in part related to area characteristics (context), in addition to the characteristics of the individuals living in those areas (composition), the cumulative effects of economic disinvestments and social decline over generations are important parts of a fuller sociological picture,[68] not least in a region such as south Wales with a rise, fall and partial regeneration that has been so dramatically compressed in time.[69]

These new developments in thinking have led to arguments for more detailed research into the 'black box' of materialist explanations for health inequalities. The continued existence and indeed widening of the health gap between wealthier and poorer people, and between advantaged and disadvantaged areas, raises all kinds of questions about the relationship between people and the social conditions in which they live and work. In order to move beyond simple restatements of the Black report's judgements on poverty, or common-sense descriptions of unhealthy behaviours, more imaginative approaches to theory and evidence are needed.

Inside the black box: understanding health inequalities

It is increasingly argued that conventional approaches to the explanation of social inequalities in health have created a 'black box', the inputs and outputs to and from which we can observe, measure and correlate, but whose interior workings – how inequality, poverty and powerlessness affect health in different social contexts – remain obscure, partly because of their resistance to easy epidemiological examination.[70] Understanding health inequalities requires a 'more micro-level examination of the pathways by which social structure actually influences mental and physical health and functioning and life expectancy', and this means adopting a 'more fine grained' approach.[71] This approach will need not just more and better statistical data and tools, but more interpretative and historical approaches, bringing together the stories of individuals and the histories of social structures in particular areas – cities, towns and communities.[72] Communities, like individuals, accumulate advantages and disadvantages over time. Inside the occasionally convoluted theorizing of the late Pierre Bourdieu is a simple message: 'The social world is accumulated history',[73] and the stories about the 'weight of the world'[74] hammer home the point that structure can be very heavy indeed, undermining individual and collective capacities and capabilities.

In trying to think of practical ways in which such approaches could be developed we need to distinguish between 'material' (decontextualized) and 'materialist' (contextualized) explanations.[75] Drawing on this distinction Frohlich has argued:

> What is missing is a discussion of the relationship between agency (the ability for people to deploy a range of causal powers), practices (the activities that make and transform the world we live in) and social structure (the rules and resources in society). Without such an understanding, factors associated with people's disease experiences within a context tend to be denuded of social meaning.[76]

How might such an analysis make sense in the context of the poor health of people in south Wales? In 1998 a report from the Coalfields Task Force argued that coalfield areas had a 'unique combination of concentrated joblessness, physical isolation, poor infrastructure and severe health problems'.[77] While it is important to keep the harsh *generic* reality of material deprivation in the forefront of any explanation of health inequalities in Wales, it is also important to recognize the way in which the *particular context* of Welsh economic and social history has shaped the people who live in certain parts of it. The bullet-point description provided by the Coalfields Task Force disguises a more complex narrative:

> [In south Wales] This was not just a case of localised economic decline but rather one of cultural crisis. The collapse of coalmining undermined a range of mechanisms of social regulation that were grounded in the politics of the workplace and the trades unions, but spread more widely into local society and politics. There was an acute sense of loss in places in which coalmines closed after decades of existence. This was typically accompanied by a period of grieving as people in these places tried to come to terms with the manifold implications of the precipitate ending of the economic *raison d'être* of their place.[78]

While the coal-mining industry in Wales had been in a state of continuous decline in the period after the Second World War, the combined economic, political and social consequences of the end of the strike of 1984–5 have had an impact on south Wales, the shock of which reverberates through economy, society and culture twenty years on.[79]

There are other contemporary examples of the way in which observable and measurable events, such as joblessness and poor housing, become episodes in the histories of places and people. Blaenau Gwent contains areas of severe deprivation, all of whose electoral wards are ranked within the 40 per cent most deprived wards in Wales – Nantyglo, Tredegar Central and West, Llanhilleth, Sirhowy and many others. It has amongst the lowest levels of earnings and house prices in Britain, a large percentage of the population with no qualifications and, as has been indicated, high levels of long-term ill health. Moreover, with low car-ownership and limited access to public transport the prospects of commuting to work are limited. Following a major strategic review in February 2001, Corus plc announced that they were going to restructure their steel enterprise and industry in Wales. One of the major casualties of this restructuring was the Ebbw Vale steelworks, situated at the heart of the Blaenau Gwent economy, which has now closed. As part of a study undertaken in the immediate aftermath of the restructuring announcement, we conducted interviews with a range of key informants not directly involved in the steel industry – health professionals, church ministers, welfare officers – to explore what had happened and was happening to the locality.[80]

Many people with deep ties to the area were only too well aware that the direct loss of jobs in steel is only part of the story. Not only do individual workers feel the harshness of redundancy, the community as a whole is undermined by these events. One health visitor working in the area said:

> People talk not only about the effect on individuals; it's the effect on the borough – everybody, regardless of whether they are employed by Corus or not. I think that there is a huge concern ... that in an area that appeared to be going downhill anyway this is the final nail in the coffin.

The nature of the work and its dominant relationship to the community – in coal and steel – generated powerful social solidarity. As the major industries have withdrawn from Blaenau Gwent the social and physical landscape has changed: 'Abertillery breaks my heart,' said the same health visitor, 'because it just was not like it looks now, it's just a dump.' Many respondents talked about the way in which the running down of the steelworks, as well as the coal mines, affected the way in which local people related to each other. Solidarity extended beyond the work into the 'social capital' of the local community. An educational welfare officer told us: 'The changes in the area over the past thirty years have been tremendous. It had a feeling all of its own thirty years ago, a very strong community of miners and steelworkers ... and now that's gone.' A district nurse who had always worked in the area spoke in similar terms, drawing attention to the impact of these changes on structures of feeling: 'That sort of comradeship has all gone. You knew who you could trust and everyone would help you, but that is disappearing, that sort of feeling is disappearing.' The nature of the work defined the quality of wider social relationships. The sights, sounds and smells associated with the steelworks imprinted themselves on the social and physical character of the surrounding towns. We see in these excerpts from interviews an understanding of the interweaving of personal narratives and social history. The sense of loss and decline in the personal or ontological narratives draws upon a wider public discourse or meta-narrative about the area.[81] Whereas in the past solidarity provided the basis for union and political action, the decline over thirty years and more has created a situation in which the 'resources for hope'[82] have been depleted.

Not only are the people of the area poorer because of the loss of work, the historical evidence of what the place was and what the people did has been taken away. In Christopher Meredith's novel about a declining Welsh steel town, one of the main characters contemplates the last slab to come out of the mill:

> Odourless invisible history would blow them all apart and they would hurtle away from each other through space and never really understand what had shifted them. Except blowing apart was the wrong idea because it was a continuing process, evolving and breaking slowly and then occasionally twitching like this. And it included everything.[83]

The personal consequences of the historical process of 'breaking slowly' and 'twitching' can be seen in this excerpt from an interview conducted with a church minister:

> In the space of six months about two years ago I buried five drug-related [deaths]. The youngest was 18 [years of age] and the oldest was a 27-year-old mother who lived in one of the streets up here. And I knew her parents fairly well, and she left a three-year old boy for her parents to look after. It's a very, very, very real problem.[84]

Poverty, inequality, social exclusion – however the distribution of resources and opportunities is conceptualized – have direct consequences for individual lives: educational failure, crime, heart disease, drugs and alcohol. Things – relationships, roles, jobs, thoughts, actions – are fractured and fragmented, no longer making sense in terms of what people understand from past experience. What our respondents spoke about were people hurtling away from each other in a process of fragmentation, personal expressions of the social conditions underlying many of the problems people face. These narrative fragments were framed within a historical analysis of decline, providing a rich context for our understanding of the way in which ill health is determined by social forces and people's responses to it.

This discussion is, of course, exploratory and provisional, but the point I want to make is this. In trying to explore the reasons for the very poor health of the people of south Wales, we see here the beginning of a whole set of themes to be explored about the way in which the history of the area is important to our understanding of the present situation. While contemporary indicators of material disadvantage are clearly crucial, the routes through which these affect behaviour and health can be seen in the extent to which people can construct a sense of identity and purpose under very difficult social and economic conditions.[85] The history of the south Wales region has a crucial bearing on this, both in terms of indicators relating to economic and social resources, but also in the sense that history is what you live, and the area, its history and the multiple interpretations of it, are things to which the people living in the area have a complex and meaningful relationship. It is not a question of converting this exploratory historical sociology into epidemiology – we already have good social epidemiology – but rather of developing these impressions into fuller sociological and historical analyses of the interrelationships between people and places over time, and using this to frame or contextualize, *inter alia*, patterns of health behaviour, health outcomes, and appropriate professional and political responses to them.[86]

Conclusion

The incontestable conclusion to any rigorous review and interpretation of the evidence on health inequalities is that: 'most of the major drivers of population health and of the distribution of health lie outside the NHS'.[87] When the world price of steel falls in the context of a strong domestic currency, thousands of people across Wales lose their jobs in places that have already experienced years of relentless de-industrialization – not something that doctors, nurses, social workers or health and social care managers can do very much about. But these economic and social changes do have consequences for physical and mental health which those health professionals and managers are expected to be able to do something about. The dilemma for those concerned with the people's health and well-being is that the more it is shown that variation in morbidity and mortality is associated with social factors of the kind I have described, the more it seems that health services of themselves can have little relevance.[88]

The post-Thatcherite Labour Governments and their official advisers in the UK have tended to respond to this dilemma in two ways. First, by acknowledging (in a way Conservative governments were unwilling to do) the importance of large-scale economic, social and environmental determinants of health and health inequalities; and secondly, by emphasizing (as Conservative governments were keen to do) an approach that seeks to persuade, exhort or cajole individuals (or communities understood as aggregations of individuals) to follow 'healthy lifestyles', supported by the 'delivery' of 'interventions' for smoking cessation, alcohol reduction, dietary change and sexual restraint. Although there has been a communitarian gloss on some of the policy documents emerging from New Labour in the UK,[89] in practical terms the focus has remained firmly upon people 'at risk' because of the lifestyles they 'adopt'.[90] There has been less evidence of sustained *sociological* thinking about the distribution of health risks in terms of how to improve the opportunity structures in local communities and environments – good housing, safe play-areas, accessible and reasonably priced food, education, and employment opportunities. This paradox makes current approaches to both health care delivery and health promotion unsustainable, inequitable and potentially destabilizing and delegitimating for welfare states.

Within its currently limited powers the Welsh Assembly Government has been innovative in its attempts both to define new parameters for the development of health policy, and in its support for new health developments and initiatives. Since 1998 the Welsh Office and then the Assembly have been involved in a process of responding to the evidence on what determines good and bad health by developing a vision and strategy for improvements in health and well-being.[91] To its credit the Assembly has strenuously insisted on placing health within a broader policy context, emphasizing the need to 'build bridges between organizations and sectors for more joint action to increase well-being across communities'.[92]

In the context of an identification of both inequalities in health experience and inequities in the distribution, access and quality of services,[93] the Welsh Assembly Government has promulgated a radical plan for health services in Wales:

> The Assembly has developed ... a number of strategies to counteract social exclusion and to create a *socially inclusive* Wales. It recognises the importance of building and supporting strong *communities* where the values of *citizenship* and collective action can grow ... This [Health] Plan builds on wide consultation over the elements that make it up and is part of the process of replacing elite policy making by *participative* policy development. Our policy here is to build on this commitment and to continue to *enhance the citizen's voice* at the heart of policy [emphases in the original].[94]

It is not my intention here to comment at any length on the state of the health services in Wales. However, it is important to recognize that, in the face of considerable political and popular pressure to shift towards an English approach, with its focus on competing foundation trusts,[95] the Assembly has continued to insist on the need to develop a sustainable health policy that refocuses on primary care, prevention and health promotion, and to put in place a formula for the equitable distribution of NHS resources to the new local health boards. This approach has been supported by an external review, conducted by a project team advised by Derek Wanless, which has further emphasized the need for 'a strategic adjustment of services to focus them on prevention and early intervention [entailing] adjusted roles for primary, secondary and social care'.[96] While recognizing the continuing need for good secondary and tertiary services to deal effectively with ill health, and for urgent action on waiting lists in the short term, Wanless argues that this can only be done sustainably by looking at new models of care as whole systems which can integrate resources across different health and social care sectors. For those with professional statuses, interests and privileges to defend, this is a most challenging agenda; as it is for public expectations of what health services will deliver. But if the health and social care services in Wales are to build programmes of service delivery that are *relevant* to the problems I have described and *sustainable* over the longer term, this is what needs to be done.

Like other government advisers before him, Wanless also emphasizes that health is too big a problem for the health and social care services alone, and that a 'step-change in individuals' and communities' acceptance of responsibility for their health is needed'.[97] However, although in his Welsh review, and elsewhere,[98] Wanless recognizes the importance of 'the range of factors which affect health', there is a tendency for the overwhelming determinants of health of the kind described in this chapter to become reduced to rather residual notions of 'personal circumstances' and 'social norms'.

In the *Eighteenth Brumaire* Karl Marx makes a statement that all doctors, nurses, health promotion officers, government health ministers and their advisers would benefit from having programmed into their electronic diaries (with suitable modification for our times, of course):

> Men make their own history; but they do not make it just as they please; they do not make it under circumstances chosen by themselves, but under circumstances directly encountered, given and transmitted from the past.[99]

Health is too important to be left to the health services alone but it is also, as I hope I have shown, too heavy with social and historical conditions for us – the academics, the professionals, the politicians, the expert advisers – to expect economically inactive individuals or socially excluded communities simply to take responsibility for it. We have to move beyond 'beer, fags, egg and chips'[100] and prescriptions for self-efficacy courses. The way forward involves the redistribution of opportunities and resources through macro-level policies but, more than this, we need a social movement with a political programme that is genuinely participative, building on the abundant social and cultural resources of 'lay knowledge'[101] or 'civic intelligence'[102] that exist in local communities and organizations; as well as the considerable social scientific knowledge about the complex effects of social inequalities in health over time and space. Any programme of this kind will have to be undertaken in such a way that power rather than dependence is rebuilt in those once powerful communities where de-industrialization and globalization have turned the world upside down.

Notes

[1] Ron Berry, *History is What You Live* (Llandysul, 1998), pp. 41–3.
[2] Hywel Francis and Dai Smith, *The Fed: A History of the South Wales Miners in the Twentieth Century* (London, 1980); (new edn. with a Centenary preface, Cardiff, 1998).

3. D. Blane, 'The life course, the social gradient and health', in M. Marmot and R. G. Wilkinson (eds), *Social Determinants of Health* (Oxford, 1999), pp. 64–78.
4. R. Hofrichter, 'The politics of health inequalities: contested terrain', in R. Hofrichter (ed.), *Health and Social Justice: Politics, Ideology and Inequity in the Distribution of Disease* (San Francisco, 2003); David Widgery, the writer and general practitioner, conveys the same message in his powerful story of a former east London docker who calls him out one Easter to a council flat near Canary Wharf and then apologises for being 'a nuisance' and 'a trouble': 'On examination he was grossly emaciated, had a collapsed lung, knobbly enlarged liver and about three weeks to live.' D. Widgery, *Some Lives! A GP's East End* (London, 1991), p. 9.
5. Francis and Smith, *The Fed*.
6. C. Thomas, 'Domestic labour and health: bringing it all back home', *Sociology of Health and Illness*, Vol. 7 (1985), 328–52.
7. D. Jones, 'Counting the cost of coal: women's lives in the Rhondda, 1881–1911' in A. V. John (ed.), *Our Mothers' Land: Chapters in Welsh Women's History, 1830–1939* (Cardiff, 1991), pp. 109–34.
8. G. H. Williams, 'Knowledgeable narratives', *Anthropology and Medicine*, Vol. 7 (2000), 135–40.
9. 'All sociology worthy of the name is historical sociology.' C. W. Mills, *The Sociological Imagination* (1959; 2nd edn, Harmondsworth, 1970), p. 162.
10. DHSS (Department of Health and Social Security), *Inequalities in Health: Report of a Working Group* (London 1980) (Black Report).
11. D. Blane, 'An assessment of the Black Report's explanations of health inequalities', *Sociology of Health and Illness*, Vol. 7 (1985), 423–45.
12. H. Graham, 'Tackling health inequalities in England: remedying health disadvantages, narrowing health gaps or reducing health gradients?', *Journal of Social Policy*, Vol. 33, no. 1 (2004), 115–31.
13. Christopher Lawrence, *Medicine in the Making of Modern Britain, 1700–1920* (London, 1994).
14. D. Greaves, 'Contrasting perspectives of inequalities in health and medical care' in Anne Borsay (ed.), *Medicine in Wales c.1800–2000: Public Service or Private Commodity* (Cardiff, 2003), p. 230.
15. D. Armstrong, 'The invention of infant mortality', *Sociology of Health and Illness*, Vol. 8 (1986), 211–32.
16. H. Graham, 'The challenge of health inequalities', in idem (ed.), *Understanding Health Inequalities* (Buckingham, 2001), pp. 3–24.
17. M. Whitehead, 'Life and death across the millennium', in F. Drever and M. Whitehead (eds), *Health Inequalities* (London, 1997).
18. T. McKeown, *The Role of Medicine* (Oxford, 1979).
19. G. Orwell, 'How the poor die' in idem, *Decline of the English Murder and Other Essays* (Harmondsworth, 1965).
20. Graham, 'Tackling health inequalities in England'.
21. Graham, 'The challenge of health inequalities'.
22. M. Marmot, 'The magnitude of social inequalities in coronary heart disease' in I. Sharp (ed.), *Social Inequalities in Coronary Heart Disease* (London, 1998).

[23] M. Marmot and M. Shipley, 'Do socio-economic differences in mortality persist after retirement? 25-year follow-up of civil servants from the Whitehall Study', *British Medical Journal*, Vol. 313 (1996), 1177–80.
[24] M. Marmot, 'Introduction' in M. Marmot and R. Wilkinson (eds), *Social Determinants of Health* (Oxford, 1999), pp. 1–15.
[25] See R. Wilkinson, *Unhealthy Societies: The Afflictions of Inequality* (London, 1996); R. Wilkinson, 'Putting the picture together: prosperity, redistribution, health and welfare', in M. Marmot and R. Wilkinson (eds), *The Social Determinants of Health*, pp. 256–74.
[26] Wilkinson, *Unhealthy Societies*.
[27] P. Boyle, S. Curtis, E. Graham, E. Moore (eds), *The Geography of Health Inequalities in the Developed World* (Aldershot, 2004).
[28] Graham, 'The challenge of health inequalities'.
[29] M. Shaw, D. Dorling, D. Gordon and G. Davey Smith, *The Widening Gap: Health Inequalities and Policy in Britain* (Bristol, 1999).
[30] C. Griffiths and J. Fitzpatrick, 'Geographic inequalities in life expectancy in the United Kingdom, 1995–1997', *Health Statistics Quarterly*, Vol. 9 (2001), 16–28.
[31] Graham, 'The challenge of health inequalities'.
[32] H. Joshi et al., 'Putting health inequalities on the map: does where you live matter, and why?', in H. Graham (ed.), *Understanding Health Inequalities*, pp 143–55.
[33] M. L. Senior, 'Area variations in self-perceived limiting long-term illness in Britain, 1991: is the Welsh experience exceptional?', *Regional Studies*, Vol. 32 (1996), 265–80; see also '"Sick man of Europe" needs a cure', *Western Mail*, 8 January 2004.
[34] Graham, 'The challenge of health inequalties'.
[35] Shaw et al., *The Widening Gap*.
[36] D. Dorling, M. Shaw and N. Brimblecombe, 'Housing wealth and community health: exploring the role of migration', in H. Graham (ed.), *Understanding Health Inequalities*, pp 186–99.
[37] Good and bad health in populations can be measured in a number of different ways. Mortality rates of various kinds, or calculations of life expectancy, are important for their precision and specificity. The Chief Medical Officer (CMO) for Wales also uses 'potential years of life lost' which assumes that everyone may live to a notional age and that younger deaths mean that more future or potential years of life have been lost. This gives a measure of the effect of premature deaths and gives added weight to younger deaths (Chief Medical Officer's Report 2001/2002). There are also important measures that count things other than mortality. These include self-reported long-term and limiting long-term illness, and reports of general health and well-being. While these are more difficult to interpret as objective biological accounts of the health of the population, in a society with relatively low overall mortality and high life expectancy such measures are often important as indicators of underlying chronic ill health and for health-service planning.
[38] G. Higgs, M. L. Senior, H. Williams, 'Spatial and temporal variation of

mortality and deprivation, 1: widening health inequalities', *Environment and Planning A*, Vol. 30 (1998), 1661–82.
39 Chief Medical Officer, *Health in Wales: Chief Medical Officer's Report, 2001/2002* (Cardiff, 2002).
40 David Gordon et al., *Wales NHS Resource Allocation Review: Independent Report of the Research Team* (Cardiff, 2001).
41 Chief Medical Officer, *Health in Wales*.
42 In the 2001 Census the LLTI rates were 23.3 per cent for Wales compared with only 18 per cent in England.
43 Senior, 'Area Variations'.
44 Ibid., 272.
45 C. Williams, *Capitalism, Community and Conflict: The South Wales Coalfield, 1898–1947* (Cardiff, 1998); Dai Smith, *Wales: A Question for History* (Bridgend, 1999); see also chapter by Steven Thompson in this volume.
46 Figures quoted are the European Age-Standardized Mortality Rates per 100,000 population.
47 Chief Medical Officer, *Health in Wales*.
48 The European Standardized Mortality Rate is used in order to make comparisons between populations that take account of the different age structures of those populations, and the figures quoted represent the rate which would occur if the population structure matched the 'European Standard Population'.
49 Wards were grouped into five categories using the Townsend Index of deprivation based on a number of key indicators.
50 Joshi et al., 'Putting health inequalities on the map'.
51 In the 1991 Census Rhondda was administratively distinct from Cynon Valley and counted separately, and came top of the LLTI league table, dropping to fifth when combined with Cynon Valley in 2001.
52 National Assembly for Wales (Statistical Directorate), *A Statistical Focus on Disability and Long-Term Illness in Wales* (Cardiff, 2003).
53 Ibid.
54 National Assembly for Wales, *Welsh Health Survey 1998* (Cardiff, 1999).
55 Ibid.
56 DHSS, *Inequalities in Health*. Notoriously, having been commissioned by the Labour Government in 1977, it was only published in photocopy format in very limited numbers by the resurgent first Conservative Government of Margaret Thatcher in 1980.
57 M. Whitehead, *The Health Divide: Inequalities in Health in the 1980s* (London, 1987).
58 G. Davey Smith, D. Blane and M. Bartley, 'Explanations for socio-economic differences in mortality: evidence from Britain and elsewhere', *European Journal of Public Health*, Vol. 4 (1994), 131–44.
59 C. Power, S. Matthews and O. Manor, 'Inequalities in self-rated health in the 1958 birth cohort: life time social circumstances or social mobility?', *British Medical Journal*, Vol. 313 (1996), 449–53.
60 Shaw et al., *The Widening Gap*.
61 Graham, 'The challenge of health inequalities'.

[62] Chief Medical Officer, *Health in Wales* (Cardiff, 2002).
[63] Shaw et al., *The Widening Gap*.
[64] M. Bartley, D. Blane and G. Davey Smith, 'Introduction: Beyond the Black Report' in M. Bartley, D. Blane and G. Davey Smith, *The Sociology of Health Inequalities* (Oxford, 1998), p. 11.
[65] D. Blane, 'The life course, the social gradient and health', p. 64.
[66] G. Davey Smith and D. Kuh, 'Does early nutrition affect later health? Views from the 1930s and 1980s' in D. F. Smith (ed.), *Nutrition in Britain: Science, Scientists and Politics in the Twentieth Century* (London, 1997), pp. 214–37.
[67] C. Power, M. Bartley, G. Davey Smith and D. Blane, 'Transmission of social and biological risk across the life course' in D. Blane, E. Brunner and R. Wilkinson (eds), *Health and Social Organization: Towards a Health Policy for the Twenty-first Century* (London, 1996), pp. 188–203.
[68] Joshi et al., 'Putting health inequalities on the map'; Shaw et al., *The Widening Gap*.
[69] For a vibrant historical interpretation of this see D. Smith, *Aneurin Bevan and the World of South Wales* (Cardiff, 1993).
[70] J. K. Shim, 'Understanding the routinised inclusion of race, socio-economic status and sex in epidemiology: the utility of concepts from technoscience studies', *Sociology of Health and Illness*, Vol. 24 (2002), 129–50.
[71] S. Macintyre, 'The Black Report and beyond: what are the issues?', *Social Science and Medicine*, Vol. 44 (1997), 723–45.
[72] J. Popay, G. Williams, C. Thomas and A. Gatrell, 'Theorising inequalities in health: the place of lay knowledge', in M. Bartley et al. (eds), *The Sociology of Health Inequalities* (Blackwell, 1998), pp. 59–84.
[73] P. Bourdieu, 'Forms of capital', in John G. Richardson (ed.), *Handbook of Theory and Research for the Sociology of Education* (London, 1988), p. 73.
[74] P. Bourdieu et al., *The Weight of the World: Social Suffering in Contemporary Society*, (Oxford, 1999).
[75] S. Macintyre, 'The Black Report and beyond'.
[76] K. Frohlich, E. Corin and L. Potvin, 'A theoretical proposal for the relationship between context and disease', *Sociology of Health and Illness*, Vol. 23 (2001), 776–97.
[77] Coalfields Task Force (CTF), *Making the Difference: A New Start for England's Coalfield Communities* (1998), para. 1.2.
[78] K. Bennett, H. Beynon and R. Hudson, *Coalfields Regeneration: Dealing with the Consequences of Industrial Decline* (Bristol, 2000).
[79] The extent to which feelings continue to run high could be felt amongst the audience in a recent BBC/Cardiff University Regeneration Institute lecture: Kim Howells MP, 'Twenty years on: the legacy of the miners' strike', 4 March 2004, Glamorgan Building, Cardiff University.
[80] P. Fairbrother et al., *Steel Communities Study*, Cardiff University: Regeneration Institute (2001) from which the quotations are taken.
[81] See for example M. R. Somers, 'The narrative constitution of identity: a relational and network approach', *Theory and Society*, Vol. 23 (1994), 605–49 for a useful methodological exposition.

82 R. Williams, *Resources for Hope: Culture, Democracy and Socialism* (London, 1989).
83 C. Meredith, *Shifts* (Bridgend, 1988), p. 211.
84 Fairbrother et al., *Steel Communities Study*.
85 J. Popay et al., 'A proper place to live: health inequalities, agency and the normative dimensions of space', *Social Science and Medicine*, Vol. 57 (2003), 55–69.
86 G. H. Williams, 'The determinants of health: structure, context and agency', *Sociology of Health and Illness*, Vol. 25 (2003), 131–54.
87 S. Macintyre, 'Prevention and the reduction of health inequalities', *British Medical Journal*, Vol. 320 (2000), 1399–400.
88 M. Blaxter, 'The significance of socio-economic factors in health for medical care and the National Health Service', in D. Blane, E. Brunner and R. Wilkinson, *Health and Social Organization*, pp. 32–41.
89 Department of Health, *Saving Lives: Our Healthier Nation* (London, 1999).
90 S. Macintyre, 'Prevention'.
91 *Better Health, Better Wales* (Cardiff, 1998).
92 Welsh Assembly Government, *Well-Being in Wales* (Cardiff, 2003)
93 NHS Resource Allocation Review, *Targeting Poor Health: Professor Townsend's Report of the Welsh Assembly's National Steering Group on the Allocation of NHS Resources* (Cardiff, 2001).
94 National Assembly for Wales, *Improving Health in Wales: A Plan for the NHS with its Partners* (Cardiff, 2001).
95 A. Pollock, D. Price, A. Talbot-Smith and J. Mohan, 'NHS and the Health and Social Care Bill: end of Bevan's vision?', *British Medical Journal*, Vol. 327 (2003), 982–5.
96 Welsh Assembly Government, *The Review of Health and Social Care in Wales: The Report of the Project Team advised by Derek Wanless* (Cardiff, 2003), p. 51. Derek Wanless had also acted as advisor to the UK Chancellor of the Exchequer on long-term health trends.
97 Ibid.
98 D. Wanless, *Securing Good Health for the Whole Population: Final Report* (London, 2004).
99 Karl Marx, 'The Eighteenth Brumaire of Louis Napoleon Bonaparte', in K. Marx and F. Engels, *Collected Works*, Vol. 2 (London, 1979), p. 103.
100 J. Popay et al., 'Beyond "beer, fags, egg and chips"? Exploring lay understandings of social inequalities in health', *Sociology of Health and Illness*, Vol. 25 (2003), 1–15.
101 Popay et al., 'Theorising inequalities in health'.
102 E. Elliott and G. H. Williams, 'Developing a civic intelligence: lay involvement in health impact assessment', Vol. 24 (2004), 231–43. *Environmental Impact Assessment Review*.

Index

AAC (Academic Assistance Council) 186, 187
Aberdare 104, 128, 133, 147
Aberdare Leader 130
Aberfan disaster 36–37
Abergavenny 225
Abersoch 73
Abertillery 301
Abertillery and District Hospital 143
Abertillery Urban District 112
abortion 110, 131–133
Academic Assistance Council (AAC) 186, 187
Acts of Union (1536 and 1543) 2
Addison's Housing Act (1919) 70
Adler, Eugen 193
agriculture
  hardship from crisis in 136
  transfer of administration in devolution process 250, 251, 252, 254, 255, 258–260, 261
  wages 72
  women's work 131
  see also farming
alcohol 303, 304
Amlwch 7
anaemia 99, 102, 108, 136
Andrews, Elizabeth 128, 134, 138n7
Angelsey 2, 32, 130, 172
antenatal clinics 127–128, 134–135
anthracite mining 18–19
anti-Semitism 184
Arab seamen 16, 89
Arfon 72

Armer, Frederick 247
Ashby, A. W. 136
Asian doctors 30
Aslett, Edward 18
Attlee government 248, 250
Australia 272, 278, 281, 284, 285
Austrian medical refugees 184, 187, 188–191, 194

Bangor
  Caernarvon and Anglesey Hospital *see* Caernarvon and Anglesey Infirmary (C&A), nurse training provider
  conference on health and society (2000) 22
  health reforms 62
  housing programmes 71–72
  Minffordd Hospital 14, 64–65, 172
  need of district hospital identified in Hospital Plan 40
  as pioneer of progressive reforms 13
  School of Nursing 166
  St David's Hospital 38–39
  typhoid epidemic 64
  University College of North Wales 9
Barry 147, 219, 227, 233
  Port Sanitary Authority 85
baths 100–101, 130–131
Bauer, Robert 187, 189
Beaumaris Port Sanitary Authority 62–63

Beck, Alfred 196
Bedwellty Urban District 104
Berger, John and Mohr, Jean: *A Fortunate Man* 213–214
Berger, Stefan 219
Bernfeld, Vernon 194, 195, 200n63
Berry, Ron 287
Bethesda 61, 62, 73
Betws 295
Bevan, Aneurin 37–38, 205, 224, 228
  opposition to devolution 248–249
  In Place of Fear 38
Beveridge, Sir William 187
birth control
  Abertillery opens first British clinic 143
  abortion practised through lack of information on 133
  attitudes to establishment of clinics/guidance centres 22–23, 133–134, 144–145
  attitudes to technology provided by clinics 151–160
  campaign propaganda 146–147
  cancer fears 152, 153
  church attitudes 144
  early clinics following government Memo 153/MCW 147–148
  female attitudes 23, 134, 150–151, 152–160, 164n84
  male attitudes 133–134, 148–151, 158, 164n84
  preference for withdrawal method 23, 146, 153–155, 157–160
Birth Control News 145, 148
birth rate 12, 22, 131
  anxiety over 135
Black, J. 217
Black Report: *Inequalities in Health* 288, 297
Black, Sir Douglas 297
Blaenau Ffestiniog 22, 64
Blaenau Gwent 42, 294, 296, 301
Blaenavon Urban District 104
Blane, D. 288–289
BMA (British Medical Association) 6, 8, 183, 189, 196, 211
Board of Celtic Studies 12

Board of Deputies of British Jews 185
Boladz, Wladzmierz 196
Borsay, Anne and Porter, Dorothy 5, 218, 221
Bourdieu, Pierre 300
Boyne, George 220, 221
Breast Test Wales 271
Brecknockshire 32, 129, 130, 227
British Medical Association (BMA) 6, 8, 183, 189, 196, 211
British Medical Journal 74, 208
Bruck, Werner Friedrich 186
Bryder, Linda 34
bubonic plague 79, 86–87
Buchan, John 187
Burnes, Jimmy 270
burns 19
Bury, C. R. 186

Caernarfon/Caernarvon
  C&A Hospital *see* Caernarvon and Anglesey Infirmary (C&A), nurse training provider
  Caernarvon and Anglesey Loyal Dispensary 165
  gradualness of reforms in 61, 62, 70–71
  infectious diseases 172
Caernarfonshire
  cancer rates 72
  criticism of County Council over response to tuberculosis 228
  death rates (1870–1939) 61, 67, 68, 71
  employment 4
  high showing of medical provision in 1931 Census 223
  housing programmes 69–74
  language spoken in 2
  local authority attitude to provision of hospitals 227
  responses to infectious diseases (1870–1939) 62–68
  social influences on health (1870–1939) 60–63
Caernarvon *see* Caernarfon/Caernarvon

INDEX

Caernarvon and Anglesey Infirmary (C&A), nurse training provider
   discipline and dismissal 169, 173–176
   examinations 169–170
   finance and patronage 176–178
   hospital as cornerstone of city health provision 65
   hygiene and cleanliness 171
   infectious diseases 172
   under NHS 178
   nursing hours 168–169, 171
   probation trial period 168, 169
   recruitment patterns 170
   role and expectations of Matron 166, 167–168, 169, 170, 174–176
   start of nurse training provision 165–167
   trainee backgrounds 167
   trainee illnesses 172–173
Caernarvonshire *see* Caernarfonshire
Caerphilly 14, 147, 294, 295, 296
   by-election (July 1968) 262
Caerphilly Miners' Hospital 224
CAJEX 194
Callaghan, James 253, 254, 255, 263
Cambrian Archaeological Society 8
Campbell, Janet M. 127
cancer
   birth control fears 152, 153
   cure claims 8
   highest rates in Europe found in Caernarfonshire 72
   mortality rates 290, 295
   screening for breast cancer 271, 284
   stomach cancer 42
Cancer Research Committee 8
Cardiff
   Cardiff City Hospital 190, 195
   Cardiff Infirmary 233
   Cardiff Naturalists Society 9
   first Chair of Tuberculosis (1920) 34
   hospital beds 32
   industry 4
   infectious diseases (1850–1950) 80–84, 86–90
   investigation into coal trimmers' lungs 18
   as a major centre of population 4, 12, 80
   male/female inter-war death rates 103, 104, 105
   medical refugees 189–191, 193
   medical schools 24, 29
   mortality rates 295
   neonatal mortality 112
   nursing intakes at King Edward VII hospital 24
   as pioneer of progressive reforms 13
   port sanitation (1850–1950) 80–90, 91–95
   seamen's boarding house conditions 92
   silicotic fibrosis in dock workers 18
   Splott clinic for birth control 148–149, 157
   St David's Hospital 196
   University College of South Wales and Monmouth 29
   University Hospital of Wales 40, 271, 276, 283
   Welsh Office established (1969) 40
Cardiganshire 32
Carey, Peter 214
Caring for the Future 277, 282
Carmarthen 9, 38, 271
Carmarthenshire 32, 130, 296
Caernarvon and Anglesey Loyal Dispensary 165
Celtic folklore 6
   see also folk medicine
Ceredigion 294, 295, 297
Chalke, H. D. 17
Chamberlain, Neville 17
Charles, Enid 155, 157
Chekhov, Anton 214
Chesterton, Laura 171
childbirth
   health effects from unremitting toil of 101, 131, 288

at home 130 *see also* maternity hospitals
  low birth weights 41
  maternal mortality in *see* maternal mortality
  miscarriages 101
  registration Act passed (1915) 125
  stillbirths 20, 101, 113–116, 125
children
  child poverty 41
  hit by infectious diseases 14
  infant mortality 20, 37, 102–103, 111–114, 290, 293
cholera
  in Cardiff (1850–1950) 80, 81–82, 83–85, 87
  cholera hospital 81
  epidemic (1849) Merthyr Tydfil 12
  European approach to epidemics 79
  as galvanizing factor in local sanitation movements 13
church
  attitudes to birth control 144
  Celtic churches and saints 6
  church background of nursing recruits at Caernarvan and Anglesey Hospital 167
  report by minister concerning drug-related deaths 302
Church Village Hospital, Glamorgan 227
circulatory disease mortality 293, 295
Citadel, The 31, 208–213, 223, 224, 228
Citizens' Charter initiative 276, 285
class formations 9, 13, 40, 70
  coronary heart disease mortality in 290
  illnesses allegedly associated with poverty and unemployment in working-class women 99
  pregnancy rates in working class 101
  social class gradient 290–293, 297, 298
  see also social conditions: of working-class Welsh women

Clement Davies Report 35, 36, 72, 74, 228, 245
  influence on Jim Griffiths 266n19
coal industry 3–4, 17–20, 36–37, 288
  Coalfields Task Force report 300
  effects on women's health 20, 100–101, 117
Coates, J. E. 186
Cochrane, Archie 19, 202, 203
Cohn, Siegfried 188
College of Medicine 276
College of Nursing 168
Collis, E. L. and Gilchrist, J. C. 18
Commission on Sanitation (1869) 79
Committee for Constructive Birth Control 148
contingency theory 220–221
contraception *see* birth control
Coombes, Bert 17
COPEC (Christian Order in Politics, Economics and Citizenship) housing survey 71
Copenhagen Declaration 284
copper mining 16
Corus plc 301
Council for Wales and Monmouthshire 249–250, 251
Cowbridge 14
Craig-y-nos 227
Crawshay, Geoffrey 230, 249
Crickhowell 225
Crickhowell House 286n5
crime 302
Cronin, A. J.
  The Citadel 31, 208–213, 223, 224, 228
  Dr Finlay's Casebook 209
Crossman, Richard 252, 253, 269n89
  Devolution Committee chaired by 257–264
Crowther, Anne 100
Crusade against Consumption, The 67–68
culture, Welsh 2
  affected by Welsh topography 2
  indigenous medical traditions *see* folk medicine

language *see* Welsh language
medical refugee contributions 195
prominent part of medical profession in 8–9
Welsh Folk Museum 8
Cummins, Lyle 69
Cummins, S. L. and Sladden, A. F. 18
Cwm Afon 187
Cyfartha 3
Cymer 27
Cymmrodorion Society 8
Cynon valley 30, 295
Czech medical refugees 184, 188–189, 191, 193, 194

Daniel, Joyce 144–145, 147
Daniel, Sir Goronwy 252
D'Arcy Hart, Philip 18, 19
Davies, Clement 73, 245
  see also Clement Davies Report
Davies, Edward 16
Davies, Elwyn 253
Davies, Helen 178
Davies, Hugh Morriston 34
Davies, Idris Naunton 27
Davies, John 217
Davies, Morgan 9
Davies, Rose 128, 133, 134
Davies, T. G. 224, 233
Dawkins, Sylvia 155
Dawson Report 244, 245
death rates
  age-specific 105–109, 112–113, 293
  in Caernarfonshire (1870–1939) 61, 67, 68, 71
  from cancer 290, 295
  from circulatory disease 293, 295
  from coronary heart disease 290, 293
  inequalities in 41–42, 71, 99, 105–106, 232, 293–294
  in inter-war England and Wales 103–106, 107, 112–113, 114–115
  maternal mortality 124, 125–126
  neonatal mortality 112–113

  regional mortality in UK 291–292
  relationship with class/health gradient 290–293
  sex-specific rates in areas of south Wales (1920–39) 103–105
  stillbirths 114–115
  from stomach cancer 42
  from tuberculosis 15, 35, 67, 68, 107–109, 136
  use in 'standard of living' debate 102
Declaration of Perth (speech by Heath) 260
Deiniolen 63
Dell, Edmund 260
Denbigh 9, 34
Denbighshire 130, 223, 227, 294
  Denbighshire Infirmary 225
dentists/dental surgeons 191, 192, 193
Department of Health 240
  see also Ministry of Health
Department of Maternity and Child Welfare 127
devolution
  debate (1945–64) 248–251
  importance of location of health administration 240–241
  legacy of First World War 241–246
  in Scotland 217, 241–242, 260–261, 263
  Welsh reconstruction during Second World War 246–247
  under the Wilson administration (1964–8) 251–257
  under the Wilson administration (1968–9) 257–264
Devolution Committee (1968–9) 257–264
diabetes 41, 290
dietary standards 17, 101–102, 136, 288, 298
  see also malnutrition; nutrition
Digby, Anne 27
Dinorwig Quarry Hospital, Llanberis 69

diphtheria 12, 14, 15, 172, 211, 215n1
dispensary establishment in England and Wales 224–226
Distress in South Wales: Health of Mothers and Babies Imperilled 21
district nurses 25
Dobry, Ales 188
docklands 88, 92
  investigation into coal trimmers' lungs 18
  ships at Cardiff hit by influenza pandemic (1918–19) 89
  see also port sanitation
doctors
  in 1931 Census 223
  Asian 30
  cultural contributions 8–9
  dependence of hospitals on GPs 28, 33
  leading role in municipal life 9
  literary portrayals 208–214
  medical refugees *see* Jewish medical refugees; refugees, medical
  pay 211
  person-centred practice 26–27
  qualified doctors in Wales in nineteenth century 7–8
  research on errors of 204–205
  training 26, 29–30
Doll, Sir Richard 201, 203
Donaldson, L. 220
Dowlais 3
drainage 12
drugs 302, 303

Earwicker, Ray 233
Ebbw Vale steelworks 43, 301
economic depression 21, 116
  relationship to health of women in inter-war south Wales 98–103, 116–117
  relationship to infant mortality and stillbirths in inter-war south Wales 111–116
  relationship to mortality of women in inter-war south Wales 99, 103–111, 116–117, 125–126, 135–136
economic regeneration 37, 283
education
  educational failure 302
  educational reform 74
  expenditure 228
  medical *see* medical education; nurse training
  transfer of administration in devolution process 245, 250, 251, 252, 254, 255, 258–260, 261
Edwards, Huw 250
Edwards, Nicholas 270
Eifionydd 72
employment 4, 5, 16, 17, 42, 73
  of girls 102 *see also* nurse training
  low-paid 66
  monopoly of MAS in medical employment 233
  see also occupational health; unemployment
England
  dispensary establishment 224–225
  English system of port sanitation 79
  health inequalities with Wales 41–42
  Health of the Nation 275, 284
  hospital provision 229–231
  infirmary establishment 224–225
  inter-war death rates 103–106, 107, 112–113, 114–115
  inter-war maternal mortality 109–111, 123–124, 125–127, 129–132
  union with Wales 2
English Consultative Council 244
enteric fever 14
epidemics
  British success at avoiding 91
  combatted by isolation 15 *see also* isolation (fever) hospitals
  combatted by provision of clean water 12, 14, 64 *see also* water supplies

INDEX

combatted by vaccination 63
control through port sanitation
  see port sanitation
European measures against 79
transmission beliefs 79
see also individual diseases
Epstein, Fred 192
European Regions for Health Network 283
European standardized Mortality Rate 295, 309n48
Evans, D. Gareth 218
Evans, Daniel 8
Evans, Emrys 185
Evans, John 8
Evans, Mills 25
Evans, Thomas (MoH) 66

family planning *see* birth control
Family Planning 144
Family Planning Association 22
farming
  affected by Welsh topography 2
  depression in the 1930s 5
  employment accidents in 17
  fresh products exchanged for tinned ones 136
  regeneration in 37
  see also agriculture
Fawcett, C. B. 244
Feiner, Alfred 187, 189, 194, 195
Fenwick, Ethel Bedford 165
Financial Times 270
Fisher, Evelyn 145, 152
Fishguard 27
Flat Holm 83, 85
Flexner, Abraham 186
Flintshire 32, 35, 223, 227
Florence, Lella Secor 155, 157–158
folk medicine 6–7, 8, 19–20, 39
food consumption 101–102
  see also dietary standards; nutrition
Foot, Michael 228
Fortunate Man, A 213–214
France, Sir Arnold 254
Fraser, Peter (MoH) 61, 63
Freud, Sigmund 192

Friendly Societies 223
Frohlich, K. 300

Gallt-y-Sil 64
Gang, Marcell 189
Gelligaer Urban District 104, 147
general practitioners *see* doctors
George, William 10
German medical refugees 183, 184, 188, 190, 194
Gill, J. 71
Glamorgan
  Church Village Hospital 227
  hospital beds 32
  iron industry 3
  male/female inter-war death rates 103, 105
  maternal mortality 124
  maternity services 128, 134
  morbidity rates 295
  mortality rates in the valleys (1970) 42, 201–202
  neonatal mortality 113
  population growth from mining industries 3, 4
  taxation 228
Glyncorrwg 42, 148, 201, 204
Gordon Walker Report 255–256, 259
Gorsed of Bards 8
Gothsmann, Kurt 189
Gottfried, Rudolph 189
Gower 7
Grant, Linda 78
Greece 291
Green, David 223, 224
Greenwood, Arthur 246
Greenwood, Major (Treasurer of SPSL) 187
Gresford colliery disaster 17
Griffiths, Cornelius 28
Griffiths Inquiry (1983) 272–273
  see also NHS: Griffiths Reforms
Griffiths, James (Jim) 18, 37, 43, 245
  appointed Minister of National Insurance 248
  The Price Wales pays for Poverty speech 35

as Secretary of State for Wales 251–252
support for devolution 248, 251, 256
Griffiths, R and Law, J. 218
Griffiths, Sir Roy 272–273
  Griffiths Inquiry (1983) 272–273
  NHS Griffiths Reforms 273–276, 285–286
Gross, Fabius 193, 218
Gurnos 295
Guttmann, Erich 187
Gwangwili Hospital, Carmarthen 38
Gwent 295
Gwyrfai 13, 61, 62, 63, 71, 73–74

Haberfeld, Erwin 189
Haldane Commission (1916) 29
Haldane Committee on the Machinery of Government 243, 244, 248
Haldane, J. S. 18
Hamadryad, HMS 81, 82–83, 225
Hamadryad VD clinic 87–88, 95
Hardy, Anne 217
Hart, Alexander Tudor 202
Hart, Julian Tudor 201–207
Hart, Nicky 113–114, 116
Heaf, Frederick 193
healing arts, traditional *see* folk medicine
health administration 34–36, 40–41, 146–147, 221–222
  of birth control advice 147–148
  criticism of local authorities 62
  devolution process *see* devolution
  management of epidemics 64–65
  in the NHS *see* NHS
  responsibilities of local authorities under 1875 Public Health Act 67
  Scottish 242
health centres for primary care 202
'health gain' currency 272, 284
health indicators
  general population health 308n37
  maternal health 111–112, 114

health inequalities 288–293
  Black Report: *Inequalities in Health* 288
  the 'health gap' 290, 299
  social determinants 296–303
  in Wales 11, 293–296
  between Wales and England 41–42, 293
  between Wales and UK 293–294
Health of the Nation 275, 284
health visitors 25–26
  antenatal care responsibilities 128
heart disease 41, 42, 290, 293, 294, 302
Heartbeat Wales scheme 41, 271, 283
Heath, Edward 260–261
Heathrow Scenarios for Nursing 282
Helsby, Sir Laurence 253
herbal remedies 8
hernias 19, 271
Hill, A. V. 183–184, 194
Hine Report 272
Hirsch, Max 187
Hodann, Max 187
Holywell 225
Hopkins, Deian 218
Hospital Plan for Wales (1962) 40
hospitals 9
  acute services 28, 229–231
  bed distribution 32, 229–231
  buildings 38–39
  cholera hospitals 81
  dependence on GPs 28, 33
  establishment of municipal hospitals 225–228
  establishment of voluntary hospitals 224–226
  facilities 9, 14–15, 33, 38–40, 271
    see also X-ray equipment
  historical patterns and processes in Wales 224–232
  hospital ships 15, 81, 82–83, 225
  isolation hospitals *see* isolation (fever) hospitals
  maternity hospitals 128, 130, 134

INDEX

Ministry of Health surveys 228–232
nationalization 38
under NHS 38–41
occupationally restricted 224
overview of services 31–35
quarry hospitals 16, 69
seamen's hospitals 81, 87–88
venereal disease clinic 87–88
voluntary provision in England and Wales 229
see also individual hospitals
Houghton, Douglas 253
housing
  boarding houses in Cardiff 92
  in Caernarfonshire (1870–1939) 69–74
  damp problems 12
  effect of industrialization and urbanization on 100
  investment 5
  on-board conditions of seamen 85–86, 92
  overcrowding 66, 69, 70–72, 74
  poor housing 35, 43, 66, 72–73, 130, 223
  public neglect of 35
Housing Acts 70
Hughes, Cledwyn 252, 255, 256, 258
Hughes, D. Arthur (MoH) 128
Hughes, Hunter (MoH) 62
Hughes, Trevor 27
Humphreys, Cerys 204
Hunt, David 275

import inspection 86
Indian doctors 30
industrialization
  legacy of health problems from 5, 12, 100–101, 222–223
  transformation of Wales through 3–4, 100
industry, extraction 111–117, 232
  effects on women's health in inter-war south Wales 100–102, 116
  effects on women's mortality in inter-war south Wales 103–108

inquiries into connection with tuberculosis 16–18
overview of occupational health in 16–20
population effects of 3, 4
workforce 45n14
see also coal industry; iron industry; slate industry
infant mortality 37, 102–103, 111–114, 293
  effects on population life expectancy 290
  neonatal mortality 20, 112–114
infectious diseases
  Caernarfonshire's responses to (1870–1939) 62–68
  children hit by 14
  false beliefs concerning 61, 68, 79
  not dealt with in mainstream nurse training 172
  notified to Port Sanitary Authority at Cardiff (1888–1909) 93
  see also epidemics (and individual diseases)
infirmary establishment in England and Wales 224–225
influenza 89–90
Information Technology 271, 273, 282, 285, 286n4
insanity 221–222
  see also mental illness
Irish immigrants 80, 89
iron industry 3
Irving, John 214
isolation (fever) hospitals 14–15, 63–64
  arrangements on island of Flat Holm 83–84, 85
  cholera hospitals 81
  hospital ships 15, 81, 82–83, 225
  seamen's hospitals 81, 87–88

Jahoda, Marie 187
Jeffcott, W. R. 254
Jenkins, P. 218
Jewish medical refugees
  British attitude to 183–187

cultural contributions 195
medical specialisms 183, 184
UK medical qualifications
    184–185, 187–189, 192
Welsh response to 187–196
John Hopkins University 29
Jones, Arthur Rocyn 7
Jones, D. Rocyn (MoH) 134, 135
Jones, Dilys M. 127
Jones, Dot 20, 101, 106, 131
Jones, Emyr Wyn 26, 38
Jones, Glyn Penrhyn 39
Jones, Ieuan Gwynedd 12, 13
Jones, Maggie Pryce 102
Jones, Merfyn 37
Jones, Naomi 143
Jones, O. Vaughan 136, 171
Jones, Rhoda 22–23
Jones, Robert 7
Jones, T. Llew 39
Jones, T. Mervyn 228
Jones, Thomas (Medical and Public Vaccination Officer of Amlwch) 7
Jones, Thomas ('T.J.', Secretary of the Pilgrim Trust) 186–187, 247
Jones, W. J. 186
Jones, Zillah 24

Kantorowicz, Myron 187
Kapp, Yvonne 190–191
Kellermann, Franz 190
Kindanstransport 184, 196
King Edward VII hospital, Cardiff 24, 28
  School of Nursing 29 *see also* Royal Infirmary
King Edward VII Welsh National Memorial Association *see* Welsh National Memorial Association
Klein, Rudolf 217
Kley, Heinz (later Henry) 190
Kurer, Jacques 193

Labour government
  devolution under Wilson administration 241, 251–264
  post-Thatcherite responses to social-related illness 304
  post-war 37
Lady of the Lake of Llyn y Fan Fach 6
Lancet Commission 168, 170
Lancet, the 40, 89, 219, 290
Landers, J. 99–100
Langlands, Sir Alan 270
language
  ascendancy of English language 2, 167
  Welsh *see* Welsh language
Last, Samuel 190
lead mining 16
Leb, Isidor 188
Lessovsky, Jerzy 195
Lewis-Faning, E. 109
life expectancy 16, 37, 41, 61, 290
  potential rates of life lost 294, 295, 308n37
  regional inequalities in Wales 294
  relationship with distribution of income, wealth and resources 291
Liverpool
  Liverpool Royal Hospital 177
  medical links with Wales 33, 249
  nursing exams for Welsh probationers held in 170
  proposed regional link with Wales 246, 249
Ljubljana Charter 272, 284, 285
Llafur 218
Llanbedr Hall 34
Llanberis 2, 62, 69, 73
Llandaff 195
Llandough Hospital 227
Llandudno 3
Llanelli 147
Llanelli and District Medical Service 224
Llanhilleth 301
Llanllechid 39
Llanrwst 61
Llantrisant 147
Llantwit Fadre 147
Lloyd George, David 9–10, 211, 223

Lloyd George, Lady Megan 253
Lloyd, William M. 128
LLTI (limiting long-term illness) rates 293, 294, 295–296
Llŷn Peninsula 72
Local Government Board 73, 87
Lomax, Rachel 271
London, Louise 184
Loudon, Irvine 110–111, 123
Lowe, R. Bruce 69
Lush, Sir Archie 253, 254

MacDonald, Ramsay 18
Mackinder, Sir Halford 244
Macmillan, Harold 250
Maerdy 295
Maesteg 148
Maggs, C. 174
malnutrition 35, 110, 136, 136–137, 298
manganese mining 16
Mardy Isolation Hospital 14–15
Marmot, M. 291
Marriott, Edward: *The Plague Race* 87
Marx, Karl 306
MAS *see* medical aid societies
maternal mortality 20–21, 37
  deaths due to abortion 132–133
  effects of malnutrition 110, 136–137
  in inter-war England and Wales 109–111, 123–124, 125–127, 129–132
  Maternal Mortality in Wales (1937 report) 110, 126, 127, 130, 132, 137
Maternity and Child Welfare Act (1918) 124, 127
maternity hospitals 128, 130, 134
Maude, Sir John 247
Maudsley hospital, London 184, 187
Maxwell, Robert 280
Mayer-von den Steinen, Runhilt 195, 200n61
McCleary, G. F. 125
McKeown, T. 290

measles 14, 79
medical aid societies 28, 33, 219, 221, 223–224, 233
  call for conversion into health clinics rejected 248
Medical Directory 7, 9
medical education 26, 29–30
  see also nurse training
medical folk traditions *see* folk medicine
medical history in Wales
  context and contingency 220–222
  historiographical approaches 216–219
  hospitals 224–232 *see also* hospitals
  primary care 223–224 *see also* primary care
  public health 222–223 *see also* public health
  Welsh effects 216, 221, 234
Medical Officer 137
medical qualifications 7, 184–185, 187–189, 192
Medical Registration Act (1858) 6–7
Medical Research Council (MRC) 18, 19
  Nutrition Committee 21
Medical Society 9
mental illness 101, 290
  historiography of insanity 221–222
  mental handicap strategy 274
Meredith, Christopher 302
Merioneth 2, 4, 32, 129, 130, 223
Merthyr Tydfil 104
  cholera epidemic (1849) 12
  free milk provision 21
  hospital beds in Merthyr 32
  male/female inter-war death rates 103, 104, 105
  maternal and infant welfare studies 21–22
  morbidity rates 295–296
  mortality rates 112, 113, 294, 295
  neonatal mortality 112, 113
  satisfactory showing in Ministry of Health hospital survey 232

tuberculosis death rates 107–109, 136, 223
Michael, Pamela 219
Michaelis, Moritz 190
midwifery 25, 26, 128–129
  antenatal care by midwives 128
  untrained midwives 129
Midwives Acts
  1902 Act 128
  1918 Act 124, 128
  1936 Act 138
Minffordd Hospital, Bangor 14, 64–65, 172
Minffordd Isolation Hospital *see* Minffordd Hospital, Bangor
mining 3, 4, 16–20
  see also industry, extraction
Ministry of Health 11, 70, 89, 240
  1919 Act 242
  assessment of maternal mortality 125, 126–127
  formation (1919) 124
  hospital surveys 228–232
  intransigence over devolution 240–241 *see also* devolution
  Report of the Committee of Inquiry into the Anti-Tuberculosis Service in Wales and Monmouthshire 130
  Report on Maternal Mortality in Wales (1937) 110, 126, 127, 130, 132, 137
miscarriages 101
Monaghan, Steven 284, 286n8
Monmouthshire
  age-standardized mortality rates 294
  cancer mortality 295
  low showing of medical provision in 1931 Census 223
  male/female inter-war death rates 103, 105
  maternal mortality 124
  maternity services 128, 134
  neonatal mortality 113
  opposition to birth control clinics 148
  population growth from mining industries 3, 4
Montgomeryshire 32
morbidity rates 42, 291–293, 296
  LLTI (limiting long-term illness) rates 293, 294, 295–296
  potential rates of life lost 294, 295, 308n37
Morgan, Kenneth 218, 228, 250, 258
Morgenstern, Christian 195
Morris-Jones, John 10
mortality rates *see* death rates
Mountain Ash 104, 112, 132, 148
Mountain Hare 15
MRC *see* Medical Research Council
Museum of Welsh Life 8
Myddfai traditions 6
Mynyddislwyn 210
Mynytho 73

Nantlle valley 2, 62, 73
Nantyglo 301
NAPT (National Association of the Prevention of Consumption and other forms of Tuberculosis) 66
National Assembly for Wales 1, 274
National Audit Office 283, 284
National Birth Control Council/Association 147–148
National Birthday Trust Fund 21, 137, 142n68
National Health Insurance (NHI) scheme 223, 242
National Health Service *see* NHS
national identity 2, 195
  see also nationalism
National Insurance Act (1911) 9–10, 34, 47–48n47, 66, 211
National Sailors' and Firemen's Union 86, 92
nationalism
  Cledwyn Hughes' warnings on playing into hands of Welsh Nationalists 256
  George Thomas' concerns on losing Labour support to nationalists 260, 261

INDEX 325

nationalist sentiment 36, 241, 242, 244
Wilson's response to growing threat of 252, 256
nationalization of hospitals 38
Nazism 187, 188
  see also Jewish medical refugees; refugees, medical
NBCA (National Birth Control Association) 147–148
Neath 8, 12, 14, 296
Nefyn 73
neonatal mortality 20, 112–114
Neuwirth, Ludwig 189
New Statesman and Nation 106
New Zealand 272, 278, 281, 284, 285
Newport
  hospital beds 32
  industry 4
  late foundation of hospital 225
  male/female inter-war death rates 104, 105
  neonatal mortality 112
NHS
  2010 Project 281–283
  alignment with Health for All campaign 275, 283
  appointment of GPs 212
  benchmarking and targets following 1990 health reforms 278, 281–282, 283
  Caring for the Future 277, 282
  Citizens' Charter initiative 276, 285
  collaboration with industry and private sector 271, 276
  criticism of commodity approach 206
  Director and Directorate of NHS Wales 270, 272–274, 280
  effect on hospital funding structure at C&A 178
  European links 278, 283–284
  expense to Welsh Office (1969) 240
  Griffiths Reforms 273–276, 285–286
  health strategy under 1990 health reforms 275–279, 283–285
  information systems *see* Information Technology
  links to social care 274, 279, 282
  management (1984–94) 271–272, 273, 276–279
  Memorandum of Understanding 280, 282–283
  negligible consideration of Wales in planning for 246
  Organization Development Review in NHS Wales 279–281
  overview 38–41
  overview of innovations, progress and problems in Wales (1984–94) 271–272
  primary care at start of 202, 205
  Project 2000 272, 285
  response to medical refugees 196
  see also Jewish medical refugees
  in Scotland 222, 246
  Strategic Intent and Direction of NHS Wales 277–279, 283–285
  Wales as a Region 233, 246
  Wales Staff College 272, 281
  Welsh Assembly's insistence on equitable distribution of resources 305
Nicholl, Edward 92
nickel mining 16
Nightingale, Florence 24, 165
North Wales Sanatorium, Denbigh 34
Northern Ireland 1, 294
Norway 281, 285
Nuffield Provincial Hospitals Trust 283
nurse training 25, 29
  at Caernarvon and Anglesey Infirmary 165–179 *see also for detail* Caernarvon and Anglesey Infirmary (C&A), nurse training provider
  Project 2000 272, 285
nursing profession 24–26
  antenatal care 128

refugee nurses 189–190
training *see* nurse training
nutrition 21, 101–102, 116
  neonatal mortality as indicator of female nutritional status 111–112
  stillbirth rate as indicator of female nutritional status 114

obstetrical care 20, 110, 129
  see also antenatal clinics; maternity hospitals
occupational health
  in Caernarfonshire (1870–1939) 68–69
  class/health gradient 290–293 *see also* class formations
  of dockers 92
  overview 16–20
  restricted hospitals 224
  of seamen 81–90, 92
Ogmore and Garw Urban District 14, 126, 148
Ogwen valley 39, 61, 74
Olson, T. 174
Osler, Sir William 2, 6, 29
Owen, Buddug 39
Owen, Sir Isambard 9

Paine, H. J. (MoH) 80, 81, 82, 92–93
pandemic, influenza 89
Parry, Robert Hughes 28
Patients' Charter 278
Patterson, Sidney 192
Pawson, R. and Tilley, N. 220
Peart, Fred 259
Pembrokeshire 32, 130
Pen-y-Waun 295
Penybont 112
People Strategy 272
Peretz, Elizabeth 21
Phillips, Marion 131
Physicians of Myddfai 6
Pierce, Evelyn 168
Pilgrim Trust 135, 186–187
Pitt, Susan 26
plague 79, 86–87, 90

Plaid Cymru 245, 253
plants, medicinal 8
Polish medical refugees 184–185, 189, 193, 194, 196
Political and Economic Planning (PEP) Report (1937) 224
pollution 14
Pontardawe 14, 148
Pontypool 148
Pontypridd 134, 144, 148
Poor Law (rate-aided provision) 33, 64, 219, 228
Poor Law Infirmary 65
population
  Cardiff as major centre of 4, 12, 80
  distribution problems for health services 32
  population health indicators 308n37
  problems of increasing birth rate and 12
  redistribution through industrialization 3–4
  of Wales 1
port sanitation 78–80, 90–91
  in Cardiff 80–90, 91–95
  English system 79
  port sanitary authorities 63, 79–80, 82, 85, 86–88
Port Talbot 148, 296
Porthmadog 22
postnatal care 128, 282
poverty 108, 117, 223, 298
  abortion stemming from 131
  connection with tuberculosis 35
  the 'health gap' 290, 299 *see also* health inequalities
  The Price Wales pays for Poverty speech by Jim Griffiths 35
  relationship to health of women in inter-war south Wales 98–103, 116–117
  relationship to infant mortality and stillbirths in inter-war south Wales 111–116
  relationship to mortality of women in inter-war south

Wales 99, 103–111, 116–117, 136–137
see also malnutrition
Powell Duffryn Workmen's Hospital, Aberbargoed 224
Powell, Martin 217
Powys 294
pregnancy 116, 128
  accidental 154
  frequent 101, 131
  work during 101, 131
  see also abortion; miscarriages; obstetrical care; stillbirths
Price, Annie 134
Price, E. O. 64, 69
primary care
  acute and primary hospital services 28
  early effects of NHS on 202, 205
  funding 211
  health centres for 202
  historical patterns and processes in Wales 223–224
  work of Julian Tudor Hart in 201–207
Prince of Wales Orthopaedic Hospital, Rhydlafar 25
Project 2000 272, 285
prostitution 88
Prys-Davies, G. 39
public health
  in Caernarfonshire (1870–1939) 61–69, 74
  in Cardiff (1850–1950) 80–84, 86–90, 93, 95
  historical patterns and processes in Wales 222–223
  overview 11–16
  public health movement (emergence 1830–1860) 289
  of women in inter-war south Wales 100–109
  see also death rates; infectious diseases; sanitation
Public Health Acts 33, 66
  1849 Act 80
  1872 Act 79
  1875 Act 67, 227
  1948 Act 12
puerperal mortality *see* maternal mortality
puerperal sepsis/fever 110, 111, 123, 125, 129, 130
  deaths due to abortion 132–133
Pwllheli 9, 22, 71, 73

qualifications *see* medical qualifications
quarantine 79, 82, 84–85
  see also isolation (fever) hospitals
quarry hospitals 16, 69
Quastel, Juda/Joseph 190

racial issues 88–89, 93
Racker, Efraim 190
Radnor 129, 130
Radnorshire 227
RAF 192, 193
rats 87, 90
Rat and Mice (Destruction) Act (1919) 89
Rees, Hugh (MoH) 60, 64
Rees, Hugh 67
Rees, J. Kenneth 186
refugees, medical 30, 185
  Jewish *see* Jewish medical refugees
registration
  of apothecaries (1815) 6
  of births 125
  of doctors (1858) 6–7
  of nurses 170
  of stillbirths 125
religion
  of nursing recruits at Caernarvon and Anglesey Hospital 167
  as possible factor in delay of establishing voluntary hospitals in Wales 233
  see also church
Report of the Committee of Inquiry into the Anti-Tuberculosis Service in Wales and Monmouthshire 130
Report on Maternal Mortality in Wales (1937) 110, 126, 127, 130, 132, 137

Rhoden, Edgar 189
Rhondda Cynon Taf 42, 294, 296
Rhondda Fach Scheme 19, 203
Rhondda Urban District
  female mortality 126
  inter-war death rates 104
  maternity services 148
  Medical Officer report (1910) 8
  neonatal mortality 112, 113
  opposition of councillors to birth control clinics 133
  tuberculosis death rates 107–108
Rhondda valley
  female mortality 106
  literary portrayal of Rhondda Fawr by Ron Berry 287–288
  maternity services 128, 130
  public health problems 12, 102
  stillbirths 115
  valleys transformed by coal industry 4
Rhydlafar 25
Rhyl 3
Rhymney valley 42
Rhys, Sir John 6
Rice, Margery Spring 131
Richardson, F. A. 88
Roberts, Alun 30
Roberts, Bob 210
Roberts, Fflorens 24
Roberts, Glynne 13
Roberts, Lord Wyn 274
Roberts, Mills 69
Roberts, Robert 70
Robinson, Kenneth 254, 255, 256, 261, 269n89
Rockefeller Foundation 186–187, 190
Rookwood Ministry of Pensions hospital, Llandaff 195
Rose, Richard 220
Ross, J. S. 222
Ross, Willie 256, 263
Rotenstein, Hynek 189
Rothschild, Paul 183
Rowland, Sir John 247
Royal Commission on Labour (1893) report 72

Royal Commission on the Civil Service 243
Royal Infirmary 29, 190
rural areas
  cottage hospitals 224
  criticism of rural authorities over response to tuberculosis 228
  dietary standards 136
  farming *see* farming
  home and unlicensed medicinal treatments 8
  housing 69, 72, 130
  lack of antenatal clinics 128
  rural deportation 3
  slowness of health improvements in 62
Ruthin Castle clinic 192, 193, 225

sailors, as potential source of infection 62, 80, 87–88
  see also port sanitation
Salzberg, Peter 188
Samet, Bernard 192
Samet, Paul 192
Samet, Vilma 192
sanatoria 17, 34–35, 66–67, 225–227, 230
sanitation 12
  Commission on Sanitation (1869) 79
  improvements in Caernarfonshire (1870–1939) 60, 61, 74–75
  of ports *see* port sanitation
  see also sewerage; water supplies
scarlet fever 14, 61, 79
Schlesinger, Rudy 192
Scotland
  devolution in 1, 217, 241–242, 260–261, 263
  exceptional policies 220
  health administration 242, 249
  Jewish medical refugee policy 187, 188
  mortality comparisons with Wales 293–294, 295
  National Health Service in 222
  tuberculosis death rates 67

INDEX

Welsh intake of Scottish doctors 30
Scottish Consultative Council 244, 245, 246
Scottish Economic Conference 250
Sebba, Alice Elfriede 189
Sekulich, Milosh 193
Senghennydd colliery disaster 17
sewerage 12, 60, 209–210
Sexton, Reggie 202
Sharpe, L. J. and Newton, K. 221
Shaw, George Bernard 215n1
Sherman, Alan J. 184
shipping, as potential source of infection 62, 78–79
  inspection of ships 85–86, 94
  see also port sanitation
Shore, Peter 260
sickness rates *see* morbidity rates
Signposts to the New Wales 251, 255
silicosis 17, 18
  compensation schemes 36
Simchowitz, H. G. 190
Simonsen, J. L. 186
Sirhowy 301
Sklarz, Ernst 188
slate industry 3, 4, 16
  empty houses available through depression in 73
  tuberculosis exacerbated by 17, 68–69
smallpox 13, 15, 79
  in Caernarfonshire (1870–1939) 61, 63
  in Cardiff (1850–1950) 82
Smith, Dai 218
smoking 204, 297, 304
social care 274, 279, 282, 304–305
social conditions 35, 43, 58n186, 135, 287–289
  in docklands 88, 92
  in inter-war south Wales 100–102, 135–136
  link with tuberculosis 35, 107–109, 222–223
  on-board conditions of seamen 85–86, 92

social class gradient 290–293, 297, 298
social determinants of health inequalities 296–303
social exclusion 302, 305
social fragmentation 303
sociological approach to health policy 304–306
  of working-class Welsh women 99, 101, 116–117, 130, 135–137, 146
  see also economic depression; housing; poverty; unemployment
Socialism 227–228
Socialist Medical Association 187
Society for the Protection of Science and Learning (SPSL) 186
South Wales and Monmouthshire Alliance of Medical Aid Societies (SWMA) 224
South Wales Gazette 144
South Wales Sanatorium, Bronllys 227
South Wales Sanatorium, Talgarth 34, 230
Spain 284
spiritual degeneration 71
Spriggs, Sir Edmund 192
SPSL (Society for the Protection of Science and Learning) 186
St Asaph, Union Workhouse 38
St David's Hospital, Bangor 38–39
St David's Hospital, Cardiff 196
St Louis (ship) 194
standardized mortality rates (SMRs) 292, 295, 309n48
  see also death rates
Stastny, Frantisek 188
State Registration of nurses 170
Stead, W. T. 8
steel industry 301–302, 303–304
Stephens, Arbour 227, 228, 232
Stewart, John 217, 222
stillbirths 20, 101, 113–116
  registration Act passed (1927) 125
Stopes, Marie 23, 148, 151, 155, 158–159

caravan clinic 144–145, 149, 151, 162n20
Cardiff birth control clinic 148–149, 157
streptococcal infection 110
stroke mortality 290
Sully Sanatorium 227
surgery at home 28
Swansea
  hospital beds 32
  industrial development 3, 4
  infirmary 225
  male/female inter-war death rates 103, 104, 105
  move from dispensary to hospital 225
  need of district hospital identified in Hospital Plan 40
  neonatal mortality 112
  sanitation schemes 12
Sweden 284, 291
Symonds, Anthea 25

Tausig, Walter 188
taxation 228
Teleky, Ludwig 187
Tennenbaum, Michael 190
Thatcher reforms 275, 284
Thomas, D. Lleufer 72
Thomas, George 258–259, 260, 263
Thomas, Gwyn 27
Thomas, Hugh Owen 7
Thomas, Owen 27
Thomas, W. E. 133
Thompson, Steven 13
Times, The 264
Tomos, David 26–27
topography of Wales 1–2
traditional healing arts *see* folk medicine
training
  medical 26, 29–30
  nursing *see* nurse training
transport
  access limitations 43, 301
  links 2
Tredegar 301
  riots 184

tuberculosis 15–16
  in Caernarfonshire 65–69, 228
  in Cardiff (1850–1950) 89
  Clement Davies Report on anti-tuberculosis services *see* Clement Davies Report
  death rates from 15, 35, 67, 68, 107–109, 136
  inquiries into connection with extraction industries 16–18
  link with social conditions 35, 107–109, 222–223
  national rates 36
  Report of the Committee of Inquiry into the Anti-Tuberculosis Service in Wales and Monmouthshire 130
  sanatoria 17, 34–35, 66–67, 225–227, 230
  services 34–35
  WNMA control of services for 230, 243
Twynyrodyn 14
typhoid 13, 14, 61
  in Caernarfonshire 64
  in Cardiff (1850–1950) 81

UKCC (United Kingdom Central Council) 2010 Commission 282
unemployment 21, 42, 43, 117, 201
  in the 1930s 5, 223
  relationship to infant mortality and stillbirths in inter-war south Wales 111–116
  relationship to women's health and mortality in inter-war south Wales 98, 99, 101–102, 109, 110, 117
  through sickness 296
University College of North Wales 9
University College of South Wales and Monmouth 29
University Hospital of Wales 40
  Medicentre 271, 276, 283
University of Wales 186
Urbanek, Zdenek 188
urbanization 3, 100, 222
  effects on immune system 69

legacy of health problems from 12
USA 291

vaccination 63
venereal disease 87–88, 93

Wade, T. W. 17
Wales and Medicine 5
Walford, Edward (MoH) 84
Walker, Patrick Gordon 253–255, 256
  Gordon Walker Report 255–256, 259
Wanless, Derek 305–306
Warner, Morton 284, 286n7
water supplies 12, 14, 60
Webster, Charles 102, 217
Weis, Max 194–195
Weisl, Hanus 196
Wellisch, Erich 187
Welsh Assembly 240
Welsh Assembly Government health policy 30, 304–305
Welsh Board of Health 11, 32, 34, 127, 219, 233
  devolutionist goal for 241
  diminished function following dissolving of WNMA 249
  failings of board mechanism 243
  formation (1919) 124, 242–243
  Ministry of Health's negative assessment of 247
  recast as Health Division of the Welsh Office 264
  Thomas Jones' negative assessment of 247
Welsh Consultative Council on Medical and Allied Services in Wales 28, 31, 32, 244–245
Welsh Council for Labour 251
Welsh Day debates 246, 248
Welsh Folk Museum 8
Welsh Health Common Services Authority (WHCSA) 283, 286n5
Welsh Health Development International 283

Welsh Health Planning Forum 277, 278–279, 283, 284
Welsh Health Technology Forum 276
Welsh Hospital Board (formerly Welsh Regional Hospital Board) 249
Welsh Housing Association 72
Welsh language
  decline in speaking of 2–3
  exceptional policies grounded on language 220
  sense of separate identity sustained through 2, 195
Welsh medical history *see* medical history in Wales
Welsh National Insurance Commission 242
Welsh National Memorial Association (WNMA) 34, 35, 66–67, 218, 219, 227
  control of hospital provision for tuberculosis 230, 243
  The Crusade against Consumption 67–68
  dissolved during devolution debate 249
  Ministry of Health's verdict on 247
  upheld as devolutionary model 243
Welsh National School of Medicine 29–30, 185, 188–189
Welsh Office 40, 240–241, 304
  Memorandum of Understanding with NHS Trusts 280, 282–283
  transfer of responsibilities under Wilson administration 251–256, 258–264
Welsh Reconstruction Advisory Council 246
Welsh Regional Hospital Board (later, Welsh Hospital Board) 38, 249
Western Mail 88, 144, 184
Whitehead, M. 297
whooping cough 61
Williams, Eliza 128, 130, 134

Williams, Herbert: *A Severe Case of Dandruff* 35
Williams, Jane 24
Williams, Lady Juliet Rhys 132–133
Williams, Megan Lloyd 178
Williams, R. Llewellyn 132
Williams, Raymond 2
Williams, Sir John 8–9
Williams, William Carlos 214, 215n3
Willink, Henry 224
Wilson government 241
   devolution and the Wilson administration (1964–8) 251–257
   devolution and the Wilson administration (1968–9) 257–264
Wilson, Harold 252, 253
   Wilson's Devolution Committee 1968–9 under Crossman 257–264
Winter, J. 99
WNMA *see* Welsh National Memorial Association
Wolpert, Ilta 188
women's health
   effects of coal industry 20, 100–101
   effects of excessive child-bearing 101, 131, 135, 288 *see also* abortion
   female mortality 103–111, 135 *see also* maternal mortality
   heavy toil 100–101, 131, 288
   in inter-war south Wales 100–109, 111–117, 135–138 *see also* maternal mortality: in inter-war England and Wales
   overview 20–23
Working-Class Wives: Their Health and Conditions 131
Working for Patients (White Paper 1989) 40
working hours
   of nurses 168–169, 171
   of women in inter-war south Wales 100
Workmen's Compensation Acts 36
World Bank 272, 283, 284
World Health Organization (WHO)
   Collaborating Centres in health promotion and strategy 271, 283
   Health for All by 2000 283
   Ljubljana Charter 272, 284, 285
   NHS links 271, 283–284
Wrexham 4, 12, 40
   Gresford colliery disaster 17
   move from dispensary to hospital 225
   need of district hospital identified in Hospital Plan 40
   Polish medical refugees 193, 196
   Ysbyty Maelor incubation unit 271, 283

X-ray equipment 16, 28, 38, 223

yellow fever 79, 81
Ysbyty Glan Clwyd 271
Ysbyty Maelor 271, 283
Ystradgynlais 196